Alcohol
and Speech

Alcohol
and Speech

Steven B. Chin
and David B. Pisoni
Department of Psychology
Speech Research Laboratory
Indiana University
Bloomington, Indiana
and
Department of Otolaryngology–Head and Neck
Surgery
DeVault Otologic Research Laboratory
Indiana University School of Medicine
Indianapolis, Indiana

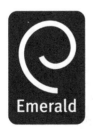

United Kingdom – North America – Japan – India – Malaysia – China – Australasia

JAI Press is an imprint of Emerald Group Publishing Limited
Howard House, Wagon Lane, Bingley BD16 1WA, UK

First edition 2007

British Library Cataloguing in Publication Data
A catalogue record for this book is available from the British Library

ISBN: 978-0-12-172775-8

Awarded in recognition of
Emerald's production
department's adherence to
quality systems and processes
when preparing scholarly
journals for print

INVESTOR IN PEOPLE

Contents

CHAPTER 7

Research Review III: 1985–1996   167

Preface

This monograph is intended primarily for researchers working on alcohol and for speech scientists. Alcohol researchers may be interested in one of the specific effects that this drug has on human performance and behavior, whereas speech scientists may be interested in how and why the speech signal changes in response to alcohol. Additionally, we hope that researchers in other fields, such as health professionals, psychologists, psychiatrists, speech and language pathologists, forensic scientists, legal professionals, human factors scientists, and safety engineers, will find this monograph useful in understanding the relationships between drugs and behavior through in-depth examination of the relationship between a specific drug and a specific behavior, in this case, speech motor control, articulation, and acoustics.

We address a wide diversity of disciplines in this work because that approach reflects the many different researchers who have contributed to the study of the effects of alcohol on speech. For any researcher approaching the subject from a single discipline, it is not always obvious where to find the relevant literature and, once there, how to interpret it. With this book as an initial guide, we hope to remedy that situation in two ways. First, we have attempted to account, as fully possible, for the relevant literature on alcohol and speech since the beginning of the 20th century. To some extent we used a fairly narrow definition of *speech* in our selection of research for discussion, excluding a number of works dealing with alcohol effects on pragmatic and social aspects of speech (by the same token, we narrow *alcohol* to mean ethanol used in beverages). Second, we have provided two introductory chapters, one on alcohol and another on speech, to provide some necessary background material for those readers unfamiliar with either alcohol characteristics or speech science. These chapters are not at all comprehensive, but we hope they will make the literature on alcohol and speech more accessible to many researchers.

In working toward our goal of providing a comprehensive overview of research on alcohol and speech, we have been aided in various ways by a number of people whose assistance we wish to acknowledge here. First, we thank our colleagues in alcohol and speech research who generously offered their ideas and suggestions, who shared with us their own work in this area, and who kept us apprised of the very latest research: Kathleen E. Cummings (Georgia Institute of Technology, Atlanta); Harry Hollien (University of Florida, Gainesville); Keith Johnson (The Ohio State University, Columbus); F. Klingholz (Munich, Germany); and Hermann J. Künzel (Bundeskriminalamt, Wiesbaden, Germany). We are additionally grateful to the many authors and publishers who gave us permission to reproduce various tables and figures from their research.

We also thank a number of our colleagues at Indiana University who assisted us in interpreting various aspects of this research: Robert F. Borkenstein, Professor Emeritus of Forensic Studies (College of Arts and Sciences); Ann R. Bradlow, National Institutes of Health (NIH) Postdoctoral Research Fellow (Department of Psychology, College of Arts and Sciences); Joe C. Christian, Professor of Medical and Molecular Genetics (School of Medicine); J. Alexander Tanford, Professor of Law (School of Law); and Ting-Kai Li, Distinguished Professor of Medicine and of Biochemistry (School of Medicine).

For their assistance in preparing the manuscript, including locating and obtaining sometimes obscure books and articles, we are very much indebted to Jennifer L. Jack (Indiana University Bloomington; now at University of Maine); Luis R. Hernández S. (Indiana University Bloomington); Jon M. D'Haenens (Indiana University Bloomington); Linette Caldwell (Indiana University School of Medicine); and the staff of the Document Delivery Service at the Indiana University Libraries (Bloomington, Indiana).

Finally, for her multitude of talents as the most able administrative assistant ever, we are especially indebted to Darla J. Sallee of the Speech Research Laboratory at Indiana University.

Preparation of this work was supported, in part, by grants to Indiana University from the Alcoholic Beverage Medical Research Foundation; the United States Public Health Service, National Institutes of Health/National Institute on Deafness and Other Communication Disorders, Training Grant (T32) DC00012; and the United States Public Health Service, National Institutes of Health/National Institute on Alcohol Abuse and Alcoholism, Alcohol Research Center Grant AA07611.

CHAPTER 1

Introduction

For many years it has been known that alcohol affects speech in a wide variety of ways. These changes include both the *content* of what someone says *and* its acoustic *form* as expressed physically by the articulation of speech and the resulting acoustic signal produced by the vocal tract of the talker. Despite firsthand knowledge and direct observations by laypeople and researchers that alcohol has some effect on speech, surprisingly little scientific research has actually been carried out to study this problem in the laboratory to understand the neural mechanisms in speech that are affected by alcohol and how they are related to other changes in an individual's behavior.

A number of specific questions arise when we consider the effects that alcohol has on speech. What cues might the speech signal contain that would indicate whether a talker is sober or intoxicated? What degrees of changes in the speech signal might indicate whether a talker is more or less intoxicated? What cues in the speech signal indicating intoxication are readily available to a listener, and what cues are recognizable only with instrumental acoustic analysis? How reliable are these cues, either auditory or acoustic, in determining whether or not a talker is intoxicated? What other types of impairment might be inferred from a speech signal that indicates intoxication? All of these questions have been studied in the modern literature on alcohol and speech, but they have been addressed by researchers from different disciplines, using quite diverse theoretical frameworks, often with diverse research goals. These various disciplines have included psychology, linguistics, forensic science, speech science, speech pathology, human factors, and medicine.

This book is about alcohol and speech. Specifically, our goal has been to bring the diverse research literature that exists on this topic together in

1

one place and to interpret and try to understand how alcohol affects speech production and the mechanisms that control phonation and articulation. In carrying out this task, we have adopted a particular research orientation that reflects the background and research experiences of the two authors. Steven Chin is a linguist with special interests and expertise in clinical phonology and phonetics; David Pisoni is a psychologist who has worked in speech perception and speech acoustics for over 25 years. The orientation of this book is therefore decidedly analytic, with a particular emphasis on laboratory-based research in the field of acoustic-phonetics and speech science. One of our goals is to review and interpret the published literature on alcohol and speech and summarize what is currently known about how alcohol affects speech. A second goal is to identify what areas need further investigation in future research on alcohol and speech. In addition to reviewing research findings that have appeared in the published literature, which was based on our own exhaustive search of journals and books going back to the beginning of the 20th century, we also report new findings on the analysis of speech from our own research program at Indiana University and several other laboratories currently working on these problems. These new results demonstrate how the effects of alcohol can be studied using several novel speech analysis techniques from the fields of electrical engineering and digital signal processing (DSP). Specifically, the use of modern DSP techniques has provided a way of extracting acoustic features and parameters from the speech waveform that are affected by alcohol as well as other factors that mediate the control of respiration, phonation, and articulation of speech. Thus, we hope this book also serves as a vehicle for increasing the scientific knowledge base about the effects of alcohol on speech.

Another more practical goal of this book is to relate these "scientific" findings to a number of applied problems in the field. One important area of alcohol research that has received a great deal of attention in recent years concerns the problem of physically measuring intoxication and impairment. The question here deals with the extent to which the speech production behavior of a talker can be used as a means or method for measuring and assessing physical and psychological impairment in a human operator. Although this problem may at first glance appear to be related to a variety of issues in the field of human factors and performance assessment, the forensic relevance of these types of measurements of speech becomes immediately obvious when one attempts to assess the degree of impairment of a human operator after an accident involving complex equipment or in a variety of human–machine interactions. Indeed, it was precisely within this forensic context that one of the authors served as an expert witness in the case of the *Exxon Valdez* oil spill. In this case, speech analysis techniques were used for the first time to analyze and measure an audiotape that contained samples of Captain Joseph Hazelwood's voice to determine if he was intoxicated at the time of the oil spill in Prince William Sound. An additional goal of this book is to review and analyze this particular case to determine the extent to which current speech analysis techniques can be used in forensic settings to assess the degree of impairment from alcohol and other drugs from samples of speech. Testimony by expert witnesses for both the plaintiffs and the defense in this case identified a number of important areas in which additional basic research on alcohol and speech is needed before a complete scientific understanding would be possible so that this new methodology could be used confidently in forensic situations. In the process of giving expert testimony during pretrial deposition, it became clear that wide gaps currently exist in our basic understanding of how alcohol affects speech and the many physiological, cognitive, and behavioral parameters that are controlled by the human talker during the course of speech production. Because this is a novel area of research in speech science and acoustic-phonetics, many issues have surfaced over the last few years that would not typically be considered in standard laboratory studies in speech science.

There are a number of good reasons why our knowledge of certain areas related to alcohol and speech is so limited at this time. First, most researchers who work in speech science are concerned with processes of normal speech production and acoustics or applications of these principles to clinical populations with neurogenic speech and learning disorders. Only rarely have speech researchers ventured beyond these traditional areas to explore the effects of variables like alcohol or other drugs on speech production. Historically, studies of this kind have not been of interest to speech science, acoustic-phonetics, or linguistics. Second, researchers working on alcohol and impairment have not been interested in speech production or perception. Moreover, and perhaps most importantly, these researchers typically do not have specialized training and experience in linguistics, speech science, acoustic-phonetics, or electrical engineering, which would provide them with the necessary tools, methodologies, and conceptual framework to study speech production in a scientific way.

In some sense, one can say that in the past the study of alcohol and speech has more or less fallen between the cracks separating two rather diverse areas of research. Each discipline has its own research history and traditions, and each area has its own experimental protocols, methodologies, and research agendas that specify the problems to be studied within the respective conceptual and theoretical frameworks. There simply has been little if any direct communication between these two diverse fields of research until just recently when the theories and methods of speech science and acoustic-phonetics were used systematically and applied to study how alcohol affects speech, specifically, how alcohol affects speech motor control, articulation, acoustics, and perception (Pisoni, Yuchtman, & Hathaway, 1986).

Speech is a form of human behavior like any other behavior that has been studied in the laboratory and in applied settings in the field. For historical reasons (e.g., the relatively late development of instrumentation for speech analysis), the study of speech and alcohol has not received the attention it deserved despite the reliance on subjective judgment of an individual's speech when determining probable cause in driving sobriety tests. Given the importance of operator-impairment problems in modern society, we hope this book serves the broad purposes outlined above. A critical review and interpretation of the past literature on the effects of alcohol and speech and a discussion of areas for future research will no doubt serve several valuable purposes. First, we hope this book will be used as the definitive source for determining what is and what is not known about the effects of alcohol on speech. Second, we have identified several important new areas for future research on alcohol and speech that are worthy of investigation. Finally, we hope the research and issues identified in this book unite speech scientists and alcohol researchers to solve a set of common problems. Each group of researchers has something unique to contribute to the understanding of how alcohol affects speech. As in many other areas of scientific research, it is not surprising that the most important and difficult problems for future research on alcohol and speech lie at the intersection of both of these research disciplines, and it is here that the greatest gains in knowledge can be made over the next few years.

This monograph provides psychologists, linguists, forensic scientists, speech pathologists, speech scientists, and jurists with a comprehensive review and interpretation of past research on the effects of alcohol on speech, as well as a comparison of the different theoretical concerns that inform such research. This work integrates the diversity of research in this area under a single, unifying perspective and serves as a basic reference source. Our intended audience is wide, encompassing both practitioners and theoreticians alike. Primary attention is given to speech motor effects evident in the acoustic record, but other effects such as reaction times, speech communication strategies, and perceptual judgments are also considered.

Chapter 2 deals with the nature and pharmacology of alcohol. This chapter includes discussion of the chemistry of alcohol, and its absorption, distribution, and elimination. Also included is a discussion of the effects of alcohol on the brain and other structures of the central nervous system (CNS), particularly the cerebellum.

In order to achieve a degree of self-containment in this monograph, as well as to set the various types of research into a coherent, meaningful framework, Chapter 3 reviews the basics of speech production and speech acoustics. The discussion of speech production derives from the view of alcohol as a CNS depressant with its most highly salient effect on speech being a degradation of peripheral speech motor control. In this chapter, we discuss the anatomy and physiology of the vocal tract, as well as articulatory phonetics, that is, the movements and placements of articulators that are necessary to produce speech. The section on speech acoustics considers speech as an acoustic signal that can be described by a well-defined sound source. Discussed here is the source–filter theory of speech production, as well as modern instrumental acoustic techniques for the analysis of speech, including waveform displays, filtering techniques, and spectral analysis.

Chapter 4 is devoted to a discussion of the different research methodologies employed in previous studies investigating the effects of alcohol on speech. Of concern here is how these various methodologies differ, how they have developed, and how their employment may affect results in specific studies. Examples of differing methodological procedures include (1) the use of clinical versus experimental evidence; (2) the differential use of human subjects (e.g., chronic alcoholic versus acute nonalcoholic subjects, or untrained listeners versus trained listeners); (3) the differential use of measurement techniques to control for level of intoxication, for example, the measurement of blood-alcohol concentration (BAC) as an experimental control; (4) the use of different behavioral measurements to ascertain the presence and extent of an effect of alcohol upon speech, for example, reaction times, number of speech errors, changes in the acoustic waveform.

Three central chapters review and interpret approximately 80 years of research on alcohol and speech. In the first period covered, with boundaries represented by Dodge and Benedict (1915) and Dunker and Schlosshauser (1964), the general approach was that changes in speech were considered within a constellation of symptoms indicative of alcohol intoxication. Articles published during this period generally appeared in psychological, psychiatric, or medical journals.

The second period began with Stein (1966) and ended with Sobell, Sobell, and Coleman (1982). During this period, research dealt specifically with effects of alcohol upon speech. Behavioral evidence was wide ranging and included articulatory errors and speech dysfluencies, response latencies, amounts of verbalization, syntactic complexity, disinhibition of verbal behavior, and changes in the acoustic record between sober and intoxicated conditions. Journals containing research during this period were equally varied and included publications in the fields of speech pathology, linguistics, psychology, psychiatry, and alcohol studies.

The third period, initiated by Pisoni, Hathaway, and Yuchtman (1985) and continuing to Dunlap, Pisoni, Bernacki, and Rose (1995) and Cummings, Chin, and Pisoni (1996), represents laboratory-based research heavily dedicated to instrumental acoustic analysis. Two main theoretical themes, human factors and forensic science, were introduced during this period.

Citations from this period also reflected these growing applied themes: in addition to literature found in medical, psychological, psychopharmacological, alcohol, and speech journals, articles during this period also began to appear in volumes devoted to engineering and human factors and in the forensics literature.

The eighth chapter constitutes a case study of the implications for, and applications of, research on alcohol and speech to a real-world situation. In 1989, the oil tanker *Exxon Valdez* ran aground in Alaska and eventually released over 1.2 million barrels of crude oil into the waters of Prince William Sound. There was some speculation that the captain of the ship was intoxicated at the time, but the only physical evidence from the time immediately surrounding the grounding was audiotape recordings of radio transmissions between the ship and the U.S. Coast Guard Vessel Traffic Center. A number of researchers were asked by the National Transportation Safety Board to analyze those recordings and to determine if signs of alcohol intoxication were present in the speech of the *Exxon Valdez* captain. Some of those researchers were subsequently retained as expert witnesses in various legal proceedings that followed the grounding. Chapter 8 discusses the protocols used to analyze the voice recordings as well as the status of those types of analysis in terms of their admissibility as scientific evidence in court.

The final chapter of the book provides a summary of past research and the foregoing discussion, and ends with an examination of potential applications of the research and directions for future research on alcohol and speech in a number of different disciplines.

The Nature and Pharmacology of Alcohol

2.0 INTRODUCTION

This chapter contains a brief summary of the characteristics of alcohol and alcoholic beverages and brief discussions of the pharmacokinetics and pharmacodynamics of alcohol. In the last case, our comments are limited to the effects of alcohol on the central nervous system (CNS), given our primary concern here with the effects of alcohol on speech. Much more detailed treatments of these topics can be found in the three-volume work edited by Kathryn E. Crow and Richard D. Batt (1989), *Human Metabolism of Alcohol*, as well as in the references cited therein. Also useful as synopses of current research on these areas of alcohol, especially as they relate to alcohol abuse and alcoholism, are the special reports on alcohol and health issued periodically by the U.S. Secretary of Health and Human Services (e.g., *Eighth Special Report*, 1993; *Seventh Special Report*, 1990). Older reference works include the three-volume *Biology of Alcoholism*, edited by Kissin and Begleiter (1971, 1972, 1974); and the two-volume *Actions of Alcohol*, by Wallgren and Barry (1970).

2.1 CHARACTERISTICS OF ALCOHOL

2.1.1 Properties of Alcohol

Scientifically, the term *alcohol* refers generically to compounds with a hydroxyl group (one oxygen and one hydrogen [−OH]) bonded to a carbon

7

molecule; such compounds include methanol, butanol, and ethanol. As used in this book, however, the unmodified term *alcohol* refers specifically to *ethanol*, CH_3CH_2OH, also called *ethyl alcohol* or *grain alcohol*. This is the specific compound found in alcoholic beverages.

Ethanol is a small ($M = 46.07$), polar molecule and at room temperature is a clear, colorless liquid that is highly volatile and flammable. Its specific gravity (compared to water) is 0.7939; the boiling point of absolute ethanol is 78.4°C and for 94.5% ethanol (ordinary pure distillation), 78.2°C.

2.1.2 Alcoholic Beverages

Alcohol used in the preparation of beverages is formed through fermentation of carbohydrates (starches and sugars) in various organic substances, mostly plant products (e.g., grain and potato mashes, fruit juices, sugar cane molasses), but also some animal secretions (e.g., milk, honey). The raw materials for the production of alcoholic beverages are generally of two types: (a) those containing high concentrations of natural sugars, and (b) those containing other carbohydrates (starches) convertible to sugars by enzymes. In the former case, enzyme-containing yeasts are added to the sugar-bearing carrier (e.g., fruit juice), breaking down the sugars into alcohol and carbon dioxide. In the latter case, when starchy raw materials (e.g., grains) are used, an initial enzymatic step converts the starches into sugars. An example of these enzymes are the amylases, which occur naturally when grains, such as barley, sprout. The source of alcohol in beverages is thus the result of enzymatic conversion of starches to sugars and then of sugars to alcohol and carbon dioxide (among other products). Modern alcoholic beverages are generally divided into five categories (Leake & Silverman, 1971): beers, table wines, dessert or cocktail wines, liqueurs or cordials, and distilled spirits.

In the production of beer, cereal grains, such as barley (and, less commonly, other grains such as maize and rice) are malted, or steeped in water and allowed to germinate. Germination of the grain produces enzymes that convert the grain starches into sugars. Water is then used to extract soluble substances, including the fermentable sugars, in a mixture called the wort. The wort is boiled with hops, the cone-shaped female flowers of the vine *Humulus lupulus,* which adds the characteristic bitterness to beer. The wort is then cooled and allowed to ferment by action of added yeast. After fermentation, the "green" beer is held in tanks and undergoes clarification and filtering. The beer is then carbonated and bottled or canned. The alcohol content of bottom-fermented beers (lager) is approximately 3–6% by volume, while that of top-fermented beers (ale, stout) ranges from 3–8% (or more) by volume.

Whereas the production of beer from cereal grains requires initial conversion of starches to sugars, the production of table wine begins with grapes, which already contain high concentrations of natural sugars. In the making of grape wine, subsequent to harvest, the grapes are first crushed, and the juice separated from the skins and seeds for white wine; in the making of red wine, the juice, skins, and seeds are all fermented together. Either the separated juice or the mashed grapes are referred to as *must* prior to and during fermentation. As in the production of beer, yeasts are used to ferment the sugars in the must. Wines are then clarified, aged, and bottled. Sparkling wines (champagnes) undergo a second fermentation through the addition of sugar, producing excess carbon dioxide kept in solution under pressure. Before the second fermentation, sparkling wines are typically around 10% alcohol by volume, and after, approximately 12%. All table wines typically contain alcohol concentrations in the range of 10–14% by volume, or approximately 12% on average for American and European wines.

Dessert and cocktail wines are wines to which additional alcohol has been introduced to achieve alcohol concentrations above 14%. These typically consist of brandy or neutral spirits made from wine or, less commonly, neutral grain spirits. The added alcohol prevents the fermentation of all of the sugar in the starting wine, resulting in a sweeter beverage. Beverages in this category include sherry, port, madeira, muscatel, marsala, and vermouth. Alcohol content is higher for these "fortified wines" than for the wines from which they are made and range from 17–18% by volume for vermouths to nearly 20% by volume for port and sherry.

The class of liqueurs or cordials originated as medieval medicinal preparations produced by distillation. The original recipes were based on mixtures of herbs. Modern preparations use fruits, flowers, herbs, seeds, bark, roots, peels, berries, juices, or other natural flavoring substances or extracts derived from them. They are typically sweet (as high as 50% sugar by weight), with alcohol concentrations ranging from 20–60% by volume.

Distilled spirits are made from fermented mixtures but have an alcohol concentration above the original mixture. The process that increases the alcohol concentration is called distillation and is based on the fact that alcohol and water have different boiling points. Whereas the boiling point of alcohol is 78.5°C, the boiling point of water is 100°C. If a fermented liquid containing alcohol is heated to a temperature between 78.5°C and 100°C, the vapor from the process will contain more alcohol than water. If this vapor is then condensed, the alcohol concentration of the condensate will be higher than that of the original mixture. Distilled spirits can be made from any number of products, as long as they contain sugar or a carbohydrate that can be converted to sugar; these include fruits, cereals, potatoes, and molasses. Broad categories of distilled spirits include brandy (from wine), whiskey (from grain), rum (from molasses), and vodka (from a variety of substances).

There are a number of ways in which the concentration of alcohol in beverages is expressed. Two of these are percent by weight (% w/w) and percent by volume (% v/v). The former is not temperature-dependent, whereas the latter is; however, practical considerations of the basis for retail sales and beverage service have made % v/v expressions the more common. The Gay-Lussac system, a fairly straightforward metric expression of % v/v, is used in a number of European countries. There are differences, however, based on different standard reference temperatures. In some English-speaking countries, proof scales are used. Historically, *proof* meant that a solution contained more ethanol than water; it was demonstrated that gunpowder soaked in a questionable beverage would burn if the alcohol concentration was greater than 50% and would not if the concentration was lower. There are differences, however, in the use of proof scales. The British proof scale uses a reference point of 57.15% v/v at 15.56°C, which is designated 100° proof. Alcohol concentrations of beverages are thus expressed as degrees over or under proof, and one degree proof is 0.57% v/v, and 1% v/v is 1.75° proof. Thus, a beverage that is 20° under proof (i.e., 80% proof) is 46% v/v, and a beverage that is 25% v/v is 56° under proof. The proof system used in the United States is more straightforward, in that one degree of proof equals 0.5% per volume at 15.56°C. Thus, a beverage that is 100° proof is 50% v/v, and a beverage that is 25% v/v is 50° proof.

2.2 PHARMACOKINETICS OF ALCOHOL

2.2.1 The Absorption of Alcohol in the Body

Alcohol is a small, weakly charged molecule that passes easily through membranes of the body by a process of simple diffusion. Because alcohol is polar and completely water soluble, the distribution of alcohol is largely determined by the water content of the organs and tissues of the body. Because of its use as a beverage and thus its oral administration, alcohol can be absorbed anywhere in the gastrointestinal tract. Absorption is most rapid in the duodenum and jejunum (the first two sections of the small intestine) and is lower but still appreciable through the mucosa of the stomach and the large intestine. Conversely, there is only minimal absorption in the mouth. Considering only the stomach and small intestine, in the average case, 80% of consumed alcohol is absorbed in the intestine, and only 20% in the stomach.

The rate of absorption of alcohol in the gastrointestinal tract depends on a number of factors, including food, dilution, composition of the beverage, and the presence of other drugs. For instance, it is a commonplace observation that the neurological effects of alcohol are slower to arise on a full stomach than on an empty one. This is explained by the fact that presence of food in the stomach delays emptying of the stomach through the pyloric valve into the duodenum. Thus, food in the stomach will also delay passage of alcohol from the more slowly absorbing stomach into the more rapidly absorbing duodenum.

Immediate absorption of alcohol in the mouth can be either through the oral mucosa into the blood circulating in the buccal tissues or through inhalation of the vapors into the lungs. If the alcohol is swallowed, however, very little remains available for absorption by either of these routes. Skin appears to be a barrier to absorption of alcohol unless it is broken. Finally, parenteral administration of alcohol is often used in laboratory experiments with both human and animal subjects. Both intraperitoneal and intravenous injection produce more uniform blood-alcohol levels than oral administration, because the variables associated with gastrointestinal uptake are avoided.

2.2.2 The Distribution of Alcohol in the Body

As mentioned above, alcohol readily permeates membranes in the body and is furthermore hydrophilic, that is, readily miscible in water; thus, it can go anywhere in the body that water can go. Additionally, there do not appear to be active uptake mechanisms for alcohol, and absorption, distribution, and elimination of alcohol appear to be explainable by a simple diffusion model, although this would be difficult to prove conclusively *in vivo* (Batt, 1989).

Simple diffusion alone would be a relatively slow process for distribution of alcohol in the body; the distribution of alcohol in the body occurs so rapidly because of vascularization and blood flow. That is, alcohol is distributed via the blood to the water compartments of body tissues and fluids. Using blood as a transport, alcohol will diffuse into body tissues as long as the concentration of alcohol in the blood is higher than the concentration in the tissue. The point of equilibration will occur sooner in those tissues with dense vascularization and a relatively greater blood supply. Equilibration will occur later in those that receive a lower percentage of output from the heart. The liver, the lungs, the kidneys, and the brain all equilibrate relatively rapidly (within a matter of minutes after consumption of alcohol), whereas skeletal muscle is slower to equilibrate. At the other end of the scale are bone and fat, which take up very little alcohol.

Although the equilibration rate varies from tissue to tissue and fluid to fluid on the basis of relative blood flow, the concentration of alcohol in each of these at equilibrium depends on the relative water content of each.

Various body tissues and fluids have been examined experimentally for their alcohol concentrations, as well as for the relation of those concentrations to tissue water or to blood-alcohol concentrations (BACs). Among the fluids and tissues that have been examined experimentally are blood, bile, cerebrospinal fluid, urine, saliva, and vitreous humor; and brain, kidney, liver, muscle, myocardium, spleen, and testes. In fact, however, results from such studies have been quite variable (Dubowski, 1985; Kalant, 1971).

Because it is blood that transports alcohol to the brain, BAC is the standard expression of alcohol in the body. It is important to note, however, that not all components of blood exhibit the same alcohol concentration, and this again is dependent on water content. Thus, plasma (the liquid portion of blood) shows a higher alcohol concentration than the suspended cells, and by the same token, both serum (the fluid remaining after coagulation) and plasma show a higher concentration than whole blood. Furthermore, the Mellanby Effect (Mellanby, 1919) describes the lower concentration of alcohol in venous blood compared to arterial blood during active absorption and before equilibration (see Forney, 1971; Forney, Hughes, Harger, & Richards, 1964; Harger & Hulpieu, 1956).

In research on behavioral effects of alcohol (including effects on speech), as well as in forensics, breath-alcohol analysis is now the most common form of chemical testing (Dubowski, 1991). Alcohol passes easily from blood through the alveolar membrane into air in the lungs. Whereas direct measurement of alcohol concentration in whole blood is taken on venous blood, expired alveolar air represents arterial blood. Because BAC has been the traditional measurement used for scientific, clinical, and forensic purposes, much research has been conducted since the 1930s to determine the exact relationship between BAC and breath-alcohol concentrations (BrAC). It does not appear that a single ratio or conversion factor can be applied uniformly to all individuals, but on the basis of earlier research, a blood to alveolar air partition ratio of 2100 : 1 has been used as a population mean for a number of purposes. These include the calibration of breath-alcohol analysis devices in grams of alcohol per 210 L of breath, as well as statutes specifically mentioning both grams of alcohol per 100 ml blood or per 210 L breath. More recent research, however, shows that a partition ratio of 2300 : 1 for healthy men is probably more accurate (A. W. Jones, 1989).

2.2.3 The Elimination of Alcohol from the Body

Alcohol is eliminated from the body in two ways: metabolism, which accounts for between 90 and 98% of ingested alcohol, and direct excretion, which accounts for the remaining 2–10%.

Metabolism of alcohol is a stepwise enzymatic oxidation process ultimately resulting in carbon dioxide and water. Although a relatively small amount of ethanol can be metabolized in the stomach, the majority of ethanol is metabolized in the liver. Alcohol is absorbed from the gastrointestinal system into the circulatory system, which transports alcohol-containing blood to the liver via the portal vein.

As mentioned above, the metabolism of alcohol through oxidation occurs in a number of steps. The first step is the conversion of ethanol to acetaldehyde. The primary enzyme involved as a catalyst in the metabolism is alcohol dehydrogenase (ADH), which is found in a number of living organisms, from lower bacteria to higher mammals, including humans. Different forms of ADH, called isoenzymes, occur in the human stomach and liver and can differ in the types of alcohol that they preferentially oxidize, the amount of alcohol that must accumulate before isoenzyme activity is initiated, and the maximal rate at which they oxidize alcohol (*Eighth Special Report*, 1993). Although the majority of alcohol metabolism takes place through oxidation by ADH, some alcohol may be oxidized within a complex called the microsomal ethanol-oxidizing system (MEOS); alcohol stimulates the microsomes when adequate chronic dosing occurs. Another system that can oxidize alcohol involves the enzyme catalase, which also appears to be stimulated at high alcohol concentrations.

The second step in the metabolism of alcohol is the oxidation of acetaldehyde to acetic acid by another enzyme called aldehyde dehydrogenase (ALDH). ALDH occurs in a number of body tissues, but metabolism of acetaldehyde occurs mainly in the liver, where the majority of ALDH synthesis occurs. In the oxidation of both alcohol and aldehyde, a single molecule of the reduced form of nicotinamide adenine dinucleotide (NADH) is produced from the oxidized form NAD^+, which serves as a coenzyme in these processes. The rate of metabolism depends to an extent on the regeneration of NAD from NADH. In the final stage of metabolism, acetic acid is oxidized to carbon dioxide and water.

A small amount of ethanol (i.e., no more than from 2–10%) can be excreted from the body through all of its body fluids; that is, unchanged, unmetabolized alcohol can be passed from the body through those routes by which water leaves the body. The bulk of unmetabolized elimination is through urine and breath, although negligible amounts may be found in tears, sweat, and saliva.

2.2.4 Specifications of Alcohol Concentrations in Blood and Breath

In the literature on alcohol and speech, the two main ways of reporting alcohol concentrations in the body are BAC and BrAC. Of these two, BAC enjoys some primacy, and in fact, BrAC is very often converted to an expression of equivalent BAC.

Following usual practice in chemistry, the common way of expressing BAC is by the weight of the quantity of alcohol contained in a given volume of blood. A common method used in the United States is expression of percent weight by volume (% w/v), which means grams of alcohol per 100 ml of blood (g/ml). In parts of Europe (e.g., The Netherlands, Austria) and in Japan, BACs are commonly reported as per mille weight by volume (‰ w/v), which means milligrams alcohol per milliliter of blood (mg/ml) or grams alcohol per liter of blood (g/L), which are equivalent proportions. In clinical usage and, for instance, Great Britain, a common expression of BAC is milligrams of alcohol per 100 milliliters of blood (mg/100 ml), sometimes expressed as mg% (although Wallgren and Barry [1970] say that the expression mg% is "inappropriate and should be abandoned"). All of these expressions are related to each other in the decimal system, so that the mg% (mg/100 ml) scale is 100 times the per mille scale and 1000 times the percent scale, and the per mille scale is 10 times the percent scale. Some different scale expressions of equivalent concentrations are given in Table 2.1.

In some jurisdictions (especially in Europe), statutory concentrations are expressed as unit weight of alcohol per unit weight of blood (1 ml whole blood weighs 1.055 g). Thus, in the Scandinavian countries of Sweden, Denmark, and Norway, statutory per se alcohol limits for operation of a motor vehicle are 0.20 mg/g, 0.50 mg/g, and 0.80 mg/g, respectively. In Germany, the statutory per se alcohol limit is 0.80 g/kg, which is equivalent to Norway's 0.80 mg/g.

Broadly, there are two ways of expressing the concentration of alcohol in expired air. The first is to convert the BrAC to an equivalent BAC, using

TABLE 2.1   Unit Equivalents in Measures of Blood Alcohol Concentration

Percent (%) = g/100 ml	Per mille (‰) = mg/ml or g/L	Milligrams percent (mg%) = mg/100 ml
0.001	0.01	1
0.01	0.1	10
0.02	0.2	20
0.05	0.5	50
0.07	0.7	70
0.08	0.8	80
0.1	1.0	100
0.15	1.5	150
0.2	2.0	200
0.3	3.0	300
0.4	4.0	400
0.5	5.0	500
1.0	10.0	1,000
10.0	100.0	10,000

a predetermined conversion factor; in this case, the units of expression will be those of BACs. The second is to report directly the concentration of alcohol in the breath; in this case, expression is almost uniformly in terms of unit weight of alcohol per unit volume of expired breath. A common weight by volume specification is milligrams alcohol per liter of expired air; the statutory per se alcohol limit in Norway and Japan, for instance, is 0.25 mg/L, in Sweden 0.10 mg/L, and in Austria 0.40 mg/L. The Netherlands and Great Britain both specify the unit weight of the alcohol as the microgram (μg, i.e., one-millionth of a gram) but differ in the unit volume of expired air; in the Netherlands the statutory per se alcohol limit is 220 μg/L and in Great Britain 35 μg/100 ml.

In the United States of America, each state has its own statutes regarding presumptive and per se alcohol limits for operation of a motor vehicle, including the determination of which body fluid or fluids (blood, breath, urine) may be analyzed for evidentiary use. In most cases, the 2100:1 alveolar air-to-blood partition ratio mentioned previously is used as a standard reference, but the application of this reference differs from jurisdiction to jurisdiction. In some states, presumptive and per se alcohol limits are set by statute in terms of BAC specifically. Separate statutes or procedural rules may allow the collection of other fluids (breath, urine) for analysis with provisions for converting those results into expressions of BAC for evidentiary use. On the other hand, some statutes are written so that limits are expressed both as BAC and BrAC. A common expression in the latter case is grams of alcohol per 210 L of breath. As can be seen, this is based on the 2100:1 partition ratio and renders the numeric expression of both BAC and BrAC the same (although the expression % is meaningless for BrAC in this case).

2.2.5 The Blood-Alcohol Curve

The blood-alcohol curve is an expression of the pharmacokinetics of alcohol in terms of an alcohol concentration versus time profile, subsequent to the ingestion of alcohol. An idealized, schematized blood-alcohol curve (adapted from Dubowski, 1985; Wallgren & Barry, 1970; and ultimately Widmark, 1932) is given in Figure 2.1. In Figure 2.1, the ideal Widmark blood-alcohol curve can be seen to have four phases, as indicated by clinical and experimental studies: (a) an absorption phase, (b) a plateau, (c) a diffusion equilibration phase, and (d) an elimination phase. The curve expresses the fact that two processes determine the BAC at any point after ingestion. First, there is an influx of alcohol into the blood, and second, an efflux of alcohol from the blood to tissues and fluids, that is, distribution, metabolism, and excretion of alcohol. Thus, if influx exceeds efflux, then the blood-alcohol curve will rise, as in (1) in Figure 2.1. If influx and efflux are approximately equal,

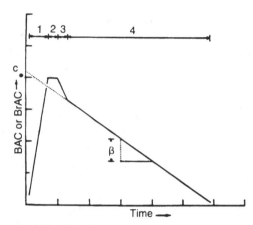

FIGURE 2.1   Theoretical blood-alcohol (BAC) or breath-alcohol (BrAC) curve (after Widmark, 1932): 1 = absorption phase, 2 = plateau, 3 = diffusion-equilibration, 4 = elimination phase. Reprinted with permission from *Journal of Studies on Alcohol*, Supplement No. 10, 98–108, 1985. © Copyright by Alcohol Research Documentation, Inc., Rutgers Center of Alcohol Studies, Piscataway, NJ 08855.

then the curve will plateau, as in (2) in Figure 2.1. And finally, when efflux exceeds influx, then the curve will descend, as in (3) and (4) in Figure 2.1. As the figure shows, absorption of alcohol is a relatively fast process (shows a steep slope), while elimination is relatively slow (shows a shallow slope), reflecting the fact that the enzymatic oxidation process by which most ingested alcohol is eliminated has a fairly low saturation threshold.

Widmark's factor β indicates the rate of descent of BAC after equilibration, that is, the slope of the descending portion of the curve. This is generally expressed as the reduction in BAC (in any of its usual expressions) per unit of time (generally either minutes (β) or hours (β_{60}). The indication C_o is the estimated or hypothetical alcohol concentration that would have obtained if ingested alcohol were immediately absorbed and instantaneously spread uniformly throughout the body water after complete absorption and distribution. This value is back extrapolated from the elimination portion of the alcohol curve. Determination of both factor β and C_o requires the elimination of alcohol from the body to follow zero-order kinetics, that is, linear elimination. We return to this point below.

An additional factor computed by Widmark, factor ρ, characterizes the distribution of alcohol in the organism. Given knowledge of the concentration of alcohol in the blood, factor ρ is the "reduced body mass" (Widmark, 1932), or the "factor by which the body weight must be reduced in order to obtain the theoretical body mass which would have the same alcohol concentration as the blood" (Watson, 1989, p. 47); additionally, the calculation of ρ is based on alcohol ingestion on a fasting stomach. Factor ρ is calculated according to the formula $\rho = A/p \times C_o$, where A is the total quantity of alcohol given and p is the weight of the organism. In fact, Widmark's calculations were based on human subjects, and mean values for ρ were 0.68 for men and 0.55 for women. Furthermore, both theoretically and empirically, there is no correlation between the factors β and ρ.

An idealized blood-alcohol curve as depicted in Figure 2.1, as well as Widmark's factors β and ρ, have provided the basis for a number of assumptions in both experimental and forensic studies. Klingholz, Penning, & Liebhardt (1988), for example, determined alcohol doses according to predicted BACs using Widmark's formula $C_o = A/p \times \rho$; it should be noted that actual achieved BACs in this instance only roughly approximated the predicted BACs. In the forensic realm, Widmark's factor ρ has also been used to estimate probable BAC after consumption of a known quantity of alcohol (see Khanna, LeBlanc, & Mayer, 1989). Widmark's factor β and the linear elimination phase on which it is based have provided the basis for back-estimation of BAC. None of these applications or their theoretical underpinnings, however, are without problems.

Widmark's estimate of the mean values for ρ differentiated males and female; however, a multiplicity of other factors have been shown to affect the shape of the blood-alcohol curve. Factors that appear to affect the rate of absorption include the presence of food in the stomach (food in the stomach slows the absorption rate); beverage composition (e.g., alcohol concentration or the presence of carbon dioxide, which appears to speed the absorption rate); consumption rate (see Dubowski, 1985); circadian rhythms (see Sturtevant & Sturtevant, 1989); the presence of drugs (see Kalant, 1971); as well as physiological characteristics including age, sex, total body weight, total body water, and general and specific metabolic disposition.

Widmark's factor ρ proposed an estimation of alcohol distribution volume on the basis of total body weight, and thus elimination rates were suggested to be a function of total body weight. However, recent research (see Watson, 1989) suggests that elimination rates are related to total body water rather than total body weight (in fact, Widmark [1932] proposed that differences in mean values of ρ for males and females were due to body fat). Perhaps the most concentrated debate regarding the elimination phase centers on the question of whether the one-compartment zero-order model first proposed by Mellanby (1919) and assumed by Widmark (1932) is the appropriate one for describing the pharmacokinetics of alcohol elimination. Lundquist and Wolthers (1958) suggested instead that alcohol metabolism followed Michaelis–Menten first-order kinetics (Michaelis & Menten, 1913). Since that time, a number of alternative models have been proposed, incorporating variations of first-order kinetics, multiple components, and multiple pathways (see von Wartburg, 1989).

Regardless of the mathematical model that best describes mean elimination patterns, or, for that matter, the mathematics of best-fit trend lines for individual elimination patterns, it is nevertheless the case that short-term fluctuations from the trend-line do occur. A number of studies reporting such irregularities and fluctuations in the blood- (or breath-) alcohol curve are cited in Dubowski (1985), and various aspects of the curve are characterized there as "unpredictable". Such fluctuations create a "steepling" effect such that there are numerous short-term but relatively sharp peaks (and troughs) all along the elimination portion of the alcohol curve. Thus, Dubowski (1985) cites three reasons for the unfeasibility of retrograde extrapolation (for at least some applications): (a) lack of knowledge regarding the timing of the alcohol concentration peak and absorption-postabsorption status, (b) lack of knowledge regarding the mathematical characteristics and mean rate of change of the individual's elimination curve, and (c) irregularities, especially short-term fluctuations from the best-fit trend line of the curve.

2.3 CENTRAL NERVOUS SYSTEM PHARMACODYNAMICS OF ALCOHOL

Alcohol exerts pharmacological effects upon a number of bodily systems in humans, including the gastrointestinal tract, the liver, the kidneys, and the cardiovascular system. However, its primary relation to speech involves its effects as a depressant on CNS functioning, which we discuss in this section.

2.3.1 Cellular and Molecular Sequelae of Alcohol Ingestion

It appears clear that alcohol has some effect on neural transmission; however, the precise molecular site or sites of alcohol's action are not clear (*Eighth Special Report,* 1990). One set of hypotheses suggests that the lipids and proteins in the cell membrane are the sites for alcohol's actions. Hunt (1985) has advanced the hypothesis that alcohol perturbs lipids in the cell membrane. Alternative hypotheses suggest that direct interactions of alcohol with a lipid-free enzyme protein explain the effects of alcohol. Whether alcohol acts on lipids or proteins, it is clear that there is alteration in the functioning of neuron-specific proteins.

Some neurotransmitters are inhibitory in their effect on electrical or chemical signals across synapses. One important inhibitory neurotransmitter, perhaps the most important in the mammalian brain, is gamma-aminobutyric acid (GABA). A number of studies have indicated that there is increased activity of the neuronal chloride ion channel that is linked to the A-type GABA receptor (GABA$_A$) during acute exposure to alcohol. These studies suggest an involvement of some of the proteins that make up the receptor in the action of alcohol. The effects of alcohol on the GABA$_A$ receptor may underlie the anxiolytic, sedative, and motor-impairing sequelae of alcohol ingestion (Givens & Breese, 1990; Suzdak & Paul, 1987). Another possible effect of alcohol involves glutamatergic neurotransmission. Glutamate is an important excitatory transmitter in the mammalian CNS. Two receptor types activated by glutamate are called the N-methyl-D-aspartate (NMDA) receptor and the α-amino-3-hydroxy-5-methyl-4-isoxazole propionic acid (AMPA) receptor. Alcohol appears to inhibit functioning of both of these receptors, and NMDA receptors appear to be more sensitive to alcohol than AMPA receptors (e.g., Dildy-Mayfield & Leslie, 1991; Lovinger, White, & Weight, 1989).

One region of the brain that shows specific effects of alcohol is the cerebellum, and in particular, the Purkinje neurons located in the cerebellar cortex. The particular sensitivity of Purkinje cells to alcohol effects have been known for some time (e.g., Chu, 1983; Rogers, Siggins, Schulman, & Bloom, 1979). Recent research has uncovered a number of alcohol effects on Purkinje cells; for example, it alters Purkinje cell electrical activity (Franklin & Gruol, 1987; Palmer, VanHorne, Harlan, & Moore, 1988); it reduces the ability of glutamate to stimulate Purkinje cell firing; and it especially potentiates responses to the inhibitory neurotransmitter GABA (Lin, Freund, & Palmer, 1991).

2.3.2 Acute Behavioral and Cognitive Sequelae of Alcohol Ingestion

We conclude this chapter with a brief discussion of various acute effects that are attributable to alcohol's depressant action on the CNS through impairment of neuronal transmission. Alcohol is an irregularly descending, general CNS depressant and produces dose-dependent effects, including decrease in the level of arousal; in this way, alcohol has effects similar to those of general anesthetics. It also produces effects that are comparable to some of those of hypnotics, sedatives, and tranquilizers. Like the sedatives, alcohol is considered to be irregularly descending, because it affects only certain functions of the nervous system, working first at the cerebral level and then descending through the cerebellar and spinal cord levels. Much of the research on the effects of alcohol has been conducted in the context of its effects on the ability to operate motor vehicles (see Starmer, 1989), and these investigations have included studies of perception (e.g., visual acuity), ocular motor functioning, psychomotor effects (e.g., reaction speed), and cognitive functioning (e.g., vigilance, memory).

Like other CNS depressants, small alcohol doses may actually improve performance on some tests of psychomotor functioning, especially in anxious subjects (Linnoila, 1974). This type of effect is observed, as mentioned, after low doses and during the rising phase of the BAC curve. These stimulatory effects are similar to those produced by stimulant drugs (e.g., amphetamines), albeit weaker. Because alcohol induces first stimulatory effects and then later depressant effects, the actions of alcohol are considered to be biphasic (Pohorecky, 1977).

Starmer (1989) reviews much of the experimental literature investigating the effects of low to moderate doses of alcohol on CNS functioning (see also the review in Chapters 6 and 7 of Wallgren & Barry, 1970), and especially those skills required for the operation of motor vehicles. Effects on visual perception include impairment of dynamic visual acuity (i.e., the ability to perceive detail in an object in motion); reduction in glare resistance (Verriest & Laplasse, 1965), and increase in recovery time after exposure to glare (Adams & Brown, 1975); impairment of color discrimination (Rizzo, 1957; Schmidt & Bingel, 1953); impaired performance on a combined tracking and visual recognition task (von Wright & Mikkonen, 1970); and increased time to perceive in a combined central visual fixation task and peripheral vision task (Huntley, 1970). Auditory perception has shown some effects from alcohol (Jellinek & MacFarland, 1940), including impairment of discrimination, although not of sensitivity (Pinkhanen & Kauko, 1962).

Also studied have been ocular motor functions, which are the most rapid and well-controlled movements performed by the human body. Effects of alcohol include decreased optokinetic fusion limit (Blomberg & Wassen, 1962); impaired accuracy of binocular coordination (Wist, Hughes, & Forney, 1967); simultaneous perception of both images (Bárány & Hallden, 1947); impaired depth perception (Chardon, Boiteau, & Bogaert, 1959); and adverse effects on both peak (Wilkinson & Kime, 1974) and mean (Guedry, Gillson, Schroeder, & Collins, 1975) saccadic eye movement velocity. A number of studies have investigated nystagmic effects of alcohol ingestion. Nystagmus is an involuntary jerking of the eyes that occurs as the eyes gaze laterally. It is a normal phenomenon, but it is exaggerated or magnified by alcohol. Positional alcohol nystagmus (PAN) occurs when the head of an alcohol-intoxicated person is placed laterally. This type of nystagmus occurs when alcohol changes the specific gravity of the blood, so that there are unequal concentrations in the blood and vestibular system, and the response of the vestibular system to gravity is thereby disturbed. Two types of positional alcohol nystagmus have been observed (Rauschke, 1954; Seedorf, 1956). In PAN I, which occurs as the BAC is increasing (i.e., alcohol concentration is greater in the blood than in the inner ear fluid), there is a slow drift of the eye upwards, followed by rapid jerks downward. In PAN II, which occurs as the BAC is decreasing (i.e., alcohol concentration is greater in the inner ear fluid than in the blood), the opposite occurs; that is, there is slow drift of the eye downward, followed by a rapid jerk upward.

Horizontal gaze nystagmus occurs as the eyes gaze to the side. In the absence of alcohol ingestion, jerking generally occurs when lateral gaze is greater than 45°, but when a subject is intoxicated, alcohol gaze nystagmus (Fregly, Bergstedt, & Graybiel, 1967) occurs at between 30° and 40°.

Research on the effects of alcohol on reaction times (RT) indicates that these effects are dependent on alcohol dose, attained alcohol concentration, and complexity of the task. Thus, effects of low alcohol concentrations will be more evident as tasks are more complex (Jellinek & MacFarland, 1940; Wallgren & Barry, 1970). Simple RTs appear to be affected by alcohol, but consistently only when large doses are administered. It has also been found that responses to auditory stimuli are more affected by alcohol than to visual stimuli (R. Martin, LeBreton, & Roche, 1957). For choice RTs, both low (Warrington, Ankier, & Turner, 1984) and moderate (Franks, Hensley, Hensley, Starmer, & Teo, 1975) doses of alcohol decrease performance. Simultaneous increases of task demands and alcohol dose appear to effect large decreases in performance; thus, RTs on a combined letter-canceling and complex RT task showed more than a two-fold increase under alcohol (Grüner, 1955, 1959).

Performance on speed and accuracy tasks also shows decrements from alcohol. In pencil and paper tests (Stone, 1984) and in clerical-task (e.g., typing) tests (Balint, 1961; Nash, 1962), alcohol affected performance. Decrements in clerical-task speed were most consistent at high alcohol doses, with somewhat less consistent results at low doses (Lawton & Cahn, 1963), but error rates consistently increased. A number of studies have been conducted that investigated the effects of alcohol on tracking. In general, it has been found that alcohol effects are greater on pursuit tracking tasks than on simple compensatory tracking tasks. In compensatory tracking tasks, studies have shown a decrease in performance corresponding to increasing BAC (e.g., Drew, Colquhoun, & Long, 1958; Newman, Fletcher, & Abramson, 1942). Although some subjects may not show performance deficits when compensatory tracking is the sole task, very often the addition of subsidiary tasks will reveal a response to alcohol. Pursuit tracking tasks appear to be more sensitive to the effects of alcohol, and a number of studies reveal a significant decrease in performance after alcohol (Hughes & Forney, 1964; Mortimer, 1963). Further degradation generally follows when other subsidiary tasks are added.

The effects of alcohol on cognitive functions have been examined in a large number of studies (Starmer, 1989; Wallgren & Barry, 1970). Selective attention appears to be impaired after low doses of alcohol, but vigilance was not impaired in a task requiring subjects to detect possible color intensity differences in six small disks presented simultaneously (Colquhoun, 1962; Docter, Naitoh, & Smith, 1966; Talland, Mendelson, & Ryack, 1964). Robust effects of alcohol on divided attention have been demonstrated in a number of studies. These include studies in which subjects were required to simultaneously perform a letter-canceling task and respond to lights in the periphery (Grüner, 1959; Grüner, Ludwig, & Domer, 1964); there was both an increase in RT to the lights and a decrease in accuracy on the cancelation task. Another study required divided attention in an auditory vigilance task (Moskowitz, Daily, & Henderson, 1979); after alcohol, performance on the vigilance task alone remained unaffected but decreased significantly when attention was divided.

In a number of studies, alcohol has been shown to affect search patterns and scanning behavior. For example, alcohol produces an increased fixation time (Moskowitz & Murray, 1976) and a decrease in the amount of time looking outside the central region of vision (Belt, 1969). In studies of visual scan patterns, significant increases in fixation time under alcohol were observed, but no effects were found on the horizontal distribution of fixations (Kobayashi, 1974; Mortimer & Sturgis, 1972).

A number of studies have investigated the effects of alcohol on memory. For instance, Rosen and Lee (1976) reported partial or complete amnesia for events occurring during a period of acute intoxication for both alcoholics and normal subjects. Goodwin, Othmer, Halikas, and Freeman (1970) examined four types of memory (remote, immediate, short-term, and recent) in subjects who consumed very high alcohol doses. Short-term memory deficits were associated with rising BACs, but only short-term memory deficit was correlated with postalcohol amnesia. Of the different types of memory, short-term memory appears to be the most easily affected (B. M. Jones, 1973; Ryback, 1971).

Alcohol intoxication presents with a number of dose-related clinical nervous system signs and symptoms. At low doses, alcohol may in some cases actually improve psychomotor performance, most likely through its anxiolytic effects (Ashton, 1987; Linnoila, 1974). Small doses appear to affect primarily mood, with a mild euphoria and a sense of relaxation. Increased doses, however, result in "ataxia, slurred speech, and eventually stupor, deep anasthesia, and coma" (Ashton, 1987, p. 178). The course of behavioral effects as a function of BAC is summarized by Santamaria (1989). Between 0.03 and 0.05%, judgment and visual acuity are impaired. Between 0.05 and 0.08%, muscle control is affected, as evidenced by increased RT and mild incoordination. As BAC rises, there is an exaggeration of these effects, as well as new ones. Around 0.10%, nystagmus develops and incoordination becomes more prominent. Articulation becomes difficult, along with performance of fine movements and skilled operations. Ataxia also emerges at this concentration. A common ataxic sign is gait abnormality (e.g., Jetter, 1938a, 1938b). Both nystagmus and ataxia are the basis for standardized field sobriety testing. Both laboratory experiments and field testing (Anderson, Schweitz, & Snyder, 1983;

Burns & Moskowitz, 1977; Tharp, Burns, & Moskowitz, 1981) established three standard field sobriety tests: walk-and-turn, one-leg stand, and horizontal gaze nystagmus.

At still higher concentrations, drowsiness, sleep, and stupor ensue, with coma appearing at about 0.30%. There is a depressed respiratory response to carbon dioxide (Ashton, 1987), and death from respiratory failure may occur at BACs above 0.40% (Ashton, 1987).

CHAPTER 3

Speech Production and Speech Acoustics

3.0 INTRODUCTION

In this chapter we discuss the process of speech production, as well as the speech signal and its measurement. Section 3.1 is a discussion of the anatomical, physiological, and neurological bases of speech production, including description of the sound segments (consonants and vowels) that serve as analytical units for much of speech science. Section 3.2 is a discussion of some of the instrumental techniques used in modern research on the analysis of acoustic signals, particularly speech. Finally, section 3.3 examines various linguistic and phonetic variables that can serve as analysis targets.

3.1 SPEECH PRODUCTION

3.1.1 Anatomy and Physiology of the Speech Organs

As will be seen, most organs used in speech have other functions not related to speech. Additionally, although the organs used in speech are interconnected physically and functionally for both speech and their other functions, it is convenient to discuss them as separate subsystems: subglottal (respiration), laryngeal (phonation), and supralaryngeal (articulation). For further discussions of the anatomy and physiology of the speech organs, see Borden, Harris, and Raphael (1994), Dickson and Maue-Dickson (1982), Kahane and Folkins (1984), and Zemlin (1988). Important anatomical landmarks in the production of speech are shown in Figure 3.1.

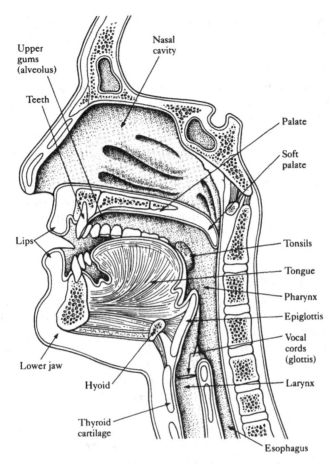

FIGURE 3.1 Vocal tract configuration with raised soft palate for articulating nonnasal sounds. (From *The Speech Chain* by Denes and Pinson. Copyright © 1993 by W.H. Freeman and Company. Used by permission.)

3.1.1.1 Respiratory Organs

The source of the airstream for the production of most speech sounds in language is the lungs. The basic biological function of the lungs is respiration, which entails an exchange of gases between an organism (in this case a human) and its environment. The important subglottal (below the larynx) respiratory organs are the lungs, where the gas exchange occurs, and the trachea, which permits communication with the upper respiratory organs and thus with outside air. Lung tissue is spongy, porous, and highly elastic. Because of a low number of smooth muscle fibers, lung tissue cannot exert force on its own. Inspiration is controlled by the intercostal muscles located between the ribs surrounding the lungs and by the diaphragm and abdominal muscles. Expiration is controlled by a combination of muscle action and elastic recoil of the lung tissue.

Phonation and speech production occur during the expiratory phase of respiration; that is, the production of speech depends on an outward-flowing airstream. However, quiet expiration is to a large extent a passive process, and this process is not sufficient to support the type of airflow necessary for speech. In order to produce an airflow that can sustain phonation and speech, a talker must use both inspiratory and expiratory processes, or muscle contractions. In the absence of this, air would flow out of the lungs too quickly, and the air supply for the production of speech would be depleted too soon. Inspiratory muscle contractions are thus used to produce an outward airflow slower than that used for quiet breathing. Once airflow due to elastic recoil has ceased, then expiratory actions further depress the chest cavity to provide more air to sustain speech.

3.1.1.2 Laryngeal or Phonatory Organs

Although the airstream exiting the lungs and trachea is necessary for most speech sounds, it is at this stage essentially undifferentiated noise. The power spectrum (see section 3.2.2.3) of air exiting the trachea is uniform across a wide range of frequencies. The larynx, modified cartilage located at the upper end of the trachea, generates the sound necessary for speech. Because it is essentially a valve at the top of the lower respiratory system, the larynx prevents both air from escaping the lungs and foreign matter from entering the lungs.

The larynx is located at the upper end of the trachea and suspended from the U-shaped hyoid bone by a number of muscles. The structural framework of the larynx itself consists of both large unpaired cartilages and smaller paired cartilages. The largest laryngeal cartilage is the thyroid cartilage, which forms most of the front and side walls of the larynx. At the top front of the thyroid cartilage is the V-shaped thyroid notch, found just above the thyroid prominence or Adam's apple. Immediately behind the tongue root and hyoid bone is a leaf-shaped structure called the epiglottis. The precise function of the epiglottis is not completely clear, although it is widely held that it prevents food from entering the trachea during swallowing by flapping down over the larynx.

The back of each side of the thyroid cartilage extends both upward and downward in superior and inferior cornua ('horns'). The superior cornua are attached to the hyoid bone by ligaments, whereas the inferior cornua articulate with the ring-shaped cricoid cartilage, located immediately above the trachea. The cricoid cartilage is smaller than the thyroid cartilage, and its articulation with the thyroid cartilage forms a pivot joint, allowing rotation of either the cricoid or the thyroid cartilage. This movement is important for changing pitch.

Located on the sloping sides of the cricoid cartilage are the approximately pyramid-shaped arytenoid cartilages. The anterior angle of each of the pair of arytenoid cartilages presents as a pointed projection called the vocal process; the vocal ligament, a part of the vocal fold, inserts on the vocal process at one end. At the other end, the vocal folds, consisting of the vocal ligament and the thyroarytenoid muscle, have a common anterior attachment below the thyroid notch. Although the vocal folds are attached to the thyroid cartilage in front and the arytenoid cartilages in back, their medial edges are free, and they project into the laryngeal cavity like shelves.

The larynx contains two pairs of joints that control adjustments of the vocal folds. The cricoarytenoid joint permits the rocking and to some extent the gliding of the arytenoid cartilages at their articulation with the cricoid cartilage, resulting in either abduction or adduction of the vocal folds. As mentioned previously, the thyroid and cricoid cartilages articulate at the cricothyroid joint, permitting rotation about a horizontal axis. This rotation results in increased tension in the vocal folds, which raises the pitch of the voice.

3.1.1.3 Supralaryngeal or Articulatory Organs

The airstream passing immediately above the glottis can be of two basic types, either with or without periodic pulsing. The former is caused by adduction of the vocal folds, whereas the latter passes through relatively abducted or widely spaced vocal folds. Once above the glottis, the airstream can be further modified and shaped by the supralaryngeal vocal tract.

The supralaryngeal vocal tract consists of the pharyngeal cavity, the oral cavity, and the nasal cavities. The lips, at the outer boundary of the oral cavity, are important in the formation of speech sounds. Both lips or only one lip can be used in the formation of speech sounds. The lower lip, because it is partially dependent on movements of the mandible (lower jaw), is more mobile than the upper lip; the formation of labiodental sounds, or sounds formed by articulating the teeth with the lips, almost always involve the upper teeth and the lower lip. The pharyngeal cavity lies within the pharynx, a tube of muscle and membrane extending from the area of the cricoid cartilage to the base of the skull. The oral cavity extends from the teeth and alveolar processes (i.e., the borders of the upper jaw [maxilla] and lower jaw [mandible] with sockets to hold teeth) in front and the palatoglossal arch in back; the top boundary of the oral cavity consists of the hard and soft palates, and the bottom boundary consists of the floor of the mouth, mostly taken up by the tongue. Within the oral cavity, important structures in the articulation of speech include the tongue, the teeth, the alveolar ridge, the hard palate, and the soft palate or velum.

Biologically, the tongue allows humans to taste, chew, and swallow food. Its role in the articulation of speech sounds is no less important, and in fact it is considered the preeminent articulatory organ, playing a major role in the production of both vowels and consonants. In the production of vowels, the tongue is the major shaping organ of the vocal tract, and in the production of consonants, it is the most active articulator. The tongue is a three-dimensional mass of muscle fiber and consists of a dorsum, which constitutes the majority of the tongue's mass, and a blade, toward the front of the tongue. The dorsum, also called the tongue body, consists of a front portion and a back portion, which are at very nearly right angles to each other. The very front of the blade is the tip, located near the front teeth. The blade itself lies below the alveolar ridge, the front under the hard palate, and the back under the soft palate. All of these portions of the tongue are used in speech sound articulation.

Tongue movements are executed by means of both external and internal paired musculature. In general, the external musculature determines movement of the tongue as a whole, and the tongue is capable of movement as a mass up and back, down and back, and up and forward. The genioglossus muscles are the largest extrinsic muscles. They originate on the inside of the mandible, run through the tongue, and attach to the hyoid bone; contraction of these muscles pulls both the hyoid bone and tongue forward. The styloglossus muscles originate at the styloid processes in the temporal bones and then insert into the sides of the tongue; contracting these muscles pulls the tongue back and up. The palatoglossus muscles originate in the soft palate and insert into the sides of the tongue; contracting these muscles either lowers the soft palate or raises the back of the tongue. Finally, the hyoglossus muscles originate from the hyoid bone and insert into the sides of the back of the tongue; contracting these muscles depresses and retracts the tongue.

The shape of the tongue, especially its surface, is determined by four intrinsic muscles. The superior longitudinal muscle runs down the middle of the tongue from back to front; contracting this muscle shortens the tongue, effectively curling the tip upward. On the underside of the tongue is the inferior longitudinal muscle; contraction of this muscle curls the tongue downward. The transverse muscle originates in the middle of the tongue and radiates laterally; contraction of this muscle narrows and elongates the tongue. Finally, the vertical muscle originates in the dorsum and courses downward; contraction of this muscle flattens the tongue.

Human dentition consists of four types of teeth: incisors, cuspids (canines), bicuspids (premolars), and molars. Important in the articulation of speech are the incisors, located in the front of the mouth, which can be used in various articulatory configurations. Additionally, articulation of the tongue with the molars is also used in the production of speech sounds.

The palate is formed of a bony plate in the front and a muscular valve in the back. Additionally, the very front of the palate is referred to as the alveolar ridge, a series of bony sockets in the upper jaw that hold the teeth. Both the alveolar ridge and the hard palate are fixed and rigid; the formation of speech sounds with these involves raising of the tongue to articulate with them. However, the posterior portion of the palate, called the soft palate or the velum, consists of muscle fibers, making it possible to raise, lower, or tense the velum. The dorsum of the tongue articulates with the velum in the formation of a number of consonant sounds; however, a perhaps even more important role of the velum is as a valve, controlling the degree of coupling between the nasal cavities and the rest of the vocal tract. Elevation of the velum effectively uncouples the nasal cavities; this configuration is used in the production of oral vowels and consonants. Lowering the velum couples the nasal cavities to the rest of the vocal tract; this configuration is used in the production of nasal vowels and consonants as well as during quiet respiration.

The nasal cavities are two narrow passages separated by the nasal septum, a vertical plate made of bone and cartilage. The nasal cavities communicate at one end with the exterior through the nostrils and at the other with the nasopharynx. The passage between the nasal cavities and the oral and pharyngeal cavities is called the velopharyngeal port. As mentioned above, elevation of the velum closes off the velopharyngeal port, effectively uncoupling the nasal cavities from the rest of the vocal tract. Conversely, lowering the velum opens the velopharyngeal port.

3.1.2 Neurological Aspects of Speech Production

Virtually all human behaviors, including language and speech, are mediated to some extent by the nervous system. Because alcohol is regarded as a central nervous system (CNS) depressant, we briefly discuss here some of the neurological aspects of speech. Discussions of this topic can be found in Borden et al. (1994), Kuehn, Lemme, and Baumgartner (1989), Love and Webb (1986), Penfield and Roberts (1959), and Zemlin (1988).

The nervous system can be divided anatomically into the CNS, consisting of the brain and the spinal cord, and the peripheral nervous system (PNS), consisting of cranial nerves that serve the head and the spinal nerves that serve all other regions of the body.

3.1.2.1 The Neuron and Neuronal Transmission

Because the neurological effects of alcohol are regarded as occurring at the cellular and molecular level, we include here a brief discussion of the basic cellular unit of the nervous system, the neuron.

The basic unit of the nervous system is a specialized cell called a neuron. Functionally, all neurons can be characterized as being either somatic (involving voluntary functions such as speech) or autonomic (involving involuntary processes such as respiration). Additionally, neurons are either efferent, conducting impulses away from the CNS, or afferent, conducting impulses toward the CNS. Structurally, a neuron consists of (a) a cell body; (b) dendrites, which carry impulses (or action potentials) to the cell body; and (c) an axon, which carries impulses away from the cell body. Each neuron has any number of dendrites but only one axon.

The action potential is carried from the cell body along the axon to the axon terminal, where the axon branches out. Conduction of the excitation depends on a plasma membrane enclosing the axon. The membrane separates the interior of the nerve fiber from the exterior, and when the nerve fiber is at rest, the interior has a negative electrical charge relative to the exterior. When the nerve fiber is excited, the membrane becomes more permeable, allowing an exchange of ions between the exterior and interior through small pores, resulting in depolarization of the nerve fiber. That is, the interior becomes positively charged relative to the exterior. Immediately after this, the fiber returns to its resting state until it is depolarized again by another impulse. As depolarization occurs at one point along the axon, this stimulates a subsequent point, and this impulse travels down the axon as long as stimulation is at a sufficient threshold.

The conduction of impulses from one neuron to another takes place at a juncture called a synapse. As an impulse reaches the axon terminal, chemical substances called neurotransmitters are released from the presynaptic neuron into the synaptic gap, a small space between neurons. At the postsynaptic side of the gap is generally a dendrite from another neuron. Contained in the dendrites are receptor molecules that recognize and bind the neurotransmitters. Some neurotransmitters are excitatory, facilitating firing of the next neuron. Conversely, other neurotransmitters are inhibitory and decrease the excitability of the next neuron.

Neural transmission is not simply the sequential passing of impulses from one neuron to another in a single, linear chain. Rather, more than one neuron can fire a single neuron, and a single neuron can fire a number of neurons, in a three-dimensional pattern. Furthermore, the axons and dendrites of numerous neurons are grouped together functionally in nerves or nerve tracts. Such nerves may be sensory, that is, having an afferent function; motor, having an efferent function; or mixed, having both afferent and efferent functions.

3.1.2.2 The Brain

The CNS consists of the brain and the spinal cord. The spinal cord is a cylindrical bundle that runs up (or down) the back, and from it emanate

31 paired nerves that innervate most body functions except those in the head. At the top of the spinal cord sits the brain, the main organ of the nervous system, which is actually continuous with the spinal cord.

The brain resembles an oval melon in shape, is gray in color, and weighs approximately 1.5 kg or about 3 lbs. Figure 3.2 is a medial view of some important structures of the brain. The greatest amount of mass invested in the brain is given over to the cerebrum, which consists of three parts: the cerebral hemispheres, the basal ganglia, and the rhinencephalon. The left and right hemispheres of the brain are roughly symmetrical in appearance, but not symmetrical in function. Communication between corresponding regions of the two hemispheres takes place across the corpus callosum, a prominent band of commissural fibers. The outer surface of the cerebrum is a layer approximately 1.5–4.5 mm thick called the cerebral cortex. The surface of the cerebral cortex contains numerous convolutions, including gyri (sg. gyrus), or elevations on the cortex, and sulci (sg. sulcus), groove-like fissures separating the sulci. The gyri and sulci form landmarks that allow identification of various regions of the cerebral cortex, most notably four lobes: the frontal, temporal, parietal, and occipital lobes. Cerebral cortex is mainly responsible for those behavioral and intellectual attributes that separate human beings from the lower animals. As well as being responsible for a number of lower functions, it is also the seat of memory, consciousness, thought, and voluntary actions. The remaining cerebral structures are embedded deeply within the cerebral hemispheres.

Located behind and at the base of the cerebrum is a considerably smaller structure called the cerebellum. As shown in Figure 3.2, the cerebellum is located between the cerebrum and the brain stem, described below. The cerebellum presents as a slightly oval, somewhat flattened structure and consists of a narrow median portion called the vermis, which connects, and is partially covered by, the two cerebellar hemispheres, which project laterally and posteriorly.

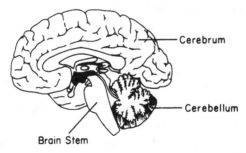

FIGURE 3.2   Medial view of the right cerebrum and cerebellum. (From Love and Webb, 1986. Copyright © 1986 by Butterworth Heinemann. Used by permission.)

Structurally, the cerebellum consists of a surface of gray matter called the cerebellar cortex, four paired subcortical nuclei, and white matter. The cerebellar cortex consists of two layers: an outer molecular layer and an inner granular layer. The molecular layer consists of small intrinsic nerve cells (basket, Golgi, and stellate cells), as well as large neurons called Purkinje cells. Purkinje cells are arranged in a single row in the deepest portion of the molecular layer; their highly arborized dendrites extend into the molecular layer, whereas their axons extend through the granular layer into the white matter, terminating in the deep nuclei. The granular layer consists of a large number of granular cells, the smallest type of neuron, which function to excite the Purkinje cells.

The cerebellum has been likened to a comparator (Zemlin, 1988), functioning to rapidly analyze a large amount of input information (from skeletal muscles) and to coordinate the timing and extent of cortically induced movements to produce smoothly coordinate voluntary muscle movement. Sensory input to the cerebellum is routed to both the cerebellar cortex and the subcortical nuclei. The most important cerebellar structures are the Purkinje cells. These are excited by climbing fibers, mossy fibers, and granule cells, and their axons terminate mainly on the subcortical nuclei. Subsequent discharge from the subcortical nuclei to the motor systems is regulated by the fact that Purkinje cells transmit exclusively inhibitory impulses, thus selectively damping the activity of the subcortical nuclei.

As the medial view in Figure 3.2 shows, the brain stem is not visible from the outside of the brain; rather, it extends from the top of the spinal cord up in between the cerebral hemispheres. The brain stem can be considered to consist of a lower brain stem, consisting of the pons and medulla oblongata, and an upper brain stem, consisting of the diencephalon and mesencephalon. The medulla oblongata is the caudal-most part of the brain and is a bulbous enlargement (it is also called the *bulb*) of the top of the spinal cord. On the anterior surface of the medulla is located a median fissure, and on either side of this are swellings called pyramids. Posterior to the pyramids are oval elevations called olives. The upper portion of the posterior of the medulla oblongata continues to the cerebellum by means of two stalks called the inferior cerebellar peduncles, which carry fibers from the spinal cord and medulla oblongata to the cerebellum. Above the medulla oblongata is a rounded structure directed anteriorly called the pons, which connects to the hemispheres of the cerebellum by means of transverse fibers located on its anterior surface. The mesencephalon (or midbrain) is a constricted segment located above the pons, and connects the pons and cerebellum with the cerebral hemispheres. The mesencephalon consists of two cerebral peduncles located lateroventrally, and dorsally, the tectum, which contains the paired superior and inferior colliculi (little hills). Above the mesencephalon is the diencephalon, which is composed of the thalamus, located ventrally, and the hypothalamus, located dorsally.

3.1.2.3 Language and Speech in the Brain

Most researchers will agree that language and speech functions are relatively well-localized in the brain; that is, certain regions of the brain bear the primary responsibility for the representation and processing of language. Specifically, in approximately 95% of the population (all right-handed and most left-handed people), language is localized in the left cerebral hemisphere. Much of the knowledge regarding the localization of language and speech (as well as of other functions) has been gained under unfortunate circumstances, when injury to the brain from either internal or external sources, either results in language impairment or does not. Until the middle of the 19th century, at least this much was known: First, injury to the brain from such external sources as weapon wounds or from such internal sources as strokes very often resulted in aphasia, that is, language impairment, which could appear in a number of forms. Second, cerebral control of various functions appeared to be contralateral; that is, each cerebral hemisphere exerted control over the opposite side of the body.

In 1861, Pierre-Paul Broca reported the case of a patient who had suffered speech loss. At post mortem examination, Broca found that the second and third convolutions of the left cerebral hemisphere were destroyed. Because the autopsy was only superficial (no cuts were made) and because even surface damage extended beyond the frontal convolutions, Broca examined another 20 cases in the next 2 years. Broca (1863) reported that speech loss typically involved frontal convolutions only on the left side, and that only speech production, rather than speech comprehension, was affected. The area identified by Broca as being responsible for speech production is now called Broca's area, and the specific type of aphasia showing production deficits is called Broca's aphasia.

Wernicke (1874) reported the identification of a second region of the brain responsible for language. A language disturbance with different symptoms from those described by Broca appeared to be related to a lesion on the first and second convolutions of the temporal lobe of the left hemisphere. Whereas the aphasia described by Broca affected predominantly motor production of speech, the disturbance described by Wernicke exhibited deficits in comprehension. Expressive speech was not lacking; in fact, it was quite abundant, but at the same time it was confused and incoherent, and there was a severe impairment in comprehension. Wernicke called this type of disturbance sensory aphasia, although it is now more generally referred to as Wernicke's aphasia. Similarly, the brain region identified by Wernicke as the site of lesions underlying this type of aphasia is called Wernicke's area.

From the identification of a second type of aphasia, one affecting comprehension rather than production, Wernicke concluded that there existed a second language center in the brain, located at the first gyrus of the left temporal lobe. Because this region was located adjacent to the primary auditory cortex, Wernicke thought it reasonable that lesions in this region would result in comprehension deficits. In addition to suggesting that language functions might be localized in the brain, Wernicke also predicted that a third type of aphasia would be evident if communication between the two regions (Broca's area and Wernicke's area) was disturbed; this type of aphasia he termed *conduction aphasia*.

More recent research has mitigated the strong view of pinpoint localization of language regions in the brain. The view proposed by Broca, however, that language is centralized in the left hemisphere (the "lateralization" of language function) has held up well, especially for right-handed persons, with some caveats necessary for left-handed persons. Besides studies of aphasics, other approaches have been taken to investigate language functions in the brain. These include the cortical stimulation studies undertaken by Wilder Penfield and Lamar Roberts in Montreal, Canada (1959). Before performing surgery for the treatment of epilepsy, the researchers used electrical stimulation to locate seizure centers but were also able to map cortical loci of a number of other functions, including speech. Newer neuroimaging techniques, such as computerized tomography (CT) scans, magnetic resonance imaging (MRI), positron emission tomography (PET), and single proton emission computed tomography (SPECT), have contributed greatly to our current understanding of language and speech in the brain (see Lemme, Kuehn, & Baumgartner, 1989, for an overview).

3.1.2.4 Motor Control of Speech Organs

Based on the work of Wolff (1979), Netsell (1982) cited the following attributes of speech production that characterize it as an instance of fine motor control:

> (1) it is performed with accuracy and speed, (2) it uses knowledge of results, (3) it is improved by practice, (4) it demonstrates motor flexibility in achieving goals, and (5) it relegates all of this to automatic control, where "consciousness" is freed from the details of action plans. (Netsell, 1982:37)

Netsell further described the motor control of speech as being comparable to that used for control of the hands and fingers in playing the violin or piano. This has far less to do with the esthetics of speech than with Netsell's assertion that speech motor control falls between the extremes of extraocular and forearm motor control (Netsell, 1982, p. 39). That is, movements for speech are slow to moderate (e.g., slower than ocular movements), typically in the 5 to 20 cm/sec range, with 30 cm/sec for fast movements. Spatial movement is precise, with single articulators rarely moving beyond 1 cm; jaw movements of 1.5 cm are extreme. Repeated tongue positioning for a single vowel sound can be within 1 mm (Gay, Lindblom, & Lubker, 1981; Netsell, Kent, & Abbs, 1980). Coordination of two articulators, such as in the production of consonant clusters, are temporally precise, as fine as 10 ms (Kent & Moll, 1975). All of this, then, occurs within the context of the act of speaking, which, according to Lenneberg (1967), requires the control and coordination of over 100 muscles at a rate of articulation of 14 phonemes (i.e., speech sounds) per second. Darley, Aronson, and Brown (1975) estimated that, conservatively, each of these 100 muscles would be composed of approximately 100 motor units (a single motor neuron and the individual muscle fibers that it innervates), so that at the rate of 14 phonemes per second, "140,000 [100 muscles x 100 motor units x 14 phonemes] neuromuscular events would be required for each second of motor speech production" (p. 17).

The frontal lobe is bounded posteriorly by the central sulcus and inferiorly by the lateral sulcus. Just anterior to the central sulcus is a gyrus called the precentral gyrus. This gyrus is particularly important, because it comprises the bulk of the motor cortex (which also includes the posterior portions of the frontal gyri), which is responsible for voluntary motor control. The motor cortex contains no granular layer, but in its fifth layer it contains giant pyramidal cells of Betz, which are the origin of the main motor pathways for voluntary skeletal muscle control, including the production of speech. The premotor area, also important in motor control, is located immediately anterior to the primary motor cortex, to which it is similar, except for the absence of giant pyramidal cells. The primary sensory area of the brain is the postcentral gyrus, which is just posterior to the central sulcus in the parietal lobe. This area involves the perception of sensation through extero-ceptive and proprioceptive afferent fibers from the thalamus and brain stem.

Three component motor systems are important for the production of speech: (a) the pyramidal pathway, (b) the extrapyramidal pathway, and (c) the cerebellar pathway. The pyramidal pathway is a direct pathway from the cerebral cortex to the spinal cord and brain stem and is responsible for all voluntary motor movements. The pyramidal pathway consists of the corticospinal tract and the corticobulbar tract. Motor impulses for the corti-cospinal tract, primarily excitatory, originate with the giant cells of Betz in the motor cortex. These impulses are carried by upper motor neurons (i.e., contained wholly within the CNS) to the cerebral peduncles in the mesen-cephalon. As the fibers enter the pons, they are mixed with pontine fibers and nuclei that communicate with the cerebellum, which modulates return impulses to the cerebral cortex. The fibers then converge at the medulla oblongata, forming the pyramids on the anterior surface of the medulla. At the medullary-cervical juncture, that is, at the point where the medulla oblongata and the spinal cord merge, between 70 and 90% (Zemlin, 1988) of the fibers decussate, or cross over to the opposite side of the CNS. The fibers that cross form the lateral corticospinal tract; the 10–30% that do not cross form the ventral (or anterior) corticospinal tract. In the spinal cord, axons from the lateral corticospinal tract terminate at synapses with lower motor neurons. Fibers from the ventral corticospinal tract decussate at the segmental level of the spinal cord. Because of decussation, cortical control of the limbs is contralateral.

The pathway followed by the corticobulbar tract is the same as the corticospinal tract until the upper brain stem. Whereas fibers of the corticospinal tract synapse with lower motor neurons in the spinal cord, corticobulbar fibers project to cranial nerves in the brain stem. The corticobulbar tract is thus an important one for speech production, because much of the involved musculature is supplied by cranial nerves. These are discussed in more detail below. Whereas the corticospinal tract exercises primarily contralateral control over innervated nerves, the corticobulbar tract contains a number of ipsilateral as well as contralateral fibers. Additionally, most of the musculature of the face, pharynx, larynx, and soft palate is supplied with bilateral innervation by the corticobulbar tract. In general, the upper part of the face is primarily represented bilaterally, whereas the lower part of the face is represented contralaterally from the motor cortex. Thus, it is possible to retract one side of the mouth, but generally not possible to wrinkle only one side of the forehead.

The extrapyramidal system can be defined as those parts of the descending motor pathway not included in the pyramidal pathway. Like the pyramidal pathway, the origins of the extrapyramidal pathway are to be found in the cerebral cortex. Whereas the pyramidal system is direct and monosynaptic (having only a single synapse at the ventral horn cell in the spinal cord), the extrapyramidal system is by comparison indirect and polysynaptic. A cerebellar circuit, for example, proceeds from the cerebral cortex to the ipsilateral pontine nuclei, then to the contralateral cerebellar cortex, then to the dentate nucleus (in the cerebellar white matter), then to the red nucleus, then to the thalamus, and then back to the cerebral cortex (Love & Webb, 1986).

Important structures in the extrapyramidal system are the basal ganglia, which consist of a number of large nuclei, and associated brain stem nuclei, including the red nucleus, the subthalamic nucleus, the substantia nigra, and the reticular formation. Extrapyramidal fibers originating in cerebral cortex descend to basal ganglia, and projections are sent from here to the brain stem. Purkinje cells in the cerebellar cortex have axons communicating with the dentate nucleus in the cerebellar white matter. Impulses from the dentate nucleus are sent to the red nucleus. Descending extrapyramidal pathways include the following:

1. The vestibulospinal pathway, which controls muscles maintaining equilibrium and posture, originates in the vestibular nucleus in the medulla oblongata and descends to the spinal cord. The vestibular nucleus receives fiber from both the vestibular apparatus and the cerebellum.

2. The rubrospinal tract, which influences coordination of postural behavior, originates in the red nucleus and descends to the spinal cord. The red nucleus relays impulses from both the vestibular apparatus and the cerebellum to the brain stem and spinal cord.

3. The tectospinal tract, which influences reflexive response to visual and auditory stimuli, originates in the mesencephalon and descends to the spinal cord.

4. The olivospinal pathways, which integrate and coordinate voluntary motor activity, originate in the olivary nucleus, which is located in the medulla oblongata, and which has fibers going to and from the cerebellum.

The cerebellum communicates with the rest of the nervous system by means of three peduncles. The superior peduncle carries nerve tracts to the red nucleus and ventrolateral nucleus. The middle peduncle carries fibers to cerebral cortex and pons, and the inferior peduncle connects the cerebellum with the spinal cord and medulla.

Most of the production of speech involves cranial nerves. These nerves originate in the brain stem and control sensory and motor information for the head. They occur in twelve pairs, are referred to both by Roman numerals and by names, and as can be seen in Table 3.1, not all have to do with speech. Cranial nerve I (olfactory) involves smell, while cranial nerves II, III, IV, and VI (optic, oculomotor, trochlear, abducent) involve vision.

Cranial nerve V (trigeminal) is the largest cranial nerve and an important one for speech production. Cranial nerve V supplies motor innervation to the jaw muscles and the tensor veli palatini muscle (allowing flattening and tensing of the soft palate), as well as sensory fibers for the anterior two-thirds of the tongue. Cranial nerve VII (facial) arises from three nuclei located in the pons. One of these, the motor nucleus, innervates those muscles involved in facial expression, including the muscles of the lips. In addition, it innervates the stapedius muscle in the middle ear, dampening excessive movement of the ossicles. Cranial nerve VIII (acoustic or vestibulocochlear) is a composite nerve consisting of the cochlear and vestibular nerves. Both carry afferent information from the inner ear to the nervous system; the cochlear nerve carries impulses related to hearing, and the vestibular nerve carries impulses related to equilibrium and orientation.

Cranial nerve IX (glossopharyngeal) arises from three nuclei located in the medulla. It carries both sensory and motor fibers, but it innervates

TABLE 3.1   Cranial Nerves

Number	Name	Function
I	Olfactory	Smell
II	Optic	Vision
III	Oculomotor	Movement of eyeball, pupil, and upper eyelid
IV	Trochlear	Rotation of eye down and outwards
V	Trigeminal	Chewing, facial sensation
VI	Abducent	Abduction of eye
VII	Facial	Movement of face (including lips); taste
VIII	Acoustic (Vestibulocochlear)	Hearing and equilibrium
IX	Glossopharyngeal	Elevation of palate and larynx, taste
X	Vagus	Innervation of pharyngeal and intrinsic laryngeal muscles
XI	Accessory (Spinal Accessory)	Movement of uvula and elevation of soft palate
XII	Hypoglossal	Innervation of intrinsic and extrinsic tongue muscles

only one muscle, the stylopharyngeus muscle, which elevates the pharynx and larynx. Sensory fibers convey taste information involving the posterior one-third of the tongue. Cranial nerve X (vagus) arises from three nuclei located in the medulla. It is extensively distributed throughout the neck and thorax, and into the abdominal cavity. Its pharyngeal and laryngeal branches serve in the production of speech. The pharyngeal branch supplies muscles and mucous membrane of the pharynx and soft palate (except the tensor veli palatini, which is innervated by cranial nerve V). The laryngeal branch includes the superior laryngeal nerve and the recurrent laryngeal nerve. The recurrent laryngeal nerve arises from the vagus below the larynx and ascends to terminate there; it supplies the subglottal laryngeal mucosa and all intrinsic muscles of the larynx except the cricothyroid, which is innervated by the superior laryngeal branch. Cranial nerve XI (accessory or spinal accessory) consists of a cranial and a spinal portion. The cranial portion arises from the medulla and supplies the uvula and levator veli palatini (which elevates the soft palate). Other fibers continue into the vagus nerve (cranial nerve X). The spinal portion arises from motor cells in the anterior horn of the spinal cord and joins the cranial portion as they pass through the jugular foramen. It innervates the sternocleidomastoid and trapezius muscles. Cranial nerve XII (hypoglossal) arises from the hypoglossal nucleus in the medulla and emerges from the brain between the pyramid and the olive. It innervates all of the intrinsic muscles of the tongue, that is, the superior longitudinal, the inferior longitudinal, transverse, and vertical muscles; as well as three of the extrinsic muscles of the tongue: the genioglossus, styloglossus, and hyoglossus.

3.1.4 Stages of Speech Production

3.1.4.1 Respiration

The formation of all speech sounds requires the movement of air through or across some articulator in the vocal tract. Furthermore, this necessary movement of air also requires a source, that is, an impetus that causes the actual movement of air. Additionally, this movement of air may occur in one of two directions, either towards the outside of the vocal tract or towards the inside of the vocal tract. In speech science, three organs have been identified as airstream sources for speech, specifically, the lungs, the glottis, and the velum, so that a speech sound can have a *pulmonic, glottalic,* or *velaric* airstream source. The direction of the airstream is designated as *egressive* if there is an outward flow, and *ingressive* if the flow is inward. Together, source and direction of airflow are an *airstream mechanism.*

Most of the speech sounds of languages of the world, and all of the speech sounds of English, rely on a pulmonic egressive airstream mechanism. That is, air originates in the lungs and flows outward through the vocal tract and out the talker's lips. In other languages, however, some speech sounds can have different airstream mechanisms, that is, different sources and directions of airflow. A pulmonic ingressive airstream mechanism, that is, an airstream mechanism involving inspiration of air into the lungs, is not used systematically for speech sounds in languages of the world. An airflow of this type may, however, occur irregularly during speech, when such emotional states as fear or surprise obtain. In other languages of the world, speech sounds may also have either a glottalic or a velaric airstream mechanism. Speech sounds formed with a glottalic source can be either egressive (forming speech sounds called *ejectives*) or ingressive (forming speech sounds called *implosives*). Sounds with a velaric source are generally ingressive, and such speech sounds are called *clicks.*

None of the research on the effects of alcohol on speech in the literature discussed here has involved investigation of any languages that do not use exclusively pulmonic egressive airstream mechanisms. It remains for future research to investigate the effects of alcohol on speech sounds produced with glottalic and velaric airstream mechanisms.

3.1.4.2 Phonation

Whereas respiration is a process vital for the maintenance of life, phonation is not, although it does play a highly important role in the formation of speech. Air emanating from the lungs and through the trachea is necessary for most speech sounds, but it is the larynx that converts what is essentially a continuous flow of air into the systematic vibratory patterns that form speech. Phonatory and other modifications of airflow can be linguistically contrastive or noncontrastive. A linguistically contrastive modification serves to differentiate one or more speech sounds in a particular language, such that replacement of one of these sounds by another, in a word otherwise the same, results in a word with a different meaning. On the other hand, modifications can result in differences that do not result in changes of meaning, for instance, the difference between normal, conversational speech and operatic singing.

The most widely observed phonatory contrast in languages of the world is the distinction between *voiced* and *voiceless* segments. In the production of a voiced speech sound, the vocal folds are held close together (adducted), so that they vibrate quasi-periodically; the initial sound in the word *zoo*, for instance, is voiced. On the other hand, if the vocal folds are held relatively far apart (abducted), so that they do not vibrate, then a voiceless sound is produced. The initial sound in the word *sue* is an example of a voiceless segment.

Although the voicing distinction is the most widely used laryngeal contrast, other states of the glottis are used in speech sound production in some of the languages of the world. In the production of *breathy voice* or *murmur* (Ladefoged, 1993), the vocal folds are held relatively far apart, as in the production of a voiceless segment; however, this position of the vocal folds is accompanied by an airflow sufficient to set them in loose vibration. Speech produced with breathy voice can indicate a variety of things, ranging from a vocal affectation to laryngeal dysfunction to a true linguistic contrast.

Phonation at an extremely low frequency is called variously *creaky voice, vocal fry, glottal fry, pulse register,* and *laryngealization.* According to Ladefoged (1993), creaky voice is produced when the arytenoid cartilages are held tightly together, and the vocal folds vibrate at the end away from the arytenoid cartilages. Laryngealization or creaky voice is used contrastively in some languages; in most languages, such as English, it is not used contrastively, but nevertheless occurs quite commonly at the ends of sentences with falling intonation.

One aspect of phonation that has been extensively researched concerns the initiation of vocal-fold vibration in the first place to form speech. By far the most widely held view of the mechanism of phonation is myoelastic aerodynamic theory, often referred to as the "classical" view of phonatory production (e.g., van den Berg, 1958; Zemlin, 1988). The theory, in essentially its current formulation, dates back to the 19th century in the work of Müller (1848). The name of the theory refers to its major components: (a) that the source of vocal fold vibration is aerodynamic (i.e., caused by air movement from the lungs and trachea), rather than neural (i.e., caused by individual nerve impulses); and (b) that vibration frequency is a function of muscular (*myo*- 'muscle') regulation of elasticity (i.e., vocal-fold length in relation to tension and mass).

3.1.4.3 Articulation

In this section we discuss the various configurations of the supralaryngeal vocal tract that form various speech sounds or segments. The broadest classification of speech segments differentiates vowels from consonants; beyond that, the following discussion should not be considered dogma, but rather a rough guide to articulatory phonetics. Those interested in pursuing further investigation of articulatory phonetics may wish to consult a number of works in which more details are proffered; these include Catford (1977), Heffner (1950), Ladefoged (1993), and Laver (1994).

The next section will also discuss the introduction at various points of alphabetic transcription symbols widely used in phonetic studies as a shorthand method of describing the articulatory characteristics that make up speech segments. These are included in square brackets close to example words illustrating speech sounds. Discussions of the issues underlying various transcription systems can be found in Abercrombie (1967, Chapter 7) and Pullum and Ladusaw (1986).

3.1.4.3.1 Vowels
Whereas consonants are formed with a relatively constricted vocal tract, so that airflow is impeded to a radical degree, vowels are formed with a relatively unconstricted vocal tract, and different vowels are formed by different shapes of the oral cavity. The most important organ in the formation of the vowels is the tongue body. Different positions of the tongue body, that is, different heights and different degrees of advancement or retraction, are sufficient to change the shape of the oral cavity and produce the different vowels. Two of the traditional descriptions and designations of vowel segments are thus the relative height and backness of the tongue body. Superimposed on, and relatively independent of, the tongue position is the shape of the lips during formation of a vowel; in some cases, the lips may be protruded in a rounded configuration, while in other cases, the lips may be spread.

Height (or closeness) and backness can be represented on a two-dimensional grid. The International Phonetics Association (IPA), for instance, recognizes four named degrees of closeness: close, close-mid, open-mid, and open; and three degrees of backness: front, central, and back. Another system, much used in the United States of America, recognizes the same three degrees of backness, but names only three heights: high, mid, and low. In addition to height, backness, and rounding, a fourth dimension, "tenseness," is used by some authors to describe the phonetic quality that differentiates, for instance, the vowels in the words *heed* (a high front tense vowel) and *hid* (a high front lax vowel).

The vowels in *heed* [i] and *hid* [ɪ] are thus high front unrounded vowels, tense and lax respectively. Mid front unrounded vowels occur in the English words *laid* ([e], tense; but see comments on diphthongs below) and *led* ([ɛ], lax). A low front unrounded vowel occurs in the English word *lad* [æ]. In English, all of the front vowels are unrounded, that is, produced with spread, rather than protruded, lips. In other languages, however, front vowels can be both rounded as well as unrounded.

English back vowels also occur at three different heights. The high back vowels, both rounded, occur in the words *Luke* ([u], tense) and *look* ([ʊ], lax). A mid back tense rounded vowel occurs in the word *boat* ([o], but see below regarding diphthongs). The vowel in some pronunciations of *bought* [ɔ] is described as a mid back rounded lax vowel by some authors, but as a low back lax rounded vowel by others. The vowel in the first syllable of the word *father* [ɑ] is definitely low and unrounded, but various sources describe it as either central or back. As can be seen, most of the back vowels of English, especially the high and mid ones, are rounded, so that in general, front vowels are unrounded and back vowels rounded. Just as other languages use front rounded vowels, it is likewise true that some languages use back unrounded vowels.

Central vowels in English are unrounded and lax. A high central vowel occurs in the final syllable of the word *citizen* [ɨ], while a mid central vowel occurs in the last syllable of the word *sofa* [ə]. Somewhat lower than the vowel just mentioned is the vowel that occurs in the word *bud* [ʌ].

All of the vowel sounds discussed thus far are *monophthongs* (from Greek *mon-* 'one, single' + *phthongos* 'voice, sound'), that is, single vowels produced in a single syllable. In some cases, vowels are produced so that a sequence of two vowels occurs in a single syllable; these combinations are referred to as *diphthongs* (from Greek *di-* 'two' + *phthongos* 'voice, sound'). A number of such diphthongs occur in English; these include the vowel sounds in the words *buy* [aɪ], *boy* [ɔɪ], and *bough* [aʊ]. Additionally, a number of authors consider all of the tense vowels in English to be diphthongal or at least to end with a vowel-like articulation called an *off-glide*. The diphthongal nature is especially clear in the mid tense vowels, both front and back, as in the words *bait* (front) and *boat* (back). Somewhat less obvious are the off-glide characteristics of the high vowels in *beat* ([ij], front) and *boot* ([uw], back).

A number of other features characterize or differentiate vowel sounds in English and other languages of the world. One distinction is between *oral* and *nasal* vowels. In the articulation of oral vowels, the velum (soft palate) is raised, so that passage to the nasal cavity is blocked, and air resonates only in the oral cavity. In the production of nasal vowels, however, the velum is lowered, allowing air to resonate in both the oral and the nasal cavities. In English, nasal vowels occur only when a vowel is followed by a nasal consonant (see below), that is, a consonant that is also produced with a lowered velum. All other vowels are oral, and in fact, no two words in English ever differ only in that one word has a nasal vowel where the other has an oral vowel. In other languages, however, the difference between oral and nasal vowels can be contrastive. Nasality is transcribed with a tilde over the relevant segment, for example, the oral vowel [o] as opposed to the nasal vowel [õ].

Another differentiating characteristic of vowels (and consonants as well) is *length*. Some descriptions of English differentiate *long* vowels from *short* vowels, for example, the difference between the vowel sounds in *bite* (long) and *bit* (short). On reflection, however, it should be clear that this difference is not one of length, per se, but rather one based on the distinction between a diphthong (as in *bite*) and a monophthong (as in *bit*). In fact, contrasts in English are never based solely on the actual duration of speech segments, but rather on other differences such as monophthong versus diphthong, or actual vowel quality (i.e., height, backness, tenseness). In other languages, however, two vowels can be distinctive only on the basis of their actual length, that is, duration, so that one vowel is temporally short, while the other is long. Length is transcribed with a [ː] (sometimes written or printed as a colon [:]) following the relevant segment.

Monophthongal vowels can thus be described according to the following parameters: (a) height, (b) backness, (c) tenseness, (d) rounding, (e) orality/nasality (if necessary; the default is oral). A diphthong, generally described as either two vowels together in a single syllable or a vowel plus an "off-" or "on-glide," can simply be considered the articulatory sum of its component segments.

Tables 3.2 and 3.3 show *primary* (front unrounded/back rounded) and *secondary* (front rounded/back unrounded) vowels respectively, with backness on the horizontal axis, height on the vertical axis, and tense preceding lax within each cell. Relevant examples from English follow Table 3.2.

3.1.4.3.2 Consonants As discussed previously, although vowels are formed with a relatively unconstricted vocal tract, consonants are formed by a constriction of one kind or another in the vocal tract. These constrictions are formed by the various articulatory organs in the vocal tract and impede the flow of air to some degree as it moves through the vocal tract toward the lips and out of the mouth. A traditional classificatory system for the description of consonants includes designations of voicing, place, and manner.

Voicing, discussed in detail in section 3.1.4.2, can have the value of either voiced or voiceless in the production of a consonant. In the formation of a

TABLE 3.2 Primary Vowels

	Front	Central	Back
High	i ɪ	ɨ	u ʊ
Mid	e ɛ	ə	o ɔ
Low	æ	ʌ	ɑ

American English examples
  [i]: vowel in the word *beat*
  [ɪ]: vowel in the word *bit*
  [e]: vowel in the word *bait* (approximately)
  [ɛ]: vowel in the word *bet*
  [æ]: vowel in the word *bat*
  [ɨ]: vowel in the last syllable of the word *citizen*
  [ə]: vowel in the last syllable of the word *sofa*
  [ʌ]: vowel in the first syllable of *butter*
  [u]: vowel in the word *boot*
  [ʊ]: vowel in the word *book*
  [o]: vowel in the word *boat* (approximately)
  [ɔ]: vowel in the word *bought* (approximately, depending on dialect)
  [ɑ]: vowel in the first syllable of the word *father*

voiced consonant, the vocal folds are tightly held and arranged relatively closely together, and there is sufficient airflow so that the vocal folds vibrate during the production of the consonant. During production of a voiceless consonant, on the other hand, the vocal folds are relatively slack and spaced farther apart, so that they do not vibrate. In many languages of the world, including English, consonant segments occur in pairs, and the only difference between the members of these pairs is that one is voiced and the other voiceless. An example of such a pair is the two words *vat* and *fat,* which differ only in the voicing of their initial segments. During production of the initial sound in the word *vat,* the vocal folds vibrate in a way characteristic

TABLE 3.3 Secondary Vowels[a]

	Front	Central	Back
High	y ʏ		ɯ
Mid	ø œ		ɣ
Low	Œ		

[a] The vowels shown in this table do not occur in standard varieties of English.

of voiced segments; during production of the initial sound in *fat,* on the other hand, that characteristic vibration is absent.

The articulatory parameter *place* (of articulation) refers to the location of the characteristic constriction in the vocal tract during production of a consonant. The formation of a constriction necessarily requires the participation of two articulators; in general, these can be designated as *active* articulators and *passive* articulators. During formation of a consonant, the active articulator will be the one that actually moves (relatively speaking), and its (relatively) stationary target will be the passive articulator. In general, the passive articulators are on the upper surface of the oral cavity, whereas the active articulators are situated such that they can move as the lower jaw moves. The major active articulator in the formation of consonant segments is the tongue, or more precisely, the various parts of the tongue. However, there are additionally a number of other active articulators that participate in the formation of the constrictions necessary for the production of consonant segments.

Beginning at the front of the vocal tract the first place of articulation is the lips. Sounds made with the two lips have a *bilabial* place of articulation, and those formed by articulating the lower lip with the upper teeth have *labiodental* place of articulation. As this last designation indicates, consonants formed with the teeth as one of the articulators have a *dental* place of articulation. In all cases involving the teeth as an articulator, the teeth are the passive articulator and the tongue tip the active articulator. The term *dental* generally refers to those segments formed by articulation between the tongue tip and the upper teeth only. However, in some languages (including English), there are consonants formed with the tongue tip protruding through the teeth, that is, articulating with both the upper and lower set, and these are designated as having an *interdental* place of articulation. Consonant segments may also be formed with an articulation between the tongue tip and the alveolar ridge, forming consonants with an *alveolar* place of articulation. Consonants formed with the tongue tip and the back of the alveolar ridge are designated as *retroflex* consonants. An articulation formed between the blade of the tongue and the back of the alveolar ridge is variously designated as *postalveolar* (International Phonetic Association, 1989), *palato-alveolar* (Ladefoged, 1993), and *alveopalatal.* Consonants formed by the articulation of the front of the tongue with the hard palate are *palatal,* whereas sounds formed by articulation of the tongue dorsum with the velum (also called the soft palate) are *velar.* Consonant sounds produced by an articulation of the tongue dorsum with the uvula are *uvular,* while sounds formed with an articulation of the tongue root and the posterior wall of the pharynx are *pharyngeal.*

The articulatory parameter *manner* (of articulation) refers to the type of articulation and degree of obstruction in the formation of a consonant. We discuss here the manners of articulation stops, fricatives, affricates, nasals, and approximants. If the passage of air through the vocal tract is completely obstructed momentarily and then released suddenly, the consonant thus formed is called a *stop* or a *plosive*. In English, stop consonants form a class of consonants formed at a number of places of articulation. These include bilabial stops (for example, the initial sounds in *bat* ([b], voiced) and *pat* ([p], voiceless)); alveolar stops (for example, the initial sounds in *den* ([d], voiced) and *ten* ([t], voiceless)); and velar stops (for example, the initial sounds in *gale* ([g], voiced) and *kale* ([k], voiceless)).

When articulators are positioned so that there is a very narrow passage between them, air passing through will create friction; consonants formed by this noisy, turbulent flow of air are called *fricatives*. As with the stops, English fricatives tend to occur in voiced/voiceless pairs at a number of places of articulation. Although other languages, such as Japanese and Spanish, use bilabial fricatives, English does not, and the foremost place of articulation of English fricatives is labiodental (for example, the initial sounds in the words *vat* ([v], voiced) and *fat* ([f], voiceless)). Next are the interdental fricatives (for example, the initial sounds in *thy* ([ð], voiced) and *thigh* ([θ], voiceless)), and then the alveolar fricatives (for example, the initial sounds in *zeal* ([z], voiced) and *seal* ([s], voiceless)). Articulated back of the alveolars are the English alveopalatal fricatives (for example, the medial sound in *vision* ([ʒ], voiced) or the initial sound in *shun* ([ʃ], voiceless)). English does not include palatal or velar fricatives in its consonant inventory, although other languages of the world do. Sometimes considered a voiceless glottal fricative is the initial sound in the word *have* [h].

Whereas *stops* (also called *plosives*) are produced by stopping the flow of air completely behind an articulatory obstruction and then releasing it suddenly, *affricates* are produced by stopping the air completely but releasing it gradually, much in the same way that a fricative is produced. English has a voiced–voiceless pair of affricates at the alveopalatal place of articulation, for example, the initial sounds in *gin* ([ʤ], voiced) and *chin* ([tʃ], voiceless). Some researchers also consider the final sounds in the words *bids* ([dz], voiced) and *bits* ([ts], voiceless) to be alveolar affricates. Other languages of the world use affricates at other places of articulation.

There are some articulatory similarities between stops and *nasals*; both involve a complete occlusion of airflow in the oral cavity. However, whereas stops are produced with the velum raised, so that air is prevented from entering the nasal cavity, nasal consonants are produced with a lowered velum. Thus, whereas stops are produced with airflow through only the oral cavity, nasals are produced with airflow through both the oral and nasal cavities. The consonant inventory of English has nasal consonants at three places of articulation. A bilabial nasal occurs as the initial sound in the word *mode* [m], and an alveolar nasal occurs initially in the word *node* [n]. English also uses a velar nasal, which, however, does not occur word-initially (or syllable-initially); the final sound in the word *sing* is a velar nasal [ŋ]. Again, other languages can have nasals at additional places of articulation.

Approximants are formed by a close positioning of articulators, but without a constriction that would either stop the flow of air completely as in stops or cause turbulence as in fricatives. Approximants are generally voiced, and the consonant segments in English included in this manner category include the initial sounds in the words *lake* [l], *rake* [r], *yoke* [j], and *woke* [w]. The term *liquid* is also applied to the class of lateral consonants (*l*-sounds) and rhotic consonants (*r*-sounds) exemplified by the initial sounds in *lake* and *rake*. The class of rhotic consonants in the languages of the world actually encompasses a wide variety of consonants with different places and manners of articulation. For instance, the American English *r*-sound that occurs initially in the word *red* is a retroflex approximant. In Spanish, the *r*-sound that occurs medially in the word *pero* is an alveolar tap, whereas the *r*-sound occurring initially in the French word *renard* is a uvular fricative or approximant. The main articulatory characteristic of *l*-sounds is that they are formed by a flow of air out the sides of the tongue in the vicinity of the molars, whereas other sounds are *central*, in that air flows through the center of the vocal tract. The initial sounds in *yoke* (palatal) and *woke* (labiovelar) are *glides* or *semivowels*. These are consonant versions of high vowels.

Although a voice-place-manner description can be used to describe a single consonant, reference to any of the categories can serve to describe more than one consonant at a time, that is, a class of consonants. The class of alveolars in English, for instance, includes the initial sounds of the words *two, due, sue, zoo, not,* and *lot*. Likewise, the class of stops in English includes the initial sounds in the words *pate, bait, Tate, date, Kate,* and *gate*. In addition to the voicing, place, and manner categories just discussed, speech scientists and linguists have defined further classes of sounds that appear to play a part in language. These categories include the following:

1. *Resonants* or *sonorants:* This class of consonant sounds includes the glides, the liquids, and the nasals.
2. *Obstruents:* This class of consonant sounds includes the stops, the fricatives, and the affricates.
3. *Sibilants:* These include the alveolar and alveopalatal fricatives, as opposed to the labiodental and interdental fricatives. The sibilants have greater acoustic energy in the high frequencies than the nonsibilants.

Table 3.4 shows a number of consonants used in the world's languages, arranged with places of articulation on the horizontal axis and manners of

TABLE 3.4   Selected Consonants[a]

	BL	LD	ID	AV	AP	PT	VL	UV	PH	GL
Stop	p b			t d		c ɟ	k g	q G		ʔ
Fric	ɸ β	f v	θ ð	s z	ʃ ʒ	ç ʝ	x ɣ	χ ʁ		h ɦ
Affr		pf bv		ts dz	tʃ dʒ		kx gɣ			
Nasal	m	ɱ		n		ɲ	ŋ	N		
Liquid				l		r				
Glide	w					j	w			

American English Examples[b] [p]: initial consonant in the word *pill* (with aspiration)
[b]: initial consonant in the word *bill*
[t]: initial consonant in the word *till* (with aspiration)
[d]: initial consonant in the word *dill*
[k]: initial consonant in the word *kill* (with aspiration)
[g]: initial consonant in the word *gill* or *go*
[f]: initial consonant in the word *fat*
[v]: initial consonant in the word *vat*
[θ]: initial consonant in the word *thigh*
[ð]: initial consonant in the word *thy*
[s]: initial consonant in the word *sue*
[z]: initial consonant in the word *zoo*
[ʃ]: initial consonant in the word *show*
[ʒ]: medial (second) consonant in the word *vision*
[tʃ]: initial consonant in the word *cheer*
[dʒ]: initial consonant in the word *jeer*
[m]: initial consonant in the word *moose*
[n]: initial consonant in the word *noose*
[ŋ]: final consonant in the word *sing*
[l]: initial consonant in the word *lake*
[r]: initial consonant in the word *rake*
[w]: initial consonant in the word *woo*
[j]: initial consonant in the word *you*

[a] BL, bilabial; LD, labiodental; ID, interdental; AV, alveolar; AP, alveopalatal; PT, palatal; VL, velar; UV, uvular; PH, pharyngeal; GL, glottal; Fric, Fricative; Affr, Affricate
[b]Symbols not listed below refer to sounds that do not occur in standard varieties of English.

articulation on the vertical. Relevant examples of these consonant segments from English follow the table proper.

3.2 SPEECH ACOUSTICS

3.2.1 The Source–Filter Theory of Speech Production

The source–filter theory of speech production describes the relationships between articulatory configurations and the acoustic speech signal. It posits a model whereby the radiated speech signal (i.e., the speech signal that exits the lips of a talker) is the result of a combination of source characteristics (i.e., the energy produced by the vibrating larynx) and filter characteristics (i.e., the resonator characteristics of the supraglottal vocal tract).

Recall from the discussion of the myoelastic aerodynamic theory above that the vibration frequency of the vocal folds is determined by the mass, the elasticity, and the tension of the vocal cords. Control over these parameters is achieved through the intrinsic and extrinsic muscles of the larynx. The effect of this vibration on passing air is to create a periodic (actually, quasiperiodic) signal. Although the generated glottal waveform is periodic, it is not a simple sine wave but rather a complex acoustic wave made up of a number of harmonic frequencies. The harmonic with the lowest frequency is called the *fundamental frequency*, and the harmonics are ideally integer multiples of the fundamental frequency. Thus, if the fundamental frequency is 100 Hz (such as for a typical male talker), there will be harmonics at 100 (the fundamental), 200, 300, 400 Hz, and so on up. Most of the energy in the glottal waveform is concentrated in the lower frequencies, so that as the frequency of succeeding harmonics increases, the corresponding intensity decreases, at approximately 6 dB per octave. A line spectrum of the glottal source would thus appear as in Figure 3.3.

According to the source–filter theory, the glottal spectrum acts as a *source function*, which is then modified (i.e., filtered) by various configurations of the vocal tract, that is, by various *transfer functions*. Depending on its specific configuration, the vocal tract will resonate at particular frequencies;

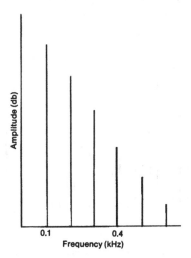

FIGURE 3.3 Spectrum of typical glottal airflow. (From Lieberman, 1977. Copyright © 1977 by Macmillan Publishing. Used by permission.)

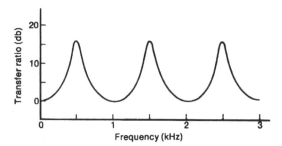

FIGURE 3.4   Transfer function of the supralaryngeal vocal tract for the vowel [ə]. For our purposes, the term *transfer ratio* is equivalent to *filter function*. Note the locations of the formant frequencies at 0.5, 1.5, and 2.5 Hz. (From Lieberman, 1977. Copyright © 1977 by Macmillan Publishing. Used by permission.)

these vocal tract resonances are called *formants*. Figure 3.4 shows the acoustic transfer function of a vocal tract configured for the vowel [ə]. As Figure 3.4 shows, the formants for the neutral vowel [ə] are equally spaced and have approximately equal amplitudes.

The application of the vocal tract filter to the glottal source thus produces an output, so that the acoustic speech signal is a product of both source and filter. Given the source spectrum in Figure 3.3 and the transfer function in Figure 3.4, the output spectrum will appear as in Figure 3.5. The glottal harmonics in the vicinity of formants in the transfer function are amplified in the output spectrum, while harmonics further removed from the formants are attenuated. Other vocal tract configurations, however, may have transfer functions with formants that are not equally spaced and that have unequal

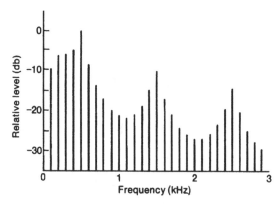

FIGURE 3.5   The spectrum that would result if the transfer function plotted in Figure 3.4 were "excited" by the glottal source plotted in Figure 3.3. The sound is the vowel [ə]. (From Lieberman, 1977. Copyright © 1977 by Macmillan Publishing. Used by permission.)

amplitudes. Figure 3.6, for instance, shows the transfer function for the vowel [i] (as in *beat*).

Whereas the source for the production of vowels is uniformly the glottis, additional sources are used for the production of consonants. The most of important of these is random acoustic noise with a broad frequency spectrum, called turbulence. Turbulence noise is of two types. The first is frication noise, which is generated at a vocal tract constriction above the glottis and which is the source for fricative consonants. In the case of source turbulence, the transfer function is a consequence of cavities that are anterior to the obstruction and, to a lesser extent, posterior to the obstruction. Frication noise may be generated as the sole source, or it may be generated in combination with a glottal source in the production of voiced consonants. The second type of turbulence is aspiration, which emanates from an open glottis with no vocal-fold vibration. Aspiration is found in the production of the sound [h] (e.g., initially in the word *hair*), as well as immediately following the release of voiceless stops, such as [p t k], in English. The posterior end of the vocal tract then constitutes the appropriate transfer function. Another source for consonant production is found in the production of stop consonants precisely at the release of the articulators and is called a transient source. During the closed portion of the stop, pressure builds in the vocal tract posterior to the closure; upon release, there is a sudden drop in pressure that creates a transient source that excites the vocal tract.

Important primary works dealing with source–filter theory include Chiba and Kajiyama (1941), Fant (1960), and Stevens and House (1955, 1961). Additionally, summary discussions can be found in Baken (1987), Borden et al. (1994), Kent and Read (1992), Stevens (1964), and Lieberman (1977).

3.2.2 Modern Instrumental Acoustic Analysis

In this section we discuss some of the instrumental methods used in the analysis of the acoustic speech signal.

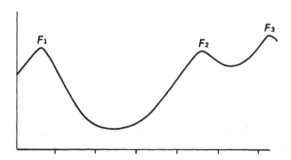

FIGURE 3.6   Transfer function for the vowel [i]. (From Lieberman, 1977. Copyright © 1977 by Macmillan Publishing. Used by permission.)

3.2.2.1 Waveform Displays

The oscillograph was developed around 1920 (Kent & Read, 1992) and displays *waveforms* of the speech signal, that is, representations of amplitude as a function of time. Vowel sounds are easily recognizable on waveform displays, due to their characteristic periodicity, and it is thus possible to measure fundamental frequency using a waveform display. Waveform displays are useful for visual identification and demarcation of spans of relatively heterogeneous acoustic phenomena, for instance, the periodicity of a sustained vowel or a silent span corresponding to stop closure. Figure 3.7 shows the waveform for a production of [ɑpɑ].

Although waveforms are useful for measuring durations and relative amplitudes, they are less useful for visually differentiating sounds within a class, such as a specific vowel or the place articulation of a stop. With a vowel, for instance, the displayed waveform is a sum of a number of different frequencies with different amplitudes. The waveform display does not permit rapid determination of these constituent frequencies. For consonants, the waveform display does not readily convey place-of-articulation information. For instance, stop consonants are characterized by complete occlusion of the vocal tract, which appears as a span of no energy on the waveform, regardless of place of articulation. Fricatives, as well, do not reveal place-of-articulation information well on waveform displays; the random noise generated appears undifferentiated for the various fricatives. For these types of determinations, the spectrogram, discussed in section 3.2.2.3, is a much more perspicuous display, and much more useful to the speech researcher.

3.2.2.2 Filtering Techniques

As discussed above, the entire supralaryngeal vocal tract acts as an acoustic filter, allowing the passage of some frequencies but suppressing others. The principle of filtering is also important in the operation of instruments for acoustic analysis. Filtering serves a number of purposes in the acoustic analysis of speech, including preemphasis and analysis itself, each of which is discussed below.

Filters are of four basic types: low-pass, high-pass, band-pass, and band-reject (or *notch*). A low-pass filter, as its name implies, passes low frequencies

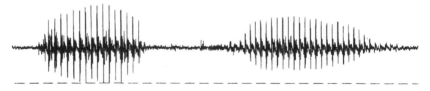

FIGURE 3.7   Waveform of [apa].

but attenuates higher frequencies, whereas a high-pass filter does just the opposite: it passes or emphasizes high frequencies while attenuating lower ones. A band-pass filter passes signals within a specified band of frequencies and attenuates those frequencies outside the specified band. Conversely, then, a band-reject or notch filter attenuates frequencies within a relatively narrow range of frequencies but allows all other frequencies to pass. Figure 3.8 shows the characteristic shapes of these four basic types of filters.

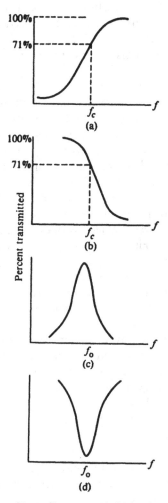

FIGURE 3.8 Characteristics of basic filter types: (A) high-pass; (B) low-pass; (C) band-pass; (D) band-reject. The cutoff frequency is f_c and the resonance frequency is f_o. (From T. D. Rossing, *The Science of Sound,* © 1982 Addison-Wesley Publishing Company Inc. Reprinted by permission of Addison-Wesley.)

As mentioned previously, energy level in the speech signal is higher in the lower frequencies than in the higher frequencies. Prior to analysis, then, a speech signal is preemphasized, that is, high-pass filtered, in order to boost the higher frequencies so that the lower frequencies will not dominate the analysis. Use of a so-called anti-aliasing filter is necessary in the analysis of digitized speech; it is a low-pass filter that attenuates all signal frequencies above the highest frequency relevant to the analysis.

Analysis using the sound spectrograph, discussed below, employs the principle of a variable band-pass filter, that is, a filter that passes specific frequencies in succession. Filters can also be used to boost the signal of relatively weak frequencies if those frequencies are of analytical interest, such as the high-frequency noise of fricative segments.

3.2.2.3 Spectral Analysis

The spectra displayed in Figures 3.3 and 3.5 show the amplitudes of the fundamental frequency and its higher harmonics, that is, the frequency components of either the glottal source waveform or the radiated signal waveform. The principle underlying our ability to derive these spectra from waveforms was discovered in the early 19th century by the Frenchman Jean Baptiste Joseph Fourier. According to Fourier's theorem, all periodic waveforms, regardless of their complexity, can be analyzed as the summation of any number (i.e., an infinite number) of component sinusoidal waves, which all have different frequencies, amplitudes, and phase relationships. The spectra displayed in Figures 3.3 and 3.5 are called *power spectra* or *amplitude spectra,* because they plot amplitude (*power*) against frequencies. The specific type of power spectrum displayed in these figures is called a *line spectrum* and represents an absolutely periodic waveform, with amplitudes plotted only for the fundamental frequency and integer multiples of the fundamental, that is, its harmonics.

Neither the glottal source waveform nor the radiated waveform, however, is completely periodic. These waveforms are best described as quasi-periodic (as opposed to either completely periodic or completely aperiodic), so that rather than showing energy at only integer multiples of the fundamental, the spectra of these signals show energy at a large number of frequencies or within a continuous range of frequencies. Thus, rather than as a line spectrum, a power spectrum of actual speech will more often appear as displayed in Figure 3.9.

A power spectrum represents the spectrum of a "slice" of the speech waveform, that is, the spectrum at more or less a single point in time. Other types of spectral representations, however, incorporate a temporal element, so that the three parameters—frequency, intensity, and time—are all incorporated into a single display. The most important of these is the *sound spectrograph* (i.e., the instrument), which displays *spectrograms* (i.e., the

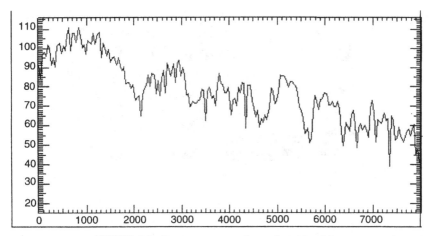

FIGURE 3.9 Power spectrum of vowel segment [a].

output, either a display on a computer screen or a printout on paper) that
are able to show the rapid spectral shifts of the speech signal. The spectrograph was developed during the 1940s (see Koenig, Dunn, & Lacy, 1946),
and although a number of technological developments (including digital
signal processing) have taken place since its initial development, the sound
spectrograph's basic analysis principles remain the same, and its use as an
analysis tool remains widespread in speech science and acoustic-phonetics.
The operation of the spectrograph is based on a variable band-pass filter
that analyzes the speech signal at various frequencies, providing intensity
information over short durations for each of the scanned frequencies.

  The spectrograph can produce either narrow-band spectrograms or wide-
band spectrograms. The production of a narrow-band spectrogram uses a
filter bandwidth of 45 Hz, whereas wide-band spectrograms are produced
using a filter with a 300-Hz bandwidth. Figures 3.10 and 3.11 illustrate

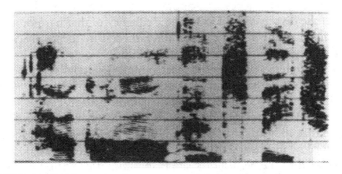

FIGURE 3.10 Narrow-band spectrogram of the phrase "alcohol and speech."

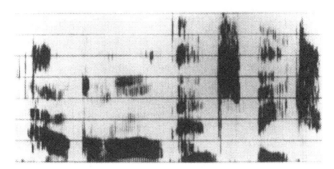

FIGURE 3.11   Wide-band spectrogram of the phrase "alcohol and speech."

narrow and wide-band spectrograms respectively for the phrase "alcohol and speech." Both of the spectrograms in Figures 3.10 and 3.11 indicate frequency on the ordinate, with lower frequencies towards the bottom and higher frequencies toward the top. In both figures, time is indicated along the abscissa, with the beginning of the utterance at the left and the end toward the right. Analog spectrographs can analyze between 2.0 and 2.5 sec of speech during a single analysis pass (depending on the particular model). Intensity is indicated by the darkness of markings on the spectrogram, that is, the darker the marking the higher the intensity. The spectrogram, itself, however, can provide only a rough indication of relative intensity.

A comparison of the narrow-band spectrogram in Figure 3.10 with the wide-band one in Figure 3.11 reveals the relative advantages of each of the two filter bandwidths. A narrow-band spectrogram, such as the one displayed in Figure 3.10, can show individual harmonics of voiced sounds. In general, narrow-band spectrograms offer better frequency resolution than wide-band ones. For example, narrow-band spectrograms can be used to track fundamental frequency. If one of the harmonics is traced through the duration of the displayed utterance, the frequency of that harmonic divided by its harmonic number will give the fundamental frequency, because harmonics are integer multiples of the fundamental.

On the other hand, wide-band spectrograms are relatively poor at frequency resolution. However, it is possible to determine fundamental frequency using a wide-band spectrogram. As indicated on Figure 3.11, each of the closely spaced lines (called *striations*) appearing during voiced portions of the utterance indicate a single glottal pulse. Fundamental frequency can be determined by measuring the time interval between two striations, which will correspond to the period of a single glottal pulse. A simpler method is to count the number of striations occurring in 100 ms and then to multiply this number by 10; this method, as well as measurements over longer temporal spans, actually provide an average fundamental frequency, but errors in measurement are also spread over a greater number of periods. Performing this type of calculation by hand is possible only if the fundamental frequency is low enough for individual glottal pulses to be visible on the spectrogram. Wide-band spectrograms also represent more clearly than narrow-band spectrograms the formants (i.e., vocal tract resonances), which appear as dark horizontal bands at lower frequencies in Figure 3.11.

The real advantage of wide-band spectrograms, however, is in temporal resolution. The wide-band filter is better adapted to showing rapid changes in the acoustic signal than the narrow-band one and thus more clearly demarcates those areas where the acoustical signal changes. Duration measures can thus be made by choosing the beginning and ending boundaries of the acoustical event and measuring the time along the horizontal axis. Various spectral characteristics are apparent for specific acoustic phenomena. Vowels are indicated by formant structure appearing as darkened horizontal bands as well as by (quasi)periodic glottal pulsing appearing as vertical striations. The apparent formant structure of vowels as indicated on a spectrogram is the result of both the particular vowel being produced and the surrounding phonetic material. On a spectrogram, the formants of a vowel may appear to be steady or to move up or to move down; movements of the formants are called *transitions.*

Stop consonants, because the airflow is blocked momentarily, will show a white span on a spectrogram indicating minimal acoustic energy or silence. The sudden release of a stop, that is, the stop *burst,* is indicated on a spectrogram by a *spike* extending across a range of frequencies. Because the frication that characterizes fricative consonants as well as the release portion of affricates is composed mainly of turbulent noise, this will appear on a spectrogram as a span of apparently random striations across a range of frequencies. The location of this frequency range will depend on the particular fricative being produced; the noise for the initial segment in *see,* for instance, will be limited to relatively high frequencies, whereas the frication noise for the initial segment in *she* will also extend into relatively lower frequencies. In the production of some stops, the burst is followed by a period of fricative-like noise prior to the onset of periodic voicing for a following vowel. This is called *voice onset time* (VOT) and corresponds roughly to the *aspiration* that follows voiceless stops in English.

3.2.2.4 Digital Signal Processing

Digital signal processing (DSP) involves the representation, storage, and analysis of a signal (such as a speech acoustic signal) in digitized form (i.e., as discrete values). The major purpose of DSP of speech is to take advantage of the capabilities of digital computers. The advantages of computer-aided analysis over older methods based on analog signal representations include increased speed and accuracy. Further information regarding DSP can be found in Karl (1989), Oppenheim and Schafer (1975), and Rabiner and Gold (1975).

The process of digitization takes a continuously varying acoustic signal and converts it into a series of numbers that can be stored and analyzed using a computer. As discussed above in section 3.2.2.1, the acoustic speech signal is a continuously changing energy wave that can be represented as a waveform, with amplitude plotted against time. Thus, two important parameters in digitizing a speech signal (or analog-to-digital conversion) are sampling and quantization. Sampling refers to the number of samples of the acoustic signal that are taken per unit of time (generally samples per second, i.e., Hz or kHz).

Normally, samples of speech are taken at a fixed, periodic rate during digitization, and an important concern is determining what that rate should be, to avoid loss of information. The simplest guideline is that the sampling rate should be twice the highest frequency of interest. This is called the Nyquist rate, which is based on Nyquist's sampling theorem. Thus, if the highest frequency of interest in the analog signal is 10 kHz, then the sampling rate must be 20 kHz (at least). Although a sampling rate higher than 20 kHz in this case would not give incorrect results, it would, however, require more computer memory without a concomitant increase in relevant information. On the other hand, a sampling rate less than twice the highest frequency of interest can lead to errors in analysis, particularly one called *aliasing*. The classic example of aliasing comes from an analogous situation in the visual realm. Under certain circumstances, a motion picture of a vehicle moving forward gives an impression of the vehicle's wheels moving backward. This visual aliasing is due to a film rate (frames per second) that is too slow to represent the forward motion of the wheels. In much the same way, a sampling rate for an acoustic signal that is too slow can lead to errors in analysis.

The second parameter in digitizing an acoustic speech signal is quantization. Whereas the sampling rate determines the number of "slices" of the signal in the time domain, quantization refers to the number of discrete units captured in the amplitude domain. The conversion of an analog signal to a digital one using discrete values gives the digital waveform a step-like appearance; however, increasing quantization levels give the waveform an appearance more like the (theoretically) smooth one of the analog signal. Visual representations aside, higher quantization levels are necessary in order to give the digital signal a more natural, less coarse quality. Analog-to-digital conversion at 8 bits, for example, which provides 256 quantization levels, is considered insufficient for capturing natural speech to be used for acoustic analysis. In most research, 12-bit quantization (4096 levels) is a minimum, with 16-bit conversion (65,536 levels) even better.

3.3 ANALYSIS TARGETS IN LANGUAGE AND SPEECH

Spoken language is highly complex and infinitely variable and is susceptible to analysis on a variety of levels according to a variety of approaches. For the researcher investigating the effects of alcohol on language and speech, it is necessary to narrow the scope of analysis if the research program is to be a realistic one. This section discusses some of the possible targets of analysis in such investigations.

Abercrombie (1967, p. 5) noted that if speech is a medium for conveying language, it is nevertheless "far from completely absorbed by being a vehicle for a specific language." That is, in addition to carrying linguistic signs, speech as a medium also carries nonlinguistic signs that reveal personal characteristics of the talker. Abercrombie continues: "A sign of this sort may be called an *index*, and the features of the medium which carry such indices may be called its *indexical* features, as distinct from its *linguistic* features" (p. 6). Thus, in the following discussion of analysis targets in the study of alcohol's effects on speech, we broadly differentiate those aspects of speech that convey linguistic information and those that carry indexical information.

3.3.1 Linguistic Properties of Speech

The structural analysis of language can occur at a number of levels, including sentences, words, morphemes (meaningful units that form words), and individual sound segments. Some of these types of analyses are discussed below.

Thus, *syntax* is the study of sentence structure, that is, how words are arranged to form sentences. The entire enterprise of syntactic analysis is based on the assumption that meaningful sentences are not simply random combinations of linguistic elements (words), but rather that the formation of sentences is rule-governed. Some of the concepts used in syntactic analysis include (a) lexical categories, that is, categories corresponding roughly to traditional "parts of speech," such as nouns and prepositions; (b) word order, that is, rules governing the sequencing of words in sentences; (c) phrasal categories, that is, units smaller than the sentence but larger than the word (e.g., the prepositional phrase "in the house").

Morphology is the study of word formation, that is, the rules that govern how words are constructed of smaller units of meaning called *morphemes.*

Two types of morphology are traditional: derivational (or lexical) and inflectional morphology. Derivational morphology deals with the construction of words by *affixation*, that is, the addition of morphemes either before or after another morpheme. Such derivational affixes can be attached either before a root morpheme (i.e., a *prefix*) or after it (i.e., a *suffix*). The word *preprocesser*, for instance, is formed from the root *process*, the derivational prefix *pre-*, and the derivational suffix *-er*. Inflectional morphology deals with affixation to indicate certain grammatical functions (e.g., singular vs. plural, past vs. present). For example, the inflectional affix *-s* can be added to *preprocessor* to indicate plurality: *preprocessors*.

The linguistic subdiscipline *phonology* is the study of sound systems of languages, that is, the function and patterning of sounds in language. The human vocal apparatus is capable of producing a wide variety of speech sounds, but in any one language, only a few of these are actually used distinctively. One goal of phonology, therefore, is to determine which sounds function contrastively, that is, serve to differentiate meaning. Such contrastive sounds are called *phonemes*. Other sounds appear only in specific phonetic environments, and their occurrence is therefore predictable (i.e., rule-governed); these are called *allophones*.

Whereas phonology is the study of the function and patterning of sounds in language, *phonetics* is the study of the sounds themselves. The study of phonetics can be approached in three ways. *Articulatory phonetics* investigates the physiological mechanism of speech production, including the roles played by the various speech organs in the production of speech. *Acoustic phonetics* is the study of the physical properties of speech sounds, especially their acoustic properties as measured by instrumentation. A third area is *auditory phonetics,* or the study of the effects that speech sounds have on the ear, on hearing, and on the perception of speech. There is necessarily a good deal of intertwining of these three approaches, and very little can be accomplished within any one of them without some reference to one or both of the others.

Other subdisciplines of linguistics include semantics, the study of meaning; pragmatics, the study of the relationship between language and the "real world"; historical linguistics, the study of language change; sociolinguistics, the study of language in social contexts; neurolinguistics, the study of the neurology of language; psycholinguistics, the study of language within the context of psychological theory. As will be seen in Chapters 5 through 7, the study of the effects of alcohol on structural aspects of language and speech has concentrated primarily on the phonological/phonetic level. There are exceptions, however, such as Collins (1980), which examines syntactic performance, and Sobell and Sobell (1972), which includes morphological categories (e.g., suffixes) in its analysis. Other studies (e.g., R. C. Smith, Parker, & Noble, 1975) examine the effects of alcohol on aspects of social communication, a sociolinguistic factor. For the most part, however, studies on alcohol and speech have been confined to the segmental, that is, the phonological or phonetic level.

3.4.2 Indexical Properties

Although Abercrombie (1967) applies the concept of *index* specifically to the study of phonetics, the term originates with the late 19th century American philosopher Charles Saunders Peirce, who incorporated the term within a theory of semiotics, or a formal theory of signs. Subsequent researchers in language and speech have also found the distinction between linguistic and indexical features useful, among them the British phonetician John Laver (1991), the British linguist John Lyons (1977), and the British/American phonetician/linguist Peter Ladefoged (see Ladefoged & Broadbent, 1957).

Abercrombie (1967, p. 7) provides the following "rough division of the indices": (a) those that indicate membership of a group, (b) those that characterize the individual, and (c) those that reveal changing states of the speaker. Indices of group membership include regional dialects and pronunciation characteristics indicating social standing. Indices that characterize the individual are, according to Abercrombie, "idiosyncratic"; that is, they enable a listener to recognize a talker on the basis of voice alone, and they arise from physical causes beyond the talker's control. Such signs may indicate age and sex, as well as physical abnormalities such as cleft palate. Abercrombie also includes in this category affected pronunciations such as lisps, which are within a talker's control. Indices that reveal changing states of the speaker are of two types. One type reveals transitory physical states, such as "fatigue, excitement, catarrh, grief, over-consumption of alcohol, nervousness" (Abercrombie, 1967, p. 9). The other type reveals mental states from which a listener can infer feeling, such as "amusement, anger, contempt, sympathy, suspicion, and everything else that may be included under 'tone of voice'" (Abercrombie, 1967, p. 9); these are referred to as "affective indices." Abercrombie contends that affective indices are more interesting than those indicating physical state, because the latter are often accompanied by other indicators of the relevant state.

A typology of index types offered by Laver and Trudgill (1979, p. 237) is similar to Abercrombie's, although one category boundary is somewhat different: (a) those that mark social characteristics, such as regional affiliation, social status, educational status, occupation and social role; (b) those that mark physical characteristics, such as age, sex, physique and state of health; and (c) those that mark psychological characteristics of personality and affective state. Laver and Trudgill refer to Abercrombie's categories as "group markers, individuating markers and affective markers" and to their own as "social markers, physical markers and psychological markers" (Laver & Trudgill, 1979, p. 237). As can be seen by comparing the two typologies, Laver and Trudgill include some indices in their physical marker category (e.g., state of health) that would have been included in Abercrombie's affective marker category.

A third consideration of indexical information appears in Lyons (1977). Lyons generally adopts the typology proposed by Abercrombie, with the exception of the third indexical subtype. Whereas Abercrombie and Laver and Trudgill specifically use the term *affective* to describe talker states for the third category, Lyons suggests that the third category be broadened to include more than affective or attitudinal (the latter term also appears in the literature) indices. For this category, Lyons suggests the terms *symptom* and *symptomatic*, defining the latter as follows:

> Any information in a sign or signal which indicates to the receiver that the sender is in a particular state, whether this be an emotional state (fear, anger, sexual arousal or readiness, etc.), a state of health (suffering from laryngitis, etc.), a state of intoxication, or whatever, will be described as *symptomatic* [italics added] of that state. (1977, p. 108.)

Thus, although Abercrombie places alcohol-affected speech only at the margin of the set of indexical signs, Lyons places it explicitly in the center.

Although talker-specific states can evidence variation in the speech signal, it is also the case that task-specific elicitation procedures under experimental conditions can leave characteristic indicators. Thus, there are differences in speaking style and thus in the speech signal, depending on whether speech is elicited in citation form (i.e., as isolated words) or in context (i.e., embedded in a phrase or sentence). Additionally, different speaking styles are used for spontaneous speech as opposed to speech that is read from a text, and between speech produced in isolation or in the presence of a discourse partner. Results across different speaking styles resulting from different elicitation procedures are thus not always comparable.

Some recent research has been directed toward quantifying the differences between various speaking styles. The work of Kathleen Cummings and her colleagues (Cummings, 1992; Cummings & Clements, 1990, 1992, 1993, 1995), for example, uses inverse filtering to extract the glottal waveform from the radiated acoustic signal. Various analyses of intensity, pitch, and glottal waveshape are applied in order to differentiate such styles as normal, clear, 50% tasking, 70% tasking, Lombard, angry, loud, soft, fast, slow, and question. The styles 50% tasking and 70% tasking refer to speech produced while the talker is performing some task; Lombard speech is produced while the talker is subjected to high levels of background noise. Cummings (1992) has identified six parameters of the glottal waveshape that can differentiate the eleven styles just mentioned: (a) closed duration, (b) opening duration, (c) top duration, (d) closing duration, (e) opening slope, and (f) closing slope. Research on speech produced under alcohol using glottal excitation analysis is in its early stages; a discussion of some of this work (Cummings, Chin, & Pisoni, 1996) is found in Chapter 7.

CHAPTER 4

Research Methodology

4.0 INTRODUCTION

One of the main problems in organizing, reviewing, and interpreting the literature on alcohol and speech is that it is widely scattered throughout journals and books from various disciplines and subdisciplines. The relevant literature having been accounted for, there still remains the problem of comparing different studies and finding generalizations. Because research into the effects of alcohol on speech has been highly eclectic, drawing from many disciplines, methodologies can vary, often widely. Results are therefore not always comparable, and in fact, up to the present time, no studies have been fully replicated within the relevant literature. This does not even take into account the fact that individuals vary widely in their physiological reaction to alcohol; it is simply the case that no two studies have approached the question in exactly the same way and with the same experimental methodology. In this chapter, we discuss a number of methodological variables that have been used in research on alcohol and speech. For more particular details of the specific methodologies employed in the various research projects investigating the effects of alcohol on speech, readers are referred to the more detailed discussion of the literature in Chapters 5, 6, and 7, or, of course, to the primary literature itself.

4.1 RESEARCH PARADIGMS

4.1.1 Case Studies

By *case studies* we mean any study that was conducted without the acquisition of new data. Only a handful of the studies discussed here fit that definition. One of the earliest studies, Romano, Michael, and Merritt (1940), reviewed five cases of apparent alcoholic cerebellar degeneration. All cases showed at least some degree of ataxia, gait unsteadiness being especially prevalent, and in two of the cases, there were speech abnormalities. A second case study was the analysis of the speech of Joseph Hazelwood, captain of the U.S. tankship *Exxon Valdez,* which ran aground in Alaska in March of 1989. In its investigation of the grounding, the National Transportation Safety Board (NTSB) retained two independent research groups to determine if audio recordings of radio transmissions indicated that the captain was intoxicated around the time of the grounding. The reports of these two groups were included as an appendix in the NTSB's report (National Transportation Safety Board, 1990), and the report from one group was later published as K. Johnson, Pisoni, and Bernacki (1990).

4.1.2 Clinical Studies

Clinical studies are those studies investigating the effects of alcohol on speech within a clinical population. By far the largest population studied in the publications discussed here is alcoholics. The effects of alcohol investigated do not always include acute intoxication.

The case study in Romano et al. (1940) was a clinical investigation, examining the relatively long-term effects of alcohol consumption in the absence of acute intoxication. Jetter (1938a) was also a clinical study, examining the connection between clinical signs of intoxication and chemical indicators of alcohol consumption in patients admitted to a hospital with diagnoses of acute clinical intoxication. Stein (1966) performed a structural linguistic analysis of the speech patterns of 11 abstinent alcoholics. Sobell and Sobell (1972) examined the effects of alcohol on the speech of alcoholics who were patients who had voluntarily admitted themselves for alcoholism treatment. Beam, Gant, and Mecham (1978) examined communication variables in alcoholics who were patients in an alcohol and drug abuse clinic. Fontan, Bouanna, Piquet, and Wgeux (1978) was an acoustic (spectrographic) study of the speech of hospitalized alcoholic patients. Collins (1980) examined syntactic and semantic ability in 39 alcoholic patients, with 39 nonalcoholic subjects serving as controls. Niedzielska, Pruszewicz, and Swidzinski (1994) examined acoustic aspects of speech in one control group and two groups of alcoholics, differing in the length of addiction.

4.1.3 Experimental Studies of Acute Intoxication in Nonalcoholics

By far the largest number of studies discussed here involve the administration of acute doses of alcohol to volunteer, nonalcoholic subjects under controlled laboratory conditions. The earliest study discussed here, Dodge and Benedict

(1915), examined the effects of alcohol on a number of neuromuscular processes in eight moderate users of alcohol and three additional subjects who were volunteer outpatients who had undergone treatment for alcoholism. In Hollingworth (1923), six male subjects remained under constant observation by laboratory staff for 7 hr on testing days. The majority of subjects, both experimental and control, in Hartocollis and Johnson (1956) were graduate students. Subjects were given either an experimental solution containing alcohol or a control beverage, identical to the experimental one except that alcohol was replaced by water. The study reported in Kawi (1961) examined psychological and physiological changes that took place at the "slurred speech threshold" in 24 patients in the psychiatric division of a county hospital. Dunker and Schlosshauer (1964) examined laryngeal irregularities in a variety of subjects, both healthy and hoarse. To examine the effects of vocal stress on laryngeal activity in a healthy person, a student was asked to yell, sing, and consume alcohol; unfortunately, the effects of vocal stress and alcohol consumption were confounded in the results.

Trojan and Kryspin-Exner (1968) examined the speech of three volunteer subjects before consumption of alcohol and then twice again after consumption of two doses of alcohol. The subjects in Zaimov (1969) were 20 volunteers who took reading and writing tests after consumption of two different doses of alcohol. In Moskowitz and Roth (1971), twelve male graduate students performed a naming task once with and once without alcohol. Lester and Skousen (1974) examined acoustic patterns of speech before consumption of alcohol and then again at regular intervals after consumption. R. C. Smith et al. (1975) examined formal aspects of verbal social communication in male–female dyads in both an alcohol and a placebo session. Andrews, Cox, and Smith (1977) used the voices of three male graduate students recorded both before and after alcohol consumption as stimuli for a perceptual response task. Sobell, Sobell, and Coleman (1982) investigated alcohol-induced dysfluency in male undergraduates, who submitted voice recordings before consumption of alcohol, after a low dose of alcohol, and after a high dose of alcohol.

A series of reports from a research group in Bloomington, Indiana (Behne & Rivera, 1990; Behne, Rivera, & Pisoni, 1991; Cummings et al., 1996; Pisoni et al. 1985, 1986; Pisoni & Martin, 1989) is based on a study undertaken with nine males as subjects; these subjects were recorded once before alcohol and a second time after consumption of alcohol. This experiment involved analysis of speech, as well as several perceptual experiments. Similarly, a series of reports from a research group working in Wiesbaden, Germany (Braun, 1991; Eysholdt, 1992; Künzel, 1990, 1992; Künzel, Braun, & Eysholdt, 1992) is based on a study involving 33 male police cadets as talkers; these subjects were recorded once before alcohol and then again at regular intervals subsequent to consumption of alcohol. This study involved linguistic, phonetic, and phoniatric analysis. A series of reports from a group of researchers working in Gainesville, Florida (Alderman, Hollien, Martin, & DeJong, 1995; DeJong, Hollien, Martin, & Alderman, 1995; Hollien & Martin, 1995, 1996) is based on experimental studies of talkers at various levels of intoxication. The study reported in Klingholz et al. (1988) involved 11 experimental talkers, 5 control talkers, and 12 listeners. Talkers produced speech both before and after consumption of alcohol. Swartz (1988, 1992) compared voice onset times (VOT) in 16 volunteer subjects, who submitted voice samples once without alcohol and once after alcohol treatment. Watanabe et al. (1994) examined the effects of alcohol on phonetic function and laryngeal morphology in both female and male subjects. Finally, Dunlap et al. (1995) examined sentence durations in speech produced with and without alcohol.

4.2 SUBJECT CHARACTERISTICS

4.2.1 Alcoholic versus Nonalcoholic versus Abstaining

None of the studies discussed in Chapters 5, 6, and 7 purposely mixed alcohol-dependent and nonalcohol-dependent subjects within the same population. When subjects from both populations were included in a single study, it was because of clinically based selection criteria, as in the case of Jetter (1938a), who examined 1159 consecutive cases with preadmission diagnoses of acute alcohol intoxication at a single hospital, or because a comparison of the two populations (or subpopulations) was intended, as in the case of Niedzielska et al. (1994), who compared acoustic results for nonalcohol-dependent, short-term alcohol-dependent, and long-term alcohol-dependent subjects. In other studies, either alcoholic or nonalcoholic subjects were studied to the exclusion of members of the other population. Sobell and Sobell (1972), for instance, investigated reading time and fluency in 16 male patients self-admitted to a state hospital. On the other hand, Pisoni et al. (1986) limited their study to male subjects who were "moderate social drinkers who were at low risk for alcoholism" (p. 132).

As Stitzer, Griffiths, Bigelow, and Liebson (1981a) pointed out, studies involving subjects with a history of alcohol abuse are generally conducted in inpatient facilities. Romano et al. (1940) examined five patients in a hospital who presented clinical symptoms indicating intracerebellar cortical atrophy, and who were alcohol-dependent. The 11 subjects discussed in Stein (1966) were all members of Alcoholics Anonymous and had been abstinent for periods ranging from 4 months to 13 years. Beam et al. (1978) examined 15 subjects who were diagnosed and self-acknowledged alcoholics. In the same year, Fontan et al. (1978) reported apparent dysarthria in 38 subjects, most of whom were alcoholic patients undergoing detoxification. Collins (1980) compared syntactic performance in alcoholic and nonalcoholic adults; the 39 alcoholic subjects were in residential alcoholism treatment programs. Other studies using alcohol-dependent persons as subjects include, as mentioned above, Sobell and Sobell (1972) and Niedzielska et al. (1994). Finally, Dodge and Benedict (1915) had originally planned to investigate the effects of alcohol "on total abstainers, occasional users, moderate users, habitual drinkers, . . . and on excessive drinkers" (p. 24). Only one subject was an excessive drinker, and his data could not be used because his pre-experimental drinking was indeterminate, and he refused to abstain from alcohol for experimental purposes.

For Dodge and Benedict (1915), certain difficulties arose from using abstainers as subjects that "were social and moral, on the one hand, and theoretical on the other" (p. 24). The social and moral problem they wished to avoid was the "small but serious risk of initiating a practice that might become habitual and excessive," and on the other hand, they were further faced with "the theoretical absurdity that after the first experimental investigation of alcohol the total abstainer had ceased to exist as such" (p. 24). In fact, no studies in the literature have used exclusively abstaining subjects.

In general, if subjects (as well as the population in general) can be characterized as being very broadly either (a) abstainers, (b) nonalcoholic users (not diagnosed as being alcoholics), and (c) diagnosed alcoholics, then by far the largest number of subjects studied in the literature of alcohol and speech fall into the second category. After eliminating total abstainers and excessive drinkers from their subject pool, Dodge and Benedict (1915) studied "occasional users, moderate users, habitual drinkers exceeding 30 c.c. of absolute alcohol a day" (p. 24). Thus, of the three groups, only abstainers have been consciously eliminated as an exclusive subject group in the research literature.

In principle, any combination of the three groups could be used in one study to produce a single set of results. Four logical possibilities are apparent: (a) all three groups, (b) abstainers and nonalcoholic users, (c) abstainers and alcoholics, and (d) nonalcoholic users and alcoholics. In point of fact, only one combination has been used as the studied population, that being the abstainers and nonalcoholic users. It is extremely difficult to imagine what a combined subject pool of all three groups would bring to bear in the way of interpretable results, and the combination of abstainers and alcoholics to the exclusion of nonalcoholic users appears patently absurd. The combination of nonalcoholic users and alcoholics makes sense as the population of "users" (either current or former), but this combination appears not to have been consciously used. The problem of identifying alcoholics and excluding them from a subject pool of nonalcoholic users is not a simple one, however, and methods used to screen potential subjects are discussed below. As stated, however, the combination of abstainers and nonalcoholic users has been used, at least in earlier research. For example, the six subjects from Hollingworth (1923) were characterized as ranging "from a total abstainer through degrees of occasional or moderate use, to the fairly regular but not excessive use of alcohol beverages" (p. 211); however, there was only one abstainer in the group. Jetter (1938b) studied 20 "young normal adults," characterized as "either occasional drinkers or, in a few instances, total abstainers" (p. 487).

As mentioned above, the largest group of subjects in the research literature on alcohol and speech come from the exclusive nonalcoholic user group; informal characterizations of this population have included "moderate users," "occasional drinkers," and "social drinkers." For instance, Hartocollis and Johnson (1956) characterized their subjects as either "casual" or "moderate" drinkers (these, in fact, designated two different groups); abstainers and "heavy drinkers" were purposely excluded from study (p. 184). The 12 male subjects in Moskowitz and Roth's (1971) study were self-described as "light," "social," or "party" drinkers (p. 970), whereas the 18 male–female dyads in R. C. Smith et al.'s (1975) study of alcohol effects on social communication excluded "abstainers from alcohol, very heavy drinkers, or users of other psychoactive drugs" (p. 1394). Whereas persons characterized as "heavy drinkers" were excluded from participation by, for example, Hartocollis and Johnson (1956), they were included among the nonalcoholic user group by Sobell et al. (1982); their subjects were characterized as "moderate or heavy social drinkers without drinking problems" (p. 317). Studies that included alcoholic subjects relied on clinical diagnoses of alcoholism, but studies in the literature prior to Sobell et al. (1982) that relied on the "moderate, social" type of designation were not explicit about the behavioral criteria for assigning potential subjects to the different categories or for inclusion or exclusion as subjects. In the absence of explicit criteria, it is, for instance, not clear what might differentiate "heavy drinkers" (Sobell et al., 1982) from "very heavy drinkers" (R. C. Smith et al., 1975), but Sobell et al. (1982) did make explicit the instruments used in screening subjects; these will be discussed next.

Pisoni et al. (1985) followed Sobell et al. in using a number of standardized screening instruments to determine the drinking patterns of their potential subjects. Other reports from the same period were somewhat less explicit regarding the specific screening procedures used; however, they generally did give some indication that criteria beyond simple informal designations were being used. Klingholz et al. (1988), for instance, eliminated speech–voice disorders and alcoholism through anamnestic and laryngologic examination. Higgins and Stitzer (1988) reported an average level of 7.2 drinks per week ($SD = 8.5$) for their six subjects. Künzel et al. (1992) used a questionnaire to determine that most of their subjects were regular users of alcohol, the remaining being irregular users.

In a few of the studies discussed in Chapters 5, 6, and 7, researchers appeared to take seriously their screening procedures. These include those that stated specifically which of the published screening instruments were used or that included a copy of assessment instruments as part of the published report. An example of the former is Sobell et al. (1982), who reported that their determination of subjects as "moderate or heavy social drinkers without drinking problems" (p. 317) was based on the Drinking Practices Questionnaire (Cahalan, Cisin, & Crossley, 1969), the brief Michigan Alcoholism Screening Test (Pokorny, Miller, & Kaplan, 1972), and the CAGE questionnaire (Mayfield, McLeod, & Hall, 1974[1]). Pisoni et al. (1985) were similarly specific and also included a table reporting scores from each of the assessment instruments for each of their subjects. Other reports from this same laboratory contained similar information (e.g., Behne & Rivera, 1990; Behne et al. 1991). Swartz (1988) included a copy of his screening questionnaire in an appendix (p. 77). This instrument included questions regarding medication, diagnosis as an alcoholic, familial alcoholism, intoxication patterns, and guilt or criticism regarding drinking habits.

4.2.2 Age and Gender

For those studies that reported age and gender of their talkers, male subjects have been used overwhelmingly. This is true both of experimental studies of acute intoxication in nonalcoholics and of clinical studies of alcoholic patients. With regard to the age of talker subjects, these have tended to be younger in the experimental studies than in the clinical studies.

The earliest work discussed in Chapter 5 is Dodge and Benedict (1915), an experimental study. In this study, there were two groups of subjects, one group of seven characterized as "normal" and another group of three who were psychiatric patients. The normal subjects ranged in age from 22 to 43 years; however, the one subject (also an author of the study) who was 43 was also the only normal subject over the age of 29 years. The three psychiatric patients ranged in age from 39 to 51 years. All of the subjects studied were male. Thus, from very early on the subject of choice in these studies has been a male, usually in his 20s or at most his 30s. Hollingworth (1923)

---

[1] The CAGE questionnaire is a four question alcoholism screening instrument. The acronym is derived from elements of the four questions: (a) "Have you ever felt you should *cut* down on your drinking?" (b) "Have people *annoyed* you by criticizing your drinking?" (c) "Have you every felt bad or *guilty* about your drinking?" (d) "Have you ever had a drink first thing in the morning to steady your nerves or get rid of a hang-over (*eye-opener*)?" (Mayfield, McLeod, & Hall, 1974, p. 1121).

established a pattern whereby subjects have been typically young adult males in their 20s and 30s. Subjects in his study were six males between the ages of 21;5 (years; months) and 29;5; in Hartocollis and Johnson (1956), 30 males between 21 and 36 years served as subjects. Moskowitz and Roth (1971) studied 12 male graduate students; Sobell et al. (1982) examined 16 male undergraduate students with an age range of 18 to 22 years, with a mean of 20 years. The Bloomington studies used up to nine males ranging in age from 21–26 years (see Behne et al., 1991). Klingholz et al. (1988) studied acoustic effects of alcohol in 16 male subjects ranging in age from 25–35 years, with a mean of 28.7 years, and the total pool of subjects for the Wiesbaden studies (e.g., Künzel et al., 1992) was made up of 33 men, with a mean age of 23.0 years ($SD = 15$ months). Dunlap et al. (1995) studied 29 male subjects, ages 21–23 years. Studies with smaller numbers of subjects included Trojan and Kryspin-Exner (1968), with three male subjects ranging in age from 26–36 years, and Andrews et al. (1977), whose stimulus voices were from "three young adult male graduate students" (p. 140).

Other experimental studies had both male and female talker subjects. Forney and Hughes (1961) used seven male and three female paid volunteers as subjects. R. C. Smith et al. (1975) specifically studied the effects of alcohol on social communication within male–female dyads; there were 18 such pairs, and members ranged in age from 21–30 years. Higgins and Stitzer (1988) studied the effects of alcohol on one female and five male volunteers with mean age of 23.8 years ($SD = 5.6$ years). Swartz (1988) used an equal number of males and females, eight of each, with ages ranging from 21–26 years. Finally, Watanabe et al. (1994) studied 11 female and 37 male subjects, ranging in age from 25–37 years.

The largest clinical study discussed here, Jetter (1938a), examined over 1000 consecutive cases with preadmission diagnoses of acute alcoholism; no age or gender data were included in the published report. Romano et al. (1940) examined five cases of alcoholic cerebellar degeneration; all patients were male and ranged in age from 36–58 years. Although Kawi's (1961) 24 subjects were not necessarily alcoholics, they were patients in a psychiatric hospital; all were male and ranged in age from 16–36 years. Stein's (1966) abstinent alcoholic subjects included 7 males and 4 females. Sobell and Sobell's (1972) study of the speech of alcoholics included 16 male patients who were being treated for alcoholism at a single hospital. The 33 alcoholic subjects of Fontan et al. (1978) were all male and ranged in age from 22–58 years.

The study of alcoholics by Beam et al. (1978) included nine males ranging in age from 30–60 years (mean 45.7 years) and six females ranging in age from 26–58 years (mean 44.8 years). Collins's (1980) comparison of syntactic performance in alcoholic and nonalcoholic adults included 39 alcoholic subjects, both male and female (proportions were not given), and ranging in age from 22–55 years (mean 39.0; SD = 7.95); control subjects were also both male and female (no proportions given), with a mean age of 39.0 years (SD = 7.95). The acoustic study by Niedzielska et al. (1994) included 30 alcoholic patients (sex and age not provided) and 10 control subjects (sex and age not provided).

In summary, subjects in experimental, acute feeding studies have generally been young adult males in their 20s. The general subject age is most likely due to conducting these experiments primarily at colleges and universities. Studies of alcoholics, however, are generally not limited to this age group. The preponderance of male subjects to the exclusion of females is likely due to a number of factors. First are social strictures on the administration of alcohol to women; this may explain the relatively late inclusion of female subjects in experimental studies, that is, around 1960. Second, epidemiological studies (e.g., Williams & DeBakey, 1992; see also *Eighth Special Report, 1993; Seventh Special Report*, 1990) would indicate a larger population of nonabstaining males than females, although males appear to be more likely to drink heavily (*Eighth Special Report*, 1993; abstainers and heavy drinkers have been purposely excluded in many of the studies on alcohol and speech). Third, and conclusive evidence of this was not available to earlier researchers, alcohol is a physical and behavioral teratogen (an agent that produces defects in offspring in utero) (*Eighth Special Report*, 1993). Published reports of a common pattern of birth defects observed in children born to alcoholic mothers first appeared in France in 1968 (Lemoine, Harouseau, Borteryu, & Menuet, 1968) and in the United States in 1973 (K. L. Jones & Smith, 1973; K. L. Jones, Smith, Ulleland, & Streissguth, 1973) and was termed *fetal alcohol syndrome* (FAS). Some researchers circumvent the problem of alcohol consumption by pregnant women simply by excluding females from the study group; others (e.g., Dunlap et al., 1995) require pregnancy tests immediately prior to the experimental procedure.

4.2.3 Sober versus Intoxicated

As will be discussed in section 4.2.5, many studies covered here obtained baseline measures of subjects' speech produced in the absence of alcohol. If speech samples from one or more nonalcohol conditions and one or more alcohol conditions are gathered in a single session, that is, on the same day, the general procedure has been to (a) record speech samples before alcohol, (b) administer alcohol, and then (c) record another set of speech samples under alcohol. If, however, nonalcohol and alcohol sessions are conducted on different days, then session order can be counterbalanced across subjects. Examples of recent single-session studies include Sobell et al. (1982), Künzel et al. (1992), and K. Johnson et al. (1993). Examples of recent multiple-session studies include Sobell and Sobell (1972), Smith et al. (1975), Andrews et al. (1977), Pisoni et al. (1985), and Dunlap et al. (1995). Section 4.2.5 includes further discussion of baseline (nonalcohol) conditions and experimental (alcohol) conditions.

In general, investigations of the speech of alcohol-dependent subjects have not involved administration of alcohol to induce acute intoxication. This holds true, for instance, in Romano et al. (1940), Beam et al. (1978), Collins (1980), and Niedzielska et al. (1994). On the other hand, the study reported in Sobell and Sobell (1972) involved 16 male alcoholic patients who had voluntarily admitted themselves to a state hospital for treatment of alcoholism. Recordings of these subjects were made once without alcohol but also under two postalcohol treatment conditions.

When the speech of alcoholic subjects is examined without acute intoxication, then it is necessary either for the study to include a separate group of control subjects for comparison or for there to be normative data from nonalcoholic subjects available. In the study reported in Collins (1980), for example, syntactic ability was assessed for 39 alcoholic subjects; the assessment instrument used for this purpose was the Developmental Sentence Scoring procedure (Lee, 1974), which was normed, but only for children. It was therefore necessary for Collins also to include 39 matched adult controls. In the absence of control subjects in a single study, comparison can be made to available normative data, either expressed or implied. In Beam et al. (1978), for instance, various aspects of communication were studied in alcoholic subjects. A variety of instruments were used, for which norms were available, including the Carrow Elicited Language Inventory (Carrow-Woolfolk, 1974) and voice measurements according to criteria established by W. Johnson, Darley, and Spriesterbach (1963). In studies using slurred speech as a diagnostic criterion, however, such as Romano et al. (1940), norms appear only to have been implied.

4.2.4 Naive Listeners versus Experienced Listeners

A few of the studies discussed in Chapters 5, 6, and 7 included a perceptual component in which a group of listeners heard speech samples from talkers and were required to make some sort of perceptual assessment or response. In some cases, these listeners could be characterized as *experienced* and in other cases as *naive*.

One type of perceptual task obviously requiring some prior training and experience is recognizing and recording speech errors and misarticulations. The main analysis in Zaimov (1969), for instance, was the recording of speech errors, including substitutions, exchanges, omissions, and repetitions. Sobell and Sobell (1972) scored speech samples according to 13 different types of speech errors, providing a measure of disfluency. A large component of the study reported in Künzel et al. (1992) was an analysis of errors of different types and at various linguistic levels.

Related to this type of study is what can be called phonetic analysis, which may take a number of different forms, all of which require some training. The study reported in Pisoni et al. (1985) and Pisoni and Martin (1989), for instance, included a phonetic transcription component, wherein two experienced phoneticians provided full narrow phonetic transcriptions. Künzel et al. (1992) included two types of phonetic analyses. The first, actually called a *phonetic analysis,* investigated such phenomena as the nasalization of oral vowels and various substitution phenomena. Another type of analysis, included in the phoniatric component of the study, involved investigations of voice characteristics. All of these measures required trained observers.

In all of the cases just described, however, listeners were not considered to be 'subjects' in the usual sense of the word; that is, the actions and responses of these listeners were not actually under study. In only a few studies were listeners actually considered subjects. In these studies, experienced listeners may be taken to mean persons who have undergone education or training to recognize differences or changes in speech or voice (not necessarily those brought on by alcohol). Naive listeners, then, are those who either are not assumed to have this type of training or for whom no assumption is made at all. In Andrews et al. (1977), for instance, listeners rated talkers on a number of scales, including "efficient" and "artistic." None of the listeners used in their study were trained to recognize precisely these characteristics, nor were they aware that some of the sentences they were listening to had been produced under alcohol conditions; nevertheless, they can be considered trained listeners, because all were advanced students of speech pathology. Likewise, in Klingholz et al. (1988), speech pathologists were asked to classify randomized speech samples presented for paired comparison as produced either when talkers were sober or when they were intoxicated. In Pisoni and Martin (1989), one group of listeners consisted of police officers, who were asked to provide absolute identification of randomized speech samples as produced while the talker was sober or intoxicated. Here, the assumption was that police officers would have had prior experience (if not explicit training) in recognizing speech samples produced under alcohol.

Among naive listeners may be included another group from Pisoni and Martin (1989), undergraduate university students. In these studies, students participated in either a paired comparison task, in which they were asked to decide which of two presented sentences was produced under alcohol, or an absolute identification task, in which they identified a single presented sentence as produced either when the talker was sober or when the talker was intoxicated. Also to be regarded as untrained listeners were the 30 clerical workers in Künzel et al. (1992), who completed an absolute identification task similar to the one used in Pisoni and Martin (1989). In both cases, university students and clerical workers were assumed not to have either the explicit training or the experience to recognize speech and voice changes.

4.2.5 Baseline Measures and Control Subjects

For purposes of comparing speech performance with and without alcohol under experimental conditions, the most common procedure has been for each subject to be tested at least twice, once with and once without alcohol. This procedure was followed as early as Dodge and Benedict (1915), who also pointed out that this procedure does not strictly furnish controls in the narrow sense, but rather baselines to which results from experimental conditions (i.e., under alcohol) can be compared. Hollingworth's (1923) subjects were given identical tests in the morning and in the afternoon. During the noon hour, subjects drank either water, a nonalcoholic beer, or an alcoholic beer. Performance could thus be compared across a number of conditions: morning versus afternoon, alcohol afternoon versus nonalcohol afternoon, and so on.

Other studies in which baseline measurements were provided by experimental subjects included Forney and Hughes (1961), Trojan and Kryspin-Exner (1968), Zaimov (1969), Moskowitz and Roth (1971), Sobell and Sobell (1972), Lester and Skousen (1974), R. C. Smith et al. (1975), Andrews et al. (1977), Sobell et al. (1982), Pisoni et al. (1985), Higgins and Stitzer (1988), Klingholz et al. (1988), Swartz (1988), Behne and Rivera (1990), Behne et al. (1991), Künzel et al. (1992), K. Johnson et al. (1993), Watanabe et al. (1994), and Dunlap et al. (1995). Although all these later studies followed the same procedure of having experimental subjects provide their own baseline measurements, procedural details were less complicated than in earlier studies, such as Dodge and Benedict (1915) and Hollingworth (1923). Whereas these earlier studies took multiple numbers of days, and all day at that, later studies in general moved much more quickly. One consideration was whether baseline measurements (i.e., without alcohol) were to be taken on the same day as measurements under alcohol. If they were, then the general procedure was to take the baseline measurement first, then administer alcohol, and then to take a second postalcohol measurement (and subsequent measurements). This procedure was followed by, for example, Künzel et al. (1992).

In other studies, sessions with alcohol and sessions without alcohol were separated by some number of days. In these studies, alcohol and nonalcohol sessions could be counterbalanced, although not all studies did this. Studies with different sessions on different days included Moskowitz and Roth (1971), in which subjects were tested once with alcohol and once with a placebo on successive days (counterbalanced); R. C. Smith et al. (1975), in which placebo and alcohol sessions occurred approximately 1 week apart in a balanced crossover design; Andrews et al. (1977), in which the first session was without alcohol and the second session, 2 weeks later, was under alcohol; Pisoni et al. (1985), in which alcohol and nonalcohol conditions were counterbalanced across two sessions; and Dunlap et al. (1995), a test–retest study in which subjects were tested in both conditions on each of two days, 12 to 16 days apart.

One study that did use control subjects in the strict sense was Hartocollis and Johnson (1956). In this study, which used a between-subjects design, 30 subjects received alcohol, and 30 subjects underwent the same tests without alcohol. Distribution of subjects between the two groups was based on careful matching of such characteristics as time of testing, usual drinking patterns, age and weight, and student or faculty status. In a similar manner, Klingholz et al. (1988) used 11 alcoholized subjects and 5 nonalcoholized subjects; the latter subjects were intended to control for effects attributable to extended use of the voice in the recording sessions. Although logistical considerations prevented them from using a separate group of control subjects, Künzel et al. (1992) pointed out in their discussion (p. 97) the desirability of using such a group, in order to control for such factors as overall fatigue, hunger, and the effects of spending hours in a sometimes smoke-filled room.

Collins (1980) compared syntactic performance in alcoholic and nonalcoholic adults. Because the instrument used, the Developmental Sentence Scoring (Lee, 1974), had been developed and normed for children, it was necessary to have both a group of alcoholic subjects ($N = 39$) and a group of nonalcoholic subjects ($N = 39$). The alcoholic subjects were all members of residential alcohol treatment programs at the time of the study, whereas the nonalcoholic subjects had never been diagnosed as alcoholics or undergone treatment for excessive alcohol consumption. The two groups of subjects were matched for age, I.Q. (using Ammons & Ammons, 1962), and years of education.

4.2.6 Other Subject Characteristics and Requirements

A number of other considerations regarding subject characteristics and requirements have been reported in the literature under discussion here. These have included the following:

Abstinence: A number of studies included provisions for subjects to fast for a period preceding the experimental session. The fasting period, that is, abstention from food or beverages, ranged from 2 hr preceding the experimental session (e.g., Higgins & Stitzer, 1988) to 4 hr (e.g., Moskowitz & Roth, 1971; Pisoni et al., 1985; Sobell et al., 1982;). In some cases, subjects were also specifically asked not to consume coffee (e.g., for 24 hr in Moskowitz & Roth, 1971) or alcohol (e.g., for 24 hr in Moskowitz & Roth, 1971, or 12 hr in Higgins & Stitzer, 1988). Jetter (1938b) specified that alcohol consumption took place "on a fasting stomach or after a light breakfast" (p. 487).

Other medications and drugs: A number of studies listed the use of other drugs and medications as contraindications to participation as a subject. Sobell and Sobell (1972) specified that subjects use "no medication concurrent with the study" (p. 862). Other studies were more specific: Higgins and Stitzer (1988) required that subject not use illicit drugs during the study; R. C. Smith et al. (1975) eliminated psychoactive drug users from their study; the subjects in Beam et al.'s (1978) study could not be taking medication that would impair speech. Collins (1980) required subjects not to take stimulants or depressants for the 12 hr preceding the study, and the subjects in Swartz (1988, 1992) could not be smokers.

Medical clearance: Some studies required general or specific medical clearance as a prerequisite for participation as a subject. Some of these general and specific requirements included no known heart, liver, metabolic, digestive or psychiatric disturbances (Hartocollis & Johnson, 1956); no encephalopathy (Kawi, 1961); no neurologic peculiarities (Trojan & Kryspin-Exner, 1968); 20/20 visual acuity (corrected if necessary) (Moskowitz & Roth, 1971); no medical contraindications (Sobell, Sobell, & Coleman, 1982); medical screening (Higgins & Stitzer, 1988); nondiabetics (Swartz, 1988).

Speech and hearing: A number of studies required that subjects have normal speech, language, hearing, or voice. These included Trojan and Kryspin-Exner (1968), Beam et al. (1978), Sobell et al. (1982), Pisoni et al. (1985), Klingholz et al. (1988), Swartz (1988, 1992), Pisoni and Martin (1989), K. Johnson et al. (1993).

Native language: A number of studies required a particular native language for participation in the study. In most of the literature discussed here, this language was specified as English or American English (e.g., Collins, 1980; Lester & Skousen, 1974; Sobell & Sobell, 1972). The study reported in Swartz (1988, 1992) included a screening procedure (based on the vowels in a standard articulation test) to ensure that all subjects were speakers of "General American" English (Swartz, 1988, p. 23). Beam et al. (1978) reported that 4 of their 15 subjects had learned English as a second language. In Trojan & Kryspin-Exner (1968; study conducted in Austria), Klingholz et al. (1988; study conducted in Germany), and Künzel et al. (1992; study conducted in Germany), the testing language was German. Other languages used for testing have been Bulgarian in Zaimov (1969), French in Fontan et al. (1978), Japanese in Watanabe et al. (1994), and Polish in Niedzielska et al. (1994).

Educational level: A number of studies required specific educational levels as requisite for participation as subjects. For instance, the study reported in Hartocollis and Johnson (1956) was limited to college-educated men, and Moskowitz and Roth (1971) used only male graduate students, this last condition to control for possible vocabulary differences in sex and education. On the other hand, Beam et al. (1978) required only that subjects be "of at least average intelligence and educational background" (p. 548). A number of studies report a fair degree of educational homogeneity in their subject groups; this is especially so for studies conducted at colleges or universities (e.g., undergraduate students in Pisoni & Martin, 1989). Authors of these studies do not always report explicitly whether these educational levels are prerequisites or simply artifacts of available subject populations.

4.3 MATERIALS ELICITATION

It is perhaps no accident that the earliest study discussed here to undertake a detailed study of speech itself under alcohol was Forney and Hughes (1961), for that work appeared just around the time that relatively high-quality audio recording equipment became generally available. Prior to Forney and Hughes, the smallest linguistic unit observed was the word, in Hartocollis and Johnson (1956), where scores were expressed as number of words produced. In the two earlier experimental studies, Dodge and Benedict (1915) and Hollingworth (1923), the real measures were in units of time, reaction times in Dodge and Benedict, time required to complete naming tasks in Hollingworth. In Jetter (1938a, 1938b) and Romano et al. (1940), speech abnormalities were noted but not further described. Beginning with Forney and Hughes, however, recording equipment made it possible to retain analog records of the actual speech samples produced by subjects and use these records for further analysis. Thus, in the various tasks requiring speech production, Forney and Hughes could analyze these productions in terms of a variety of speech errors, as well as in terms of the number of words produced.

Forney and Hughes's (1961) study established a number of protocols that continue to hold for the most very recent research on alcohol and speech. First, very few studies after Forney and Hughes failed to make audio recordings (either analog or digital) of subjects' speech. Not only did these recordings maintain a permanent record for further analysis, they also provided the opportunity to conduct perceptual experiments like those described in Klingholz et al. (1988); Pisoni and Martin (1989); Künzel, Braun, and

Eysholdt (1992); and Hollien and Martin (1995). Second, Forney and Hughes used connected speech as the basis for analysis. All responses in Hollingworth (1923), for instance, were single words. The use of connected speech afforded researchers the possibility of examining a far greater number of effects than could be observed using isolated words. Furthermore, the use of a standardized text gave researchers the opportunity to perform detailed cross-subject and cross-condition analyses.

4.3.1 Spontaneous and Semispontaneous Speech

These two types of speech are grouped together, because it is often difficult, especially under experimental conditions, to differentiate between truly spontaneous speech and speech that is in some way moved in a certain direction by an examiner. We may superficially define spontaneous speech as that use of language that normally occurs under normal, nonexperimental, everyday circumstances; this, in fact, is most likely the type of speech that people are most exposed to and most engaged in. Obviously, in discourse with others, it is incumbent upon a speaker to remain on topic and to try to make only relevant utterances. It is this requirement of discourse that blurs the line between spontaneous and semispontaneous speech under experimental conditions.

Examples of relatively spontaneous speech are male–female dyad verbal social communication examined in R. C. Smith et al. (1975) and monologue speech in Higgins and Stitzer (1988). In both cases, the direction of communication was determined by someone other than the examiner. In the case of R. C. Smith et al. (1975), the production of speech was determined by the interaction between the two members of the subject dyad; in the case of Higgins and Stitzer (1988), a lone subject determined the course of speech production. Note that in both of these studies, no attempt was made to assess linguistically the structural aspects of speech, such as phonetics or acoustics. In Smith et al., transcriptions were made of such social aspects of verbal communication as degree of acknowledgment and interruption; in the case of Higgins and Stitzer, the only measurement made was the total amount of speech produced in a 40-min session.

A third possible example of relatively spontaneous speech is the task reported in Trojan and Kryspin-Exner (1968), in which subjects were asked to "relate a self-experienced story" (p. 218). The extent of this description indicates that no further directions as to topic were given. Lester and Skousen (1974) reported that in both the alcohol and nonalcohol conditions, one speech sample consisted of "an impromptu monologue from the subject or conversation between the subject and the person administrating the experiment" (p. 233). It is unclear what instructions were given to the subjects in the study reported in Fontan et al. (1978); however, there are some indications in the text that spontaneous utterances were recorded. Last, we may consider the speech recorded from the captain of the *Exxon Valdez*, reported in K. Johnson, Pisoni, and Bernacki (1989, 1990), to exemplify spontaneous speech. Considerations in interpreting this type of speech include the fact that the speech was not uttered under experimental circumstances, that the speech was uttered in a relatively formal situation, and that the talker was aware of being tape-recorded.

Under semispontaneous speech we include speech that approximates spontaneous speech in its structure to everyday conversational speech, but which occurs within a narrower topic range, as determined by the examiner. Note that the structural requirement does not demand full sentences, either for elicited spontaneous or semispontaneous speech under experimental conditions, anymore than for everyday conversation. A prototypical example of semispontaneous speech elicitation is a description of a picture. The main reason for this type of elicitation is that it narrows both lexical and syntactic choice somewhat, permitting more cross-subject and cross-condition comparisons than does truly spontaneous speech. The speech elicited in Jetter (1938a) may be considered a type of semispontaneous speech. In that study, subjects were asked to provide simple information such as name and residence. Obviously, although the semantic and phrase-structure ranges of responses was limited, the phonetic possibilities were considerably broader. The interviews described in Stein (1966) resulted in approximately 18 hr of recorded material for 11 subjects. Questions asked by the examiner ranged from relatively narrow ones, such as questions about age and birthplace, to fairly open-ended ones, such as those regarding views about the future.

As mentioned, picture description is one way to elicit semispontaneous speech; alcohol and speech studies using this technique included Collins (1980) and Künzel et al. (1992). In the case of Collins (1980), speech was elicited using pictures from the Thematic Apperception Test (Murray, 1943), according to procedures from Wilson (1963). Because this study examined syntactic abilities, a minimum of 50 sentences or sentence attempts had to be produced by the subject, and subjects could be prompted. In Künzel et al. (1992), semispontaneous speech was elicited by means of a drawing, but results were not reported.

4.3.2 Naming

In *naming* tasks, we assume the elicited speech consists of isolated words. Elicitation can be by any number of methods, including elicitation of object names with pictures of the objects as stimuli (e.g., Moskowitz & Roth, 1971; Trojan & Kryspin-Exner, 1968); elicitation of color names with cards in those colors as stimuli (e.g., Hollingworth, 1923); or elicitation of adjectives with orthographic representations of their antonyms as stimuli (e.g.,

Hollingworth, 1923). Important in differentiating this type of elicitation from other elicitation techniques are (a) that responses consist of a single word in isolation, (b) that the subject does not hear a model of the desired response, (c) that the subject is not shown an orthographic representation of the desired response, and (d) that the range of possible responses is considerably more narrow than in spontaneous or semispontaneous speech.

In the color-naming task described in Hollingworth (1923), subjects were shown cards colored red, blue, green, yellow, or black, occurring in random order. Subjects were required to name the color of each card as rapidly as possible; subjects could not continue to the next trial until a correct response was given. Results were expressed as the total amount of time required to complete the task. Procedure for the antonym-naming task was similar, except that subjects were given a typewritten list of adjectives rather than colored cards; responses had to be exact antonyms of the stimulus adjectives. Again, subjects had to respond correctly before moving to the next trial, and scores were expressed as time required to complete the task. One of the tasks reported in Trojan and Kryspin-Exner was to provide names of objects pictured on cards. Responses were in German, and the recorded responses were used for linguistic, phonetic, and voice analysis. In Moskowitz and Roth (1971), subjects were required to name objects depicted on cards, five cards at each of six levels of word frequency (Thorndike & Lorge, 1944). Measurements were response latencies for each of the presentations.

If picture naming can be considered the prototypical naming task, then the antonym-naming task from Hollingworth (1923) is slightly removed from the prototype. Similar tasks were used by Hartocollis and Johnson (1956). Four ostensible naming tasks were administered, each placing narrower restrictions on responses than the previous one. Subjects were required (a) simply to produce words for 3 min; (b) to name words that began with a certain letter; (c) to name objects that were members of certain semantic classes such as "vegetables"; and (d) to give words with specified meanings and beginning with specified letters. In all of these tasks, scores were the number of correct responses given in a specified amount of time. In all these tasks, naming could depend on the subjects' ability to access orthographic representations and match them with meanings; however, at no point were subjects actually shown orthographic representations.

Other elicitation techniques that might be considered to fall under the rubric of naming tasks include the sentence-completion task of Kawi (1961) and the counting task in Künzel et al. (1992). In Kawi (1961), examiners read an incomplete sentence to subjects, who were then required to complete the sentence. In the published report, no examples are given, so it is difficult to determine the range of possible completions, but the two measures taken from this task were reaction time and a content analysis. In Künzel et al.

(1992), one of the tasks for subjects was to recite the numbers in German from 21 to 30.

4.3.3 Shadowing Speech

In a shadowing task, stimulus materials are presented auditorily to subjects, who then repeat what they have heard as quickly as possible. A subset of the stimuli used in the Pisoni et al. (1985) study were presented in this way. Monosyllabic word and sentence stimuli were presented over headphones with an attached boom microphone for recording responses. Subjects were told that they had a limited amount of time to respond to each stimulus and were instructed to repeat what they had heard as quickly as possible.

4.3.4 Read Speech

To elicit read speech, stimuli are presented in orthographic form to subjects. Texts for reading can consist of lists of isolated words (e.g., Behne & Rivera, 1990; Dodge & Benedict, 1915; Lester & Skousen, 1974; Pisoni et al., 1985) to isolated phrases or sentences (e.g., Behne et al., 1991; K. Johnson et al., 1993; Pisoni et al., 1985; Swartz, 1988, 1992) to entire connected passages (e.g., Andrews et al., 1985; Behne et al., 1991; DeJong et al., 1995; Künzel et al., 1992; Pisoni et al., 1985; Sobell & Sobell, 1972; Sobell et al., 1982). Examples of read words, sentences, and texts can be found in the appendices.

The mode of presentation of text for reading could also vary. In Dodge and Benedict's (1915) study, single words printed on cards were presented one at a time using a special exposure apparatus constructed for this experiment. A refined version of this type of apparatus was the Hunter Cardmaster used for presentation of pictures in Moskowitz and Roth (1971). In both cases, the time of presentation of the stimulus was controlled, and the voice of the subject stopped a timer, recording the response latency. For Moskowitz and Roth (1971), in addition to response latency, it would have been possible to record actual tokens of subjects' speech; this possibility was not practicably available to Dodge and Benedict (1915). An even more refined method of presenting single words was used by Pisoni et al. (1985). In this study, single words were presented by computer on a cathode-ray tube (CRT) monitor. Because actual speech, not response latencies, was recorded in this task, presentation rate was self-paced; subjects pressed a button on a response box when they wished the next item to be presented. The words used in Dodge and Benedict (1915) were all four letters long, a length arbitrarily chosen. This was the only study discussed here in which the selection of words was based on orthographic considerations. The words used in Lester and Skousen (1974) were one, two, four, or five syllables in length, chosen to cover the ranges of phoneme occurrence, word positions, and syllable structures. Two types of words were used in Pisoni et al. (1985):

(a) 204 monosyllabic words, which covered the range of English phonemes and partially the range of syllable structures (all words were closed syllables); and (b) 38 spondees, that is, two-syllable words with stress on both syllables (e.g., *airplane*).

The study in Pisoni et al. (1985) included elicitation of sentences produced in isolation by subjects, including sentences with multiple occurrences of identical or very similar phonemes (e.g., "Brother Sam sits on the seesaw"). The ten sentences used in Swartz (1988, 1992) were constructed to elicit five tokens each of the voiced and voiceless alveolar stops in identical immediate phonetic environments (e.g., "What did Beth do last weekend?" and "The fourth tulip is yellow," in which the target segment is preceded by a voiceless interdental fricative and followed by a high back vowel followed by a lateral liquid).

The connected text used for reading in Sobell and Sobell (1972) was a 613-word passage taken from McDavid and Muri (1967). Passages used in other studies have varied in length: the passage from Montagu (1958) used in both Andrews et al. (1977) and Sobell et al. (1982) was 73 words long. Three passages were used by Pisoni et al. (1985): the Grandfather Passage (132 words), the Victory Garden Passage (202 words), and the Rainbow Passage (332 words). In the study by Pisoni et al. (1985), however (as well as others, including Behne et al., 1991), subjects read all three passages; the summed length of all three passages is 666 words, approximately comparable in length to the passage used by Sobell and Sobell (1972). In Künzel et al. (1992), subjects read Aesop's fable "The Northwind and the Sun" in German, which is 109 words long; Künzel et al. reported that the time required to read this passage at a normal speaking rate was between 40 and 45 sec. Klingholz et al. (1988) reported that their subjects "read the beginning of a well-known fairy tale over an interval of at least 2.5 min" (p. 930), so that the reading time in this study was at least three times as long as for the subjects in the study by Künzel et al. (1992).

In summary, elicitation procedures for speech materials range from elicitation of fairly spontaneous speech in conversation with acquaintances to read speech. Read speech may consist of single words presented individually or in a list to entire paragraph-length passages. Between these two extremes are a number of other methodologies, including picture naming and shadowing. Specificity regarding the exact elicitation procedure is important, as both baseline measures and experimental measures may vary, depending on the type of speech elicited.

4.4 QUANTITATIVE NONSPEECH MEASUREMENTS OF ALCOHOL IN THE BODY

In this section we discuss the different methods that have been used to determine the amount of alcohol present in body fluids and tissues at the time of testing. Two main methods appear in the literature: prescribed dosages of ethanol and *post hoc* chemical analysis of the alcohol content of body fluids and breath.

4.4.1 Dosage Control

Except for Dunker and Schlosshauer (1964) and possibly Künzel et al. (1992), none of the experimental studies discussed here appear to have allowed unlimited, uncontrolled consumption of alcohol by its subjects. All other experimental studies controlled explicitly the amount of alcohol introduced into the bodies of their subjects. With one exception, all of these studies prescribed *per os* administration of alcohol; the exception was Kawi (1961), who administered alcohol intravenously.

Each of the oral dosage prescriptions used in the remaining studies can be characterized in one of three ways: (a) absolute amounts of alcohol or an alcoholic preparation for every subject; (b) prescribed dosage based on units of alcohol (weight or volume) per units physical attribute (usually subject's body weight) and/or a target blood- or breath-alcohol concentration (BAC/BrAC) or target window, but without subsequent chemical analysis of blood, urine, or breath; and (c) prescribed dosage based on units of alcohol (weight or volume) per units physical attribute (usually subject's body weight) and/or a target BAC/BrAC or target window with subsequent chemical analysis. Alcoholic preparations used have included pure (95%) ethanol, vodka, bourbon whiskey, liquor, beer, and wine. Vodka has been the most-used beverage, usually 40% (80-proof U.S.), and generally mixed in a carrier such as tonic water or grapefruit juice.

Two doses of alcohol were used in the study reported in Dodge and Benedict (1915): 30 cc and 45 cc of alcohol, both mixed in a carrier. Subjects in Trojan and Kryspin-Exner (1968) were tested once before alcohol consumption, once after consumption of a portion of a total prescribed amount of 13% "heavy Austrian wine," and once after consumption of the entire amount, "which determined the limit of the individual tolerance" (p. 218); it is not reported what determined either the total amount to be consumed or what exactly the "limit of individual tolerance" was. Each of the subjects in Zaimov (1969) consumed between 100 and 550 ml of a 65% alcohol solution made to taste like anise brandy. Each subject was tested on a reading task after consumption of 50 ml of the alcohol preparation and then again after consuming the entire prescribed dose; Zaimov does not cite the basis for differences in the prescribed dosages. Lester and Skousen (1974) prescribed 1 oz of 86-proof bourbon whiskey every 20 min, with speech sampling occurring immediately prior to consumption of the interval dose. Each of the three talker subjects in Andrews et al. (1977) consumed three alcoholic doses, each consisting of 1.5-oz 80-proof vodka contained in 3 oz of fruit juice and ice; total alcohol consumption was 4.5-oz 80-proof vodka. Subjects in Higgins and Stitzer (1988) were administered 0, 22-, 45-, and 67-g doses of ethanol mixed with enough water to total 8 oz in volume; this solution was then mixed with 8-oz orange juice. Two of the subjects were also given 90-g doses of ethanol.

Hartocollis and Johnson administered alcohol to their 30 experimental subjects to raise alcohol concentrations to 0.10%, based on body weight according to calculations in Haggard and Jellinek (1942). The alcoholic beverage contained 20% absolute ethanol, 20% water, 60% grapefruit juice, and two drops of peppermint oil, whereas the beverage given to control subjects was identical, except that the ethanol was replaced by water. An example of the dosage for a 150-lb subject was 56.8 cc of alcohol in a beverage with a total volume of 284 cc. Moskowitz and Roth (1971) administered alcohol as 1 oz of 80-proof (U.S.) vodka per 40-lb body weight, or 0.52 g/kg body weight, mixed with an equal volume of orange juice; this was prescribed to produce a BAC between 0.06 and 0.07%. Sobell and Sobell (1972) tested speech after 0, 5-, and 10-oz portions of 86-proof liquor, designed to produce BACs of 0, .10, and .25%. In R. C. Smith et al. (1975), subjects were given both a low and a high dose of alcohol, based on ml of pure ethanol per kg of body weight. In the low-dose session, men were given 1.0 ml alcohol/kg body weight and women .83 ml/kg. In the high-dose session doses for men and women were the same, 1.5 ml/kg. The dose was carried in a beverage consisting of 80-proof (U.S.) vodka in a peppermint-flavored carrier. Sobell et al. (1982) recorded subjects three times in a single session, at target BACs of 0, 0.05, and 0.10%. After recording without alcohol, subjects consumed a beverage calculated at 0.345-g 95% ethanol/kg body weight, consisting of 1 part 190-proof alcohol to 4 parts water. A second identical dose was administered after recording and before the third recording; the combined dosage was thus .69-g 95% ethanol/kg body weight.

A number of studies administered alcohol doses according to target BACs/BrACs or target windows and then followed up with chemical analyses of blood or breath. In Klingholz et al. (1988), target BACs were 0.01% increments between 0.05 and 0.15%. Alcohol was administered as beer (1 L of beer contained 40 g of alcohol), according to body weight and a 0.7 reduction factor. Achieved BACs as determined by blood sampling ranged from 0.067–0.159%, but not necessarily in 0.01% increments. Swartz (1988, 1992) used a standard police chart to determine the number of 12-oz beers subjects of given weights needed to consume in a specified amount of time to achieve BACs within a window of 0.075–0.100%. Subjects consumed between 40 and 71 oz (mean = 52.19 oz) of beer within time periods ranging from 1 : 18 (hours:minutes) to 4:27 (mean = 2:05); breath analysis showed BACs ranging from 0.075 to 0.099% (mean = 0.087%).

In Behne et al. (1991), target BACs were set to be at least .10%. Prescribed doses were 1-g ethanol/kg body weight, in a beverage consisting of 1 part 80-proof (U.S.) vodka to 3 parts orange juice. Actual achieved BACs, as measured by breath analysis, at the beginning of recording ranged from .10 to .19% and after recording ranged from .075 to .15%. Subjects in Künzel et al. (1992) were administered alcohol in the form of 40% vodka, which could be consumed either straight or diluted. Subjects were informed of the approximate number of 100-ml containers of the beverage needed to be consumed to reach the BrAC window that ranged from 1.0–2.0%. BrAC analysis just preceding the first alcohol-condition speech sampling showed BrACs ranging from 0.15–2.12%.

4.4.2 Alcohol Concentration in Body Fluids

Chemical tests for alcohol content in body fluids and tissues dates back to the 19th century (American Medical Association Committee on Medicolegal Problems, 1970); fluids that are susceptible to analysis include blood, urine, and saliva. The most widely used body fluid for analysis, however, is blood, based to a large part on the development by Widmark (1932) of a micromethod for determining the alcohol content of blood and his recommendation of its use. In Sweden, where Widmark worked, legislation was enacted in 1931 providing for the use of chemical tests of intoxication in traffic cases, and in the United States, chemical tests were first used around 1926 (Harger & Hulpieu, 1956). Analysis of body fluids is often expressed in terms of its relation to the alcohol content of blood, because that is the fluid that reaches the brain; however, as research establishes with more confidence the ratio between BAC and the concentration of alcohol in other body fluids, alcohol concentration is often expressed in terms of its concentration in other fluids and breath. Overviews of the history and technology of chemical analysis for alcohol content can be found in the American Medical Association Committee on Medicolegal Problems (1970), Dubowski (1986, 1991), A. W. Jones (1989), and Sunshine and Hodnett (1971).

Blood sampling has been used in a number of studies discussed here, although in the more recent literature, it has yielded somewhat to breath-alcohol analysis. Jetter's (1938a) hospital study was designed to correlate clinical and chemical indicators of intoxication, so that the blood of over 1000 subjects was tested for alcohol, and in about a third of these cases, urine samples were also drawn and analyzed. Jetter's (1938b) nonalcoholic subjects also gave blood samples at intervals of 1, 2, 3, 4, 6, 8, 12, and 24 hr after consumption of an alcoholic preparation. Klingholz et al. (1988) administered alcohol in varying doses measured to distribute 11 subjects at 0.01% BAC intervals between 0.05% and 0.15% BAC. Blood-alcohol analysis using a Perkin-Elmer F40 Gas Chromatograph revealed that the actual distribution diverged somewhat from the target distribution, and recorded BACs ranged from 0.067% to 0.159%. In the study reported in Watanabe et al. (1994), both alcohol and aldehyde levels were measured from blood at 30-min or hourly intervals for 2.5 hr.

4.4.3 Alcohol Concentration in Breath

The commercial availability of manual Breathalyzers in 1954 made measurement of alcohol in the body considerably more convenient for both law enforcement authorities and researchers in areas such as that currently under discussion. The direct determination of alcohol in the blood and other body fluids had presented a number of difficulties, which breath-alcohol analysis could overcome. These included the invasiveness of procedures for obtaining samples of blood and other body fluids, the need for qualified personnel to draw and test samples, the need for specialized laboratory facilities to test samples, and the slow turn-around time for receiving test results. Modern breath-alcohol analysis devices overcome these problems by offering a relatively noninvasive procedure for obtaining necessary samples, a need for only a minimal number of personnel, a considerably reduced technical background for personnel, a minimal requirement for test facilities, and relatively short intervals before results are available. Rapid reporting of results is especially important if there is a predetermined target BAC or BrAC level or window, and the advantages of breath sampling over blood sampling are especially clear when either relatively large numbers of experimental subjects are involved or multiple samples are taken at relatively short intervals or both. It is highly unlikely, for instance, that the level of sampling described in Künzel et al. (1992) could have been maintained had blood, rather than breath, samples been necessary. An overview of breath-alcohol technology can be found in Dubowski (1991).

Modern breath-alcohol analysis devices generally depend on one of five basic scientific principles: chemical oxidation and photometry, electrochemical oxidation/fuel cell, gas chromatography, infrared spectrometry, and solid state (semiconductor) sensing. The various models of Breathalyzers, for instance, operate on the basis of chemical oxidation and photometry, whereas the Intoxilyzer uses infrared spectrometry. Various commercial devices have been used in studies described here. Additionally, there are at least two ways of reporting results from breath-alcohol analysis. The first is to convert the results to equivalent BACs. This is generally done based on an assumed partition ratio for blood to breath of 1 : 2100. The second way is to report BrACs directly, that is, to report results as the mass of alcohol per unit volume of breath. In general practice, this is stated as grams of alcohol per 210 L of breath, although other units of concentration are used (as in Europe, e.g., in Künzel et al., 1992).

Just as they were the first to use audio recordings and connected speech in their experimental research, so too were Forney and Hughes (1961) the first to determine alcohol levels using breath-alcohol analysis. The device they used was the Borkenstein Breathalyzer, a chemical oxidation and photometric device, as mentioned above. Concentrations were reported as BACs of "approximately 100 mgm per cent" (p. 186). Among the research literature discussed here, it was another 20 years before breath-alcohol analysis was employed again. This was reported in Sobell et al. (1982), who determined alcohol concentrations using an Alco-Analyzer Gas Chromatograph (Model 1000). The results of analysis using this device revealed that in general, subjects did not achieve the target peak BACs predicted by the alcohol doses that were administered. Two target levels were the goal: a moderate dose for 0.05% BAC and a high dose for 0.10% BAC. In fact, the mean peak BAC from the moderate dose was 0.026% (range: 0.016–0.051) and from the high dose was 0.078% (range: 0.045–0.117). Higgins and Stitzer (1988) used an Intoxilyzer (CMI Corp.), which uses infrared spectrometry, to estimate BACs at three time intervals in each experimental session: before consumption of alcohol, immediately before each talking session began, and immediately after each talking session. Results from this analysis showed an orderly increase in BACs as a function of alcohol dose.

For the study reported in Behne et al. (1991), the speech of nine subjects was sampled twice, once before consumption of alcohol (.00% BAC) and once after consumption of alcohol when BAC was at least .10%. This was determined using a Smith and Wesson Breathalyzer (Model 900A), again a chemical oxidation/photometric analysis device. Results using this device showed initial BACs (i.e., before postalcohol recordings were made) to range from .10–.19% and final BACs (i.e., after postalcohol recordings were made) to range from .075–.15%. Swartz (1988, 1992) stated that for his study, alcohol level was determined using a portable breathalyzer test (PBT), although it is not clear whether *breathalyzer* here is used in a specific sense or a generic sense. The study reported in Künzel et al. (1992) used a Siemens Alcomat, which uses infrared spectrometry, to determine BrACs. Target BrACs were between 1‰ and 2‰, and actual achieved BrACs for the 33 subjects ranged between 0.15‰ and 2.12‰. Dunlap et al. (1995) used an Alco-Sensor IV (Intoximeters, Inc.), an electrochemical oxidation/fuel cell sensor, to determine if subjects were within a predetermined BrAC window in order to produce a postalcohol speech sample. The use of a portable breath-alcohol analysis device permitted retesting at regular intervals if subjects were not within the prescribed BrAC window at the first breath analysis.

Although, as mentioned above, operation of breath-alcohol analysis devices and interpretation of results require less training than for body fluid analysis, there is nevertheless a certain amount of training necessary. In

Swartz (1988), for instance, the analysis device was operated by police officers trained in the use of the device and administration of the test.

4.5 QUALITATIVE NONSPEECH MEASURES OF ALCOHOL IN THE BODY

The nonspeech measures described below were taken in a few studies to correlate them with chemical results.

4.5.1 Odor of Alcohol

The odor of alcohol on the breath was used as a clinical sign of intoxication in two studies (Jetter, 1938a, and its follow-up study, Jetter, 1938b). In both of these studies, a diagnosis of clinical intoxication was forthcoming if there was gross gait abnormality and at least two of the following: gross speech abnormality, facial flushing, dilated pupils, and alcoholic odor of breath.

4.5.2 Nystagmus

Nystagmus is an involuntary jerking of the eye (see Berkow, 1992), and although it is a naturally and normally occurring phenomenon, it is magnified or exaggerated by alcohol and other drugs. Three general categories of nystagmus are observed: (a) vestibular nystagmus, (b) nystagmus resulting from neural activity, and (c) nystagmus caused by pathological disorders. Horizontal gaze nystagmus, which occurs when the eyes gaze to the side, is used widely as a test of intoxication in law enforcement (Burns & Moskowitz, 1977).

In Künzel et al. (1992), postrotational and positional alcohol nystagmus was induced by having subjects spin around quickly three times. Postrotational nystagmus occurs because of disturbances in inner ear fluid caused by the rotation; positional alcohol nystagmus (PAN) occurs when a foreign fluid that alters the specific gravity of blood, such as alcohol, is in unequal concentrations in the blood and the vestibular system. In Watanabe et al. (1994), initial assessment of the effects of alcohol was through observation of spontaneous nystagmus, optokinetic nystagmus, and eye tracking.

4.5.3 Dexterity and Sway

In Jetter (1938a, 1938b), gross disturbances of gait were the absolute requirement for a diagnosis of clinical intoxication. In the study reported in Künzel et al. (1992), a number of neurological measures were made of gross and fine motor control. In addition to nystagmus testing, these included walk-and-turn, finger-to-finger, and path-tracing.

4.6 QUANTITATIVE LINGUISTIC AND
SPEECH MEASURES

In studying the effects of alcohol on language and speech, it is often necessary to narrow the scope of investigation to either a specific behavior or a specific linguistic level. Early studies, usually conducted by researchers other than language or speech specialists, generally used measures taken from experimental psychology, such as response latencies or task completion times. Later studies moved the scope of investigation to an analyis of the linguistic and speech signal itself; a good deal of the most recent work depends on recordings and instrumental analysis, techniques that were not available to earlier researchers. In this section, we discuss some of the measures that have been taken in the study of alcohol and speech.

4.6.1 Reaction Times/Response Latencies

The earliest research into the effects of alcohol on speech discussed here was reported by Raymond Dodge, a psychologist, and Francis Gano Benedict, a Harvard-trained chemist and director of the Nutrition Laboratory. In studying the effects of alcohol on certain neuromuscular processes, Dodge and Benedict (1915) used a relatively straightforward measure of its effects on reading, namely, reaction time. Words were presented on cards, and subjects responded by talking into a voice key. This response broke an electrical circuit and stopped a kymograph, recording the time between presentation of the word and the response.

Over 50 years later, Moskowitz and Roth (1971) reported a similar experiment, this time measuring response latencies in object naming (rather than reading printed words). Using somewhat more sophisticated apparatus, Moskowitz and Roth presented pictures to subjects, who were required to give the name of the object in the picture as quickly as possible. Stimulus presentation, responses, and response latencies were all controlled and recorded electronically.

4.6.2 Task-Completion Times

Similar to measurement of response latencies is the measurement of the time required to complete an entire task. One difference between the two is that whereas measurement of response latencies involves single trials, measurement of task-completion time involves blocks of trials. One example of this type of task measurement was used in Hollingworth (1923). In one task, subjects were presented with 100 small colored squares mounted on a large card and were required to name the card colors in order as quickly as possible. A correct response on each trial was required before proceeding to the next, and the total time to respond to all 100 stimuli was recorded, using a stopwatch. In DeJong et al. (1995), subjects performed two speech tasks at various alcohol levels: reading a text passage and repeating diadochokinetic syllables as quickly as possible. The total time required to complete each of these tasks was measured.

4.6.3 Amount of Verbalization

Included here are a number of measures, including tests of verbal fluency and measures of social communication. In the study reported in Hartocollis and Johnson (1956), as a measure of verbal fluency, subjects were required to name words in four increasingly restrictive tasks. In all four tasks, scores were the number of correct words produced in the specified amounts of time.

R. C. Smith et al. (1975) studied the effects of alcohol on formal aspects of verbal social communication. One of these measures was the amount of speech produced. This was investigated with 18 male–female dyads, who participated in free-form discussion sessions in a placebo session and two postalcohol sessions. Among other measures, the transcriber recorded the total amount of communication, the length of individual sequences of speech, interruptions and overlaps, and the degree of acknowledgment. Higgins and Stitzer (1988) also examined the effects of alcohol on amount of speech produced, but in isolated persons rather than in social dyads. A placebo and three different doses of alcohol were administered to six volunteer subjects, who were then seated facing a console in a sound-attenuated chamber. Instructions were to produce speech monologues, that is, to speak on any topic they wished and in any amount they wished, but to speak at least occasionally to indicate that they were awake. Results were expressed as the total amount of speech produced by these isolated subjects.

4.6.4 Syntactic and Morphological Measures

Syntactic and morphological measures assess sentence-formation (syntactic) and word-formation (morphological) performance. The most common type of measure is an assessment of whether or not a particular construction (sentence, phrase, word) is correctly formed. In some cases, however (e.g., Collins, 1980), constructions were compared on a scale of developmental norms.

Collins (1980) examined syntactic performance in a group of 39 alcoholic males and females and a group of 39 matched controls. Speech was elicited by means of a set of pictures, recorded, transcribed, and finally analyzed according to the Developmental Sentence Scoring (DSS) procedure (Lee, 1974). Analysis was based on eight syntactic constructions and on measures of syntactic completeness and syntactic complexity. The use of matched control subjects was necessary in this study, because although the DSS is a standard assessment instrument for syntax, it is normed only for children.

Beam et al. (1978) examined the language of 15 alcoholic subjects, using the Carrow Elicited Language Inventory (Carrow-Woolfolk, 1974). Responses were scored on such aspects as ability to complete a thought, word substitution, short-term memory for sentences, ability to complete a sentence, and ability to reproduce tenses and articles correctly. In the study reported by Trojan and Kryspin-Exner (1968), subjects were asked to relate a story from their own lives and to name objects pictured on cards before alcohol and twice after. Analysis involved tallying syntactic and grammatical infelicities, such as repetitions of words and phrases and anacolutha. Trojan and Kryspin-Exner cautioned, however, that errors arise in spontaneous and semi-spontaneous speech even when talkers are sober.

The subjects in Sobell and Sobell (1972) were alcoholics who were also acutely intoxicated for the purposes of the study. Elicitation of speech was achieved with a 613-word passage for reading, which was recorded when subjects were sober and at two degrees of intoxication. Each speech sample was scored on a number of error categories, including interjections, word repetitions, phrase repetitions, sound–syllable repetitions, revisions of single words, incomplete phrases, and broken words. The latter category included rhythm changes, and alterations in suffixes and prefixes, through omission, change, or addition.

Further studies that examined syntactic and morphological errors in read passages included Zaimov (1969) and Künzel et al. (1992). Zaimov's analysis of the speech of acutely intoxicated subjects included recording errors on a number of linguistic levels. Relevant to the present discussion were substitution, exchanges, omissions, and repetitions of words; repetitions of lines; and skipping of lines. These categories can arguably be classified at the syntactic/morphological level, although errors involving "lines" are obviously unique to printed texts. Similar categories were used in the error analysis reported in Künzel et al. (1992). In this study, the relevant error types were insertions, omissions, substitutions, and repetitions, and the relevant levels were segment/syllable, single word, word order, and line. Here too, the "line" category was tied directly to the printed passage used for speech elicitation. On the other hand, word order is a truly linguistic characteristic, as well as a specifically syntactic one.

4.6.5 Phonological Errors

The distinction between this category and the one discussed in the next section (4.6.6. Acoustic-Phonetic Measurements) is not entirely clear-cut, and some changes in speech produced under alcohol may well be classified in either category. A simple and perhaps gross distinction is that the phonological error category includes those changes perceived by untrained listeners as an error. Additionally, such errors should affect whole segments. Errors in phonetic implementation, however, are noticeable only to trained listeners or by means of instrumental analysis. A rough typology of errors is given in Künzel et al. (1992, p. 16); the error types described there are insertions, omissions, substitutions, and repetitions, and the error level relevant in the present instance is that of segment/syllable. Syllable errors are classed together with segmental errors, because in some cases, a particular error can be described as either one. This will occur in cases where a change in a single segment also alters the syllable structure of a given token; for example, if an entire syllable consists of only one segment, and that segment is omitted, then the syllable is also omitted. With these caveats in mind, we proceed to discuss some of the ways that phonological errors have been measured in the literature on alcohol and speech.

It is first of all not possible to determine if descriptions such as speech abnormality (e.g., Jetter, 1938a), thick speech (e.g., Romano et al., 1940), and slurred speech (e.g., Kawi, 1961) refer to segmental errors or errors at some other level of linguistic structure. Most likely these are questions of phonetic implementation and cases of incomplete articulations in the sense of Künzel et al. (1992 pp. 30, 38). In the earlier, non-speech-specific literature, these terms are often used without operational definitions or examples, and it is often impossible to tell what is meant by these terms. The evaluation sheet from the study reported in Forney and Hughes (1961, p. 190) is somewhat more precise about what form errors may take. In the verbal and counting tasks, errors are subcategorized as omissions, insertions, mispronunciations, spasms (stammers), prolongations, and other, but these could also characterize whole words, as well as phonological segments.

The study reported in Trojan and Kryspin-Exner (1968) was perhaps the earliest to give explicit examples of what we are calling phonological errors. These are phenomena that were included in their category phonetic disturbances (substitutions, omissions, and distortions) or decay of sounds. Included in this category were examples of such phenomena as omissions, substitutions, "weakenings," and lengthenings. Some of these, though, may fall into the category that we might call changes in phonetic implementation, for example, the weakenings and lengthenings of specific segments. Zaimov's (1969) typology classified errors as substitutions, exchanges, omissions, and repetitions, and two relevant levels that could be affected were the syllable and the letter (recall that speech was elicited by a reading passage).

Sobell and Sobell (1972) included the error categories "sound/syllable interjections" and "sound/syllable repetitions," which appear to be phonological errors. Lester and Skousen (1974) observed a number of sound substitutions, including word-final devoicing, merger of alveolar and alveopalatal fricatives, and deaffrication. Again, these may be matters of phonetic implementation, but each of the substituting segments is also a distinctive phoneme in the target language.

The study reported in Pisoni et al. (1985) included a phonetic transcription component conducted by two trained transcribers working independently. Observed errors included segment lengthening, deletions and partial articulations, deaffrication, distortions, devoicing, and palatalization. Finally, as mentioned previously, the taxonomy used for the analysis of errors in Künzel et al. (1992) included the following types: insertion, omission, substitution, repetition; in addition, errors were recorded at the following linguistic levels: segment/syllable, single word, word order, line.

4.6.6 Acoustic-Phonetic Measurements

A number of acoustic-phonetic parameters of the speech signal are amenable to instrumental measurement and analysis. Although a number of alcohol-induced changes in this realm may be auditorily perceptible, in some cases, it is only through instrumentation that these changes can be clearly observed and quantified into physical measurements. The development of high-quality audio recording equipment and the sound spectrograph (Koenig et al., 1946) made possible a broad range of analysis techniques, and the further development of digital signal processing (see Kent & Read, 1992) has opened even more possibilities. In this section, we discuss some of the phonetic and acoustic parameters that have been examined, measured, and analyzed in the research on alcohol and speech.

A very common measurement made in speech analysis is duration, which can be measured at a number of linguistic levels, from units smaller than the phonological segment to entire sentences or even passages. An early use of durational measurement can be found in Lester and Skousen (1974). Proceeding from the common observation that "drunken speech appears to be drawn out" (p. 233), as well as from the specific observation of Kozhevnikov and Chistovich (1965) that "normal slow speech displays lengthening chiefly in the vocalic segments of the syllables" (p. 233), Lester and Skousen measured durations of both consonants and vowels using an oscillographic display. Similarly, Fontan et al. (1978) used a sound spectrograph to measure durations in the speech of alcoholic patients.

Using digital signal processing techniques, Pisoni et al. (1985) measured durations of both entire sentences and individual segments or parts of segments. Voice onset time (VOT) is another durational measurement, and using digital sound spectrography, Swartz (1988, 1992) examined the effects of alcohol on VOT in both voiced and voiceless alveolar stops. Behne and Rivera (1990) measured durations of both segments and the words containing them and from these measurements also calculated segment-to-word duration ratios. In Behne et al. (1991), duration measurements were also made for monosyllabic words and spondees, isolated sentences, and sentences in connected passages. Künzel et al. (1992) measured the durations of both speech material and pauses; both appeared to increase under alcohol. DeJong et al. (1995) measured durations for two tasks, reading a passage and repeating diadochokinetic syllables; on both measures, durations increased. Finally, Dunlap et al. (1995) found a reliable increase in sentence durations at relatively low alcohol levels.

A third parameter of the speech signal that has been examined acoustically is fundamental frequency (FØ), an acoustic correlate of perceived pitch. Pisoni et al. (1985) reported only small changes in mean pitch for their subjects but a considerable increase in the variability of pitch (as measured by the standard deviation of the mean fundamental frequency) from the nonalcohol condition to the alcohol condition. Similarly, Klingholz et al. (1988) calculated the FØ distributions of 11 subjects both before and after consumption of alcohol and found that variation in fundamental frequency increased. Behne and Rivera (1990) reported that both FØ and FØ variability increased in the vocalic portions of spondees. Künzel et al. (1992) also measured FØ both before and after alcohol consumption; mean fundamental frequency increased for the majority of subjects. Furthermore, similar to findings in Pisoni et al. (1985) and Klingholz et al. (1988), standard deviations of fundamental frequency increased under alcohol in the Künzel et al. study. Whereas Künzel et al. and Behne and Rivera found a general trend for increase in FØ under alcohol, Watanabe et al. (1994) found that mean FØ decreased for both male and female talkers. Alderman et al. (1995) found a decrease in FØ for one subject group but no consistent changes for a second group. Besides standard deviations of fundamental frequency, another measure of pitch variability is "jitter," peak-to-peak perturbations of frequency and an acoustic correlate of hoarseness. In some cases using differing algorithms, the studies by K. Johnson et al. (1990, 1993), Künzel et al. (1992), Niedzielska et al. (1994), and Watanabe et al. (1994) included jitter measurements.

A further acoustic parameter that has been investigated is the frequencies of the vowel formants, or resonances of the vocal tract (see Fry, 1979; Lieberman, 1977). The most characteristic effect of the relative position of formants is the differentiation of vowel sounds, because different settings of the vocal tract give rise to formants at different places. Fontan et al. (1978) noted a compacting of vowel formants in their spectrographic study, resulting in inappropriate-sounding vowels. Klingholz et al. (1988) compared F1/F2 ratios before and after alcohol consumption, as well as profiles of the time derivatives of FØ, F1, and F2. Behne and Rivera (1990) measured the frequencies of F1, F2, and F3 both before and after alcohol.

Voicing (see section 3.1.4.2) is another phonetic parameter that can be assessed acoustically and instrumentally. For instance, Lester and Skousen (1974) measured oscillographically segments that indicated a process of final-obstruent devoicing. Likewise, Pisoni et al. (1985) found that some phonologically voiced segments were produced under alcohol as voiceless ones postvocalically. On the other hand, in their spectrographic analysis of the speech of alcoholics, Fontan et al. (1978) found evidence that some phonologically voiceless stops were being produced as voiced segments, but they also found that some voiceless plosives were being aspirated. Pisoni et al. (1985) calculated the number of voiced and voiceless frames in their acoustic analysis of sentences produced both with and without alcohol, essentially a measure of the relative durations of voiced and voiceless segments.

Manner of articulation (see section 3.1.4.3.2) also has acoustic correlates that have been examined in the studies discussed here. Among the obstruents, the three main manners of articulation are stops, fricatives, and affricates. Acoustically, stops are indicated by a period of silence, fricatives by frication or turbulence, and affricates by a silent period followed by frication. Fontan et al. (1978) found spectrographic evidence for the frication of stops in the speech of alcoholic subjects. Pisoni et al. (1985) found acoustic evidence for deaffrication, that is, incomplete closure or lack of closure during the stop portion of an affricate, which appeared acoustically as a "leak" of noise preceding the fricative release.

Amplitude, the magnitude of sound wave displacement and an acoustic correlate of perceived loudness, has been examined in just a handful of studies. Sobell et al. (1982) reported that readings under the no-alcohol condition showed significantly greater amplitude than readings under either of two alcohol conditions. On the other hand, Behne and Rivera (1990) reported that mean amplitudes were higher in the alcohol condition in the production of spondees. Furthermore, amplitude variability was also greater in the alcohol condition, although there was some individual variation. Watanabe et al. (1994) also reported mean intensity results for two of their subjects. Control of amplitude, intensity, and perceived loudness are fairly complex capabilities, involving at least control over subglottal air pressure and vocal-fold tension (Colton & Casper, 1990). Control over these parameters thus appears to be both respiratory and phonatory.

Other phonetic and acoustic parameters that have been investigated in the literature include: signal-to-noise ratio (SNR) and noise interference (e.g., Klingholz et al., 1988; Niedzielska et al., 1994); long-term average spectra (LTAS; e.g., Klingholz et al., 1988); harmonic structure (e.g., Niedzielska et al., 1994); and vowel periodicity (e.g., Niedzielska et al., 1994). The acoustic-phonetic measures discussed in this section are essentially analyses of the radiated acoustic signal, that is, the signal proceeding from a talker's lips. A recently developed type of analysis uses inverse filtering to eliminate vocal tract (transfer function) characteristics to derive only glottal (source) characteristics. Analyses of glottal excitation include intensity, pitch, and glottal waveshape, as reported in Cummings et al. (1996).

4.6.7 Measures of Respiratory and Phonatory Ability

Included here are quantitative measures of respiratory and phonatory abilities, generally originating in the clinical realm (e.g., Hirano, 1981). These include vital capacity (e.g., Eysholdt, 1992); mean flow rate (e.g., Watanabe et al., 1994); overall voice quality (e.g., Eysholdt, 1992); frequency range of phonation (e.g., Eysholdt, 1992; Watanabe et al., 1994); speaking fundamental frequency (Eysholdt, 1992); vocal attack (Eysholdt, 1992); and mean flow rate (Watanabe et al., 1994). Glottal waveform analyses (e.g., Cummings et al., 1996) may also be considered measures of phonatory ability. Visual observation of laryngeal activity is discussed in section 4.7.2.

4.7 QUALITATIVE LINGUISTIC AND SPEECH MEASURES

We include here discussions of measures that depend on the subjective judgment of observers. In section 4.7.1 we discuss a number of experiments that have been conducted to determine whether there are differences in the perception of speech when produced under alcohol and when not. In section 4.7.2 we discuss the few phoniatric studies that have involved visual observation of the speech organs.

4.7.1 Listener Judgments

A number of studies discussed here have included a perceptual component involving presentation of recordings of speech samples to listeners, who must make some kind of determination about the talker producing the speech. In most cases, the determination to be made is whether the talker producing the speech was intoxicated or not, but in one case (Andrews et al., 1974) the task was somewhat different. In that study, three talkers were recorded reading a passage in both alcohol and nonalcohol conditions. Two tapes were made for presentation to listeners, advanced speech and language pathology students, consisting of the passage as recorded by three speakers. One tape contained the passage read under alcohol and one without alcohol. A list of 114 scale characteristics was administered three times to each listener subject. On the first administration, listeners were asked to estimate the importance of each characteristic to a communicative message. On the second administration, listeners were asked to estimate the amount of the characteristic in the stimulus passage that was heard, and on the third administration to do the same for the alternate version of the stimulus. Listeners were unaware that some of the recorded utterances had been produced by talkers who had consumed alcohol. Seven of the scales were found to differentiate significantly between the two alcohol and nonalcohol conditions.

Other experiments required listeners to determine whether an utterance had been produced under alcohol or not. These studies were of two types: paired-comparison tasks and absolute-identification tasks. In paired-comparison tasks, used in Pisoni et al. (1985), Klingholz et al. (1988), and Pisoni and Martin (1989), tokens from the same talker produced both with and without alcohol were presented together; the listeners' task was to determine which of the two tokens had been produced under alcohol use. In absolute-identification tasks, used in Klingholz et al. (1988), Pisoni and Martin (1989), and Künzel et al. (1992), listeners heard only single sentences in isolation on each trial and had to determine whether each of the sentences had been produced with or without alcohol. Furthermore, for both tasks in Klingholz et al. (1988), once listeners had decided that a sentence was produced under alcohol use, an additional task was to select one or more of the following six reasons for their decision: (a) speech fluency, (b) speech quality, (c) speech errors, (d) voice quality, (e) voice instability, (f) voice effort. In the identification tasks for Pisoni and Martin (1989) and Künzel et al. (1992), listeners were also asked to rate their own confidence in their response for each trial by assigning a number from a scale to their response. In the paired comparison tasks, Klingholz et al. used trained listeners (speech therapists), while Pisoni and Martin used untrained listeners (college undergraduates). For the absolute-identification task, Klingholz et al. used the same trained listeners, Künzel et al. used untrained listeners (clerical workers), and Pisoni and Martin compared untrained listeners (college undergraduates) and trained listeners (police officers).

4.7.2 Visual Examination of Speech Organs

Three of the studies discussed here included visual inspection of the larynx. Dunker and Schlosshauer (1964) used high-speed photography and stroboscopy to examine laryngeal patterns in subjects with both hoarse and normal voices. Apparatus included a series of mirrors to direct light to the larynx, as well as images of the vocal folds back to the camera. Eysholdt (1992) and Künzel et al. (1992) reported endoscopic examination using a magnifying laryngoscope incorporating an integrated airway and an attached lighting cable. The light source could be adjusted to produce either sustained or a strobed light. Subjects in this study were not locally anesthetized, and Künzel et al. reported that videotaping had to be suspended after the first interval because of subjects' heightened pharyngeal sensitivity. Watanabe et al. (1994) included fiberscopic views of both male and female larynges both before and after alcohol consumption. Contrary to the findings from Eysholdt (1992) and Künzel et al. (1992), Watanabe et al. did find evidence of alterations in the hypopharyngeal and laryngeal mucosa, including capillary dilation, edema, and vocal-fold injection.

4.8 SUMMARY

The methodologies used in the study of alcohol and speech are thus widely varied and reflect both the disciplinary backgrounds and goals of the researchers and the development of new technologies. Studies of the effects of acute intoxication on nonalcoholic subjects have generally drawn their subjects from the population of young adult, educated males, whereas studies of alcoholic subjects have drawn on a wider range of ages, as well as both sexes. Early studies examined speech as a response mode but did not directly measure aspects of speech itself; measurements such as response latencies and task completion times reflect the study of speech within a wider context of the medical, chemical, and behavioral effects of alcohol. Intense study of the effects of alcohol on speech itself developed in parallel with developments in speech science, especially in the employment of new instrumentation. The sound spectrograph, high-quality audio recording and playback capabilities, and computerized digital analysis have all contributed greatly to our understanding of the speech signal itself and to our understanding of how alcohol affects that signal. Finally, the development of breath-alcohol analysis devices provided an accurate, fast, noninvasive method of determining the amount of alcohol in the body and has greatly facilitated research into the relationship between alcohol and speech.

CHAPTER 5

Research Review I: 1915–1964

5.0 OVERVIEW

This earliest period of research on the relationship between alcohol and speech can be characterized by a combination of clinical studies and the application of research methodology adapted from the developing field of experimental psychology. Three of the studies, Jetter (1938a), Romano et al. (1940), and Kawi (1961), drew their subjects from a clinical population. They represent a range of clinical subjects relevant to the study of alcohol and speech. Over a 3-year period, Jetter (1938a, discussed in section 5.3) drew more than a thousand patients with preadmission diagnoses of acute alcohol intoxication, investigating the relation between chemical measures of intoxication and clinical criteria for intoxication, including speech abnormalities. Romano et al. (1940, discussed in section 5.5), on the other hand, reported on just five patients, all of whom suffered from alcoholic cerebellar degeneration. In two of the five cases under investigation, Romano et al. found speech abnormalities of the dysarthric, "thick and slurred" type. Finally, Kawi (1961, discussed in section 5.8) used intravenous introduction of alcohol to bring 24 patients to the "slurred speech threshold." Once this relatively constant level was reached, Kawi investigated a number of other physiological and psychological phenomena. In a sentence-completion task, subjects showed reduced reaction time under alcohol.

Five of the remaining studies investigated alcohol effects on psychological measures, including speech. Dodge and Benedict (1915, discussed in section

5.1) investigated the effects of alcohol on a wide range of neuromuscular processes; in the particular instance of speech measures, they investigated speech response times to visually presented words. These latencies increased a small but measurable amount (approximately 3%) when alcohol had been consumed.

Whereas Dodge and Benedict investigated neuromuscular reactions, Hollingworth (1923, discussed in section 5.2) proposed that the real psychological effects of alcohol were to be found in those processes he called more "mental." Accordingly, in investigating the effects of alcohol on speech, Hollingworth required subjects to name colored squares presented randomly and to give antonyms of words presented visually. In both instances, Hollingworth found that both small and large doses of alcohol diminished performance (effected longer response times) on these tasks.

Whereas Jetter (1938a) was a clinical study of patients with a diagnosis of acute alcohol intoxication, Jetter (1938b, discussed in section 5.4) was an experimental study investigating the effects of alcohol on nonalcoholics. As in the earlier study, a set of clinical criteria for intoxication was investigated that included abnormalities of speech. In order to examine the effects of alcohol on "fluency," Hartocollis and Johnson (1956, discussed in section 5.6) used four tests differing in the restrictions that were placed on the types of words to be produced. They found that alcohol reduced fluency (the number of words produced in a given period of time) except in cases in which alcohol also appeared to affect subjects' perception of the acceptability of responses (standards of conformity). In their study of verbal and arithmetic performance under alcohol, Forney and Hughes (1961, discussed in section 5.7) also examined the effects of delayed auditory feedback. Although auditory feedback was a factor in decreasing verbalization performance, its effects were not enhanced by alcohol; Forney and Hughes concluded that verbalization remained unaffected by alcohol.

Most of the behavioral measurements employed in these earlier studies will be familiar to modern researchers, especially to experimental psychologists. Measures such as response latencies, task-completion times, number of (correct) words produced, and number of errors are all part of the experimental repertoire of modern scientists. Other measures such as content analysis (Kawi 1961) will be familiar to linguists and researchers in discourse analysis. Still others, such as the determination of speech abnormality (Jetter 1938a, 1938b) and thick and slurred speech (Romano et al., 1940) may be familiar to speech/language pathology, law enforcement, and some medical practitioners. A useful distinction to keep in mind when considering the literature on alcohol and speech is one between the form and the content of speech. *Form* refers specifically to structural characteristics, whereas *content* includes semantic and pragmatic characteristics. In general, characteristics of form are more readily quantifiable and less liable to subjective judgments than those of content.

For the speech scientist, however, none of these measures are measures of speech per se. In measuring a response latency, for instance, measurement ends at the beginning of the response word; what comes after, that is, the majority of the acoustic signal corresponding to the response word, is of no consequence. For the measurements taken by Dodge and Benedict (1915), this is quite literally true. In almost all cases of word response measures, subjects were required to provide a correct answer; so, for instance, Hollingworth (1923) measured the time to complete the entire color-naming task, but subjects were required to name a color correctly before moving on to the next. In Hartocollis and Johnson (1956), the measurement itself was the number of correct responses. In such cases, there is measurement of the response itself (rather than the time it takes to begin the response); nevertheless, this measurement (correct/incorrect) is only a gross one. More exacting in its analysis of the speech signal itself was the scoring procedure used by Forney and Hughes (1961). Here, errors in speech could be characterized as omissions, mispronunciations, spasms (stammers), or prolongations. Thus, the measurement and quantification of speech reactions can take many different forms.

A number of the studies in this chapter, however, employed qualitative rather than quantitative measures. Such measures include the speech abnormality characterizations used in Jetter (1938a, 1938b) for diagnosing clinical intoxication, the slurred and thick characterization of speech in Romano et al. (1940), and the content analysis of sentence completions in Kawi (1961). Although technically measures of speech itself, these are nevertheless subjective, rather than objective, measurements. In none of these studies were explicit, objective criteria provided for these assessments of speech.

Finally, Dunker and Schlosshauer's (1964, discussed in section 5.9) employed high-speed photography and stroboscopy to study morphological and functional differences in normal and hoarse voices. The measurements employed here are unlike any of the others discussed in this chapter. The experimenters were able to observe directly the vocal apparatus during use and to ascertain whether or not any changes had occurred due to yelling and "liberal" consumption of alcohol. One finding was that subjective impressions of hoarseness and morphological changes in the vocal organs did not necessarily co-occur.

The work summarized in this chapter, then, might well be characterized as the medical/psychological period of research on alcohol and speech. In methodology and in measurement, one finds similarities in present-day research, but not always in alcohol-speech research, which has progressed substantially from these earlier studies.

5.1 DODGE AND BENEDICT, 1915

This work reports on a large-scale study of the effects of alcohol conducted by researchers affiliated with the Carnegie Institution of Washington at the institution's psychological laboratory of the Nutrition Laboratory located in Boston, Massachusetts, during the academic year 1913–1914. The study investigated a wide range of effects of alcohol on neurological systems. Of particular interest in the present context is the experiment on speech reaction time (RT) for reading isolated words described in the third chapter. Unless otherwise indicated, all information below applies only to the speech RT experiment.

5.1.1 Subjects

For the complete study, the investigators originally sought to include subjects from five categories: "total abstainers, occasional users, moderate users, habitual drinkers exceeding 30 c.c. of absolute alcohol a day, and excessive drinkers" (p. 24). Because of the reluctance of total abstainers to consume alcohol, even for experimental purposes, no particular efforts were made to obtain subjects with this characteristic. Dodge and Benedict also noted the logical problem that after an initial dose of alcohol, no subject could truly be characterized as a total abstainer. Subjects from the last category, excessive drinkers, were also difficult to include in the investigation; the only subject included in preliminary investigations (subject XIII), refused to participate in those portions of the study requiring him to abstain from alcohol, and his results consequently could not be used.

In all, fourteen males began the experiment; the number eventually reported was only ten. Two (subjects I and V) left the experiment too early to figure statistically into the group results, and a third, subject XIII mentioned above, produced results that were eliminated from the pool because of a lack of baseline measurements. Finally, the results from Subject VIII, judged to be a total abstainer, were absent from the final data analysis. Three of the remaining ten subjects were outpatients from the Psychopathic Hospital of Boston undergoing treatment for alcoholism; at the time of the experiment, all three were considered to be abstainers. The seven nonpsychiatric subjects ranged in age from 22 years to 43 years at the time of testing; the age range for the psychiatric patients was from 39 years to 51 years.

All of the seven nonpsychiatric subjects were further required to be of legal age and to have graduated from college. Three of these seven were medical students, three were instructors or interns, and one was one of the authors of the report. Specific information regarding ages, heights, and weights of the ten subjects are given in Table 5.1.1.

TABLE 5.1.1   Subject Characteristics[a]

Subject	Age (years)	Height (cm)	Weight (kg)
II (Normal)	29	182.2	74.8
III (Normal)	25	176.5	67.5
IV (Normal)	27	181.6	73.0
VI (Normal)	25	164.0	68.0
VII (Normal)	26	177.8	67.5
IX (Normal)	22	174.0	63.5
X (Normal)	43	182.9	85.0
XI (Psychopathic)	51	161.3	55.8
XII (Psychopathic)	40	169.1	68.1
XIV (Psychopathic)	39	166.6	67.6

[a] From Dodge and Benedict (1915). Copyright © 1915 by the Carnegie Institution of Washington. Used by permission.

5.1.2 Methods

5.1.2.1 Dosage and Intervals

Dodge and Benedict administered a standard dosage of alcohol to all subjects (no adjustments were made in the dosage to reflect individual subject characteristics). Although they admitted that attempting to achieve a standard blood-alcohol concentration (BAC) would have been most satisfactory, especially as it "would appear necessary in all attempts to measure individual differences," nevertheless Dodge and Benedict "chose to follow the easier traditional usage in these experiments, and administer the alcohol in fixed doses for all subjects" (p. 29).

The standard dose was an average of what was considered a moderate dose, which, it was conceded, lacked both experimental and conventional standardization. Citing Meyer and Gottlieb (1914), who estimated the "stimulating" dose for abstaining adults at between 30 and 40 g, Dodge and Benedict fixed the standard dose (Dose A) at 30 cc (more exactly, 29.8 cc). A second, higher dose (Dose B) contained 45 cc (44.7 cc) of alcohol. The alcohol was carried in a solution made from roasted grain to render it more palatable, but there was no further attempt to mask the flavor of the alcohol, nor was there an attempt to reproduce the flavor of the alcoholic beverage in the control beverage.

Tests were administered under three conditions: normal (without alcohol), Dose A, and Dose B. For each subject, full days were devoted to measurements under each condition. For each subject, there were generally two normal days and one day each for Dose A and Dose B.

5.1.2.2 Stimuli

The stimuli consisted of 24 words, each four letters long (the specific length was arbitrarily chosen). Stimuli were printed on cards, which were inserted into the exposure apparatus by hand in random order by the experimenter. This set of 24 words was used in all experiments. All subjects were shown each of the words from the set separately before experiments on the first day; additionally, the psychiatric patients were shown each word separately before experiments began on each day.

5.1.2.3 Instrumentation
Instrumentation for speech RT in reading isolated words included an exposure apparatus, a voice-reaction key, and a kymograph to record response latencies. Both the exposure apparatus and reaction key were developed by the Nutrition Laboratory; the kymograph was a standard Blix-Sandström model.

Unlike with a tachistocope, the purpose of the exposure apparatus was not to expose stimuli (in this case printed words) for extremely short periods of time, but rather to allow exposure of the stimuli without eye movements, and thus to duplicate normal eye fixation in reading. Rapid movement of the visual field, however, was deemed necessary, as well as placing fixation marks and stimuli on the same surface. Important here was that the stimuli move rapidly toward the fixation point and then stop suddenly, becoming legible only at the point of stopping. Using a pendulum stop, the researchers were able to overcome problems of noise and vibration.

The voice-reaction key consisted of a short brass tube 4 cm in diameter. The tube was fitted at one end with a hard-rubber ring across which a rubber membrane was stretched. The membrane pressed against a light spring against a contact point within the tube. At equilibrium, the spring and contact point touched lightly. Increases in air pressure within the tube, such as that caused by speaking into the open end, broke contact between the spring and the contact point and thus broke an electrical circuit. There was an instrumental latency (for both the exposure apparatus and the voice-reaction key) of approximately 37 ms.

5.1.2.4 Procedure
Subjects were seated upright; the voice-reaction key was held in the left hand, while the left arm rested either upon a table or on a support in the subject's lap. Subjects were instructed (a) to hold the voice key firmly against the upper lip; (b) to say the word appearing on the exposure apparatus as soon as possible after its appearance; (c) in the case of misreadings or mispronunciations, to resay the word as soon as possible. The interstimulus interval was 10 sec, and stimuli were changed by the operator by hand.

With the kymograph turning in a circular motion, the experimenter inserted one of the stimulus cards into the exposure apparatus. Shortly (2.0 to 2.5 sec) before stimulus exposure, the experimenter changed the motion of the kymograph from a circular to a spiral motion. As the kymograph revolved, an offset on its shaft engaged a circuit breaker, to which the voice key, the kymograph marker, and the electromagnets on the exposure apparatus were attached. This first break in the circuit exposed the stimulus card to the subject; the circuit was then closed again, but the card remained exposed. A second break in the circuit was caused by input into the voice key. The kymograph thus recorded two breaks in the circuit: the first (approximately) at the time of stimulus exposure, the second when the subject reacted by speaking into the voice key. Measurement between these two circuit breaks on the kymograph record thus indicated the response latency.

5.1.3 Results

For normal subjects, the average recorded RT in the normal condition (without alcohol) was 455 ms (range 402–486 ms); for the psychiatric patients, average recorded reaction time was higher at 590 ms (range 567–700 ms).

After alcohol Dose A, the average recorded RT for normal subjects was 444 ms (range 410–498 ms). For psychiatric patients, average RT was 597 ms (range 508–689 ms). Alcohol Dose B was not administered to the psychiatric patients, but for the group of nonpsychiatric subjects, average recorded RT after Dose B was 487 ms (range 411–542 ms). The effect of Dose A on RT was negligible to the point of being nonexistent (a decrease of 11 ms); for Dose B, however, there was a small but consistent increase in latency (a mean increase of 32 ms). For both doses considered together, then, the average increase in latency after ingestion of alcohol was approximately 3%.

5.1.4 Discussion

This study was representative of a number of earlier studies discussed in this chapter (e.g., Hollingworth, 1923; Jetter, 1938a, 1938b), in which speech was examined among a larger group of psychological and neurological markers of intoxication. As mentioned previously, the specific measurement made in this study was not a measure of the speech signal per se, but rather of the processing time it took to initiate speech after presentation of a visual stimulus.

One question raised by Dodge and Benedict themselves was what type of speech reaction (movement of air) would be necessary to break the circuit in the voice key and so record the response latency. As they correctly pointed out, different words would have sufficient air movement in different places, so that the reaction key would not always record the exact commencement of the word. However, Dodge and Benedict defended the type of instrument used on the grounds that as long as the stimulus words were always the same across conditions, total measurements from one condition to another should be valid.

A second concern had to do with the way dosages were calculated. Although at the time of this experiment, it was known that an important variable in determining intoxication was the alcohol content of blood (Dodge & Benedict, 1915, p. 29), Dodge and Benedict nevertheless chose the somewhat more expedient method of selecting three standard doses, more or less based on estimates of a stimulating dose. What is interesting is that standard doses were absolute amounts of alcohol in a beverage; that is, there was no attempt to estimate standard doses based on subjects' body weights. In this regard, it may be important that the range in weight among the normal subjects was from a low of 63.5 kg to a high of 85 kg, and in the psychiatric subjects the range was from 55.8 kg to 68.1 kg. For the normal subjects, then, this meant that the heaviest subject weighed over a third more than the lightest.

Dodge and Benedict thus examined speech response latencies without alcohol and with two doses of alcohol. The smaller dose of alcohol (30 cc) had no appreciable effect on speech reactions, whereas the larger dose (45 cc) brought about a small but consistent increase in latencies over the no-alcohol condition.

5.2 HOLLINGWORTH, 1923

This study was similar to Dodge and Benedict (1915) in that it investigated the effect of alcohol on a number of processes, subjects having been required to undergo a battery of tests during the course of the investigation. A major difference, however, is that whereas Dodge and Benedict (1915) investigated fairly superficial effects (i.e., neuromuscular processes), including a number of reactions characterized as reflexes, Hollingworth also investigated the effects of alcohol on complex reactions, those he termed *mental*. Of the nine measures made in this study, the following required verbal responses: Control of the speech mechanism, Mental calculation, and Logical relations. We confine our discussion below to the first and last of these. At the time this article appeared, H. L. Hollingworth was affiliated with Barnard College (Columbia University) in New York, New York.

5.2.1 Subjects

The subjects examined in this study were six males, ranging in age from 21;1 (years; months) to 29;5. They ranged in weight from 106–180 pounds and in height from 64–74.5 inches. Specific information for each of the six

TABLE 5.2.1   Subject Characteristics[a]

Subject	Sex	Age (years;months)	Weight (lbs)	Height (feet-inches)
1	Male	29;5	139	5–10
2	Male	25;6	106	5–4.5
3	Male	25;1	147	5–7.5
4	Male	22;11	182.5	6–2
5	Male	22;7	147	6–0.5
6	Male	21;5	149	5–9.5

[a] From Hollingworth (1923)

subjects, including age, height, and weight are included in Table 5.2.1. One abstainer was included in the group (subject 3); the remaining subjects ranged in alcohol consumption from occasional to regular (although not excessive) users. Subjects were compensated if they completed the series of experiments.

5.2.2 Methods

5.2.2.1 Procedure

The course of the experiment was run over 12 days during the period from Friday, 6 June 1919, through Thursday, 19 June 1919, inclusive. During this period, experimentation was carried out on all days except Sundays. Each of the experimental days was committed to one of the following conditions: Practice, Blank (no beverages were ingested except water), Control (a nonalcoholic beer-like beverage was ingested), and Beer (an alcoholic beer was ingested), Dinner (subjects ate a large meal but consumed no alcohol).

The general procedure for each day included a battery of seven tests plus recording of the pulse rate. A ninth test, the Memory for Paired Associates, was conducted only on the last 3 days. Each experimental day began at 9:00 A.M., and all tests (plus recording of pulse rate) were run at 30-min intervals between 9:00 A.M. and 11:30 A.M. (six trials per morning). From 12:00 to 1:00 P.M., the subjects ate lunch, including a beverage that depended on the condition for that day (either water, the control beer, or the standard beer). After lunch, commencing at 1:00 P.M., subjects were again run through the same tests as in the morning, at 30-min intervals until 3:30 P.M. (again, six trials in the afternoon). Tests were conducted in separate rooms, so that during the course of a 30-min period, subjects moved from room to room. The entire battery of eight tests required the full 30-min period.

5.2.2.3 Dosages

Dosages were measured as multiples of a bottle containing 370 cc (12.5 fluid oz) of either a standard beer (approximately 2.77% alcohol by weight or 3.55% by volume) or a control beer (no alcohol). In all, there were 5 days on which alcoholic beer was consumed. Dosages were different for each of these days, and additionally, the fifth day included standard dosages before noon, but relatively uncontrolled drinking during the noon hour. For each of the first 4 beer days, consumption of the alcoholic beverage was confined to the noon hour. On the first beer day, each subject drank six 12.5-oz bottles, on the second four bottles, on the third five bottles (except for subject 2, who became ill after three bottles), and on the fourth day three bottles.

On the fifth (final) beer day, subjects completed three rounds of testing and then, at 10:45, consumed one bottle of standard beer. At 11:15 a second bottle was consumed after a fourth round of testing. A fifth round of testing ended at 11:50, when subjects drank a third bottle of beer and then completed a sixth testing round. The lunch period began at 12:30; during this hour, subjects ate lightly and consumed as much beer as possible during the 1-hr period. Thus, subjects differed in the amount of beer they consumed during the entire course of the day; individual consumption was as follows: subject 1, eight bottles total; subject 2, six bottles total; subject 3, seven bottles total; subject 4, seven bottles total; subject 5, nine bottles total; and subject 6, nine bottles total.

5.2.2.4 Materials

5.2.2.4.1 Control of Speech Mechanism   For this test, the experimenters used the Woodworth-Wells Color Naming Test (Woodworth & Wells, 1911), consisting of a large card with 100 printed colored squares, 20 each of red, blue, green, yellow, and black. The squares occurred in random order, and the card could be turned to create multiple randomizations. The task was to name the colors as rapidly as possible in the order in which they occurred on the card. Subjects were required to name each square's color correctly before proceeding to the next square; in the event of an incorrect utterance, the experimenter said "No," and the subject was required to give the correct color before proceeding. The total amount of time to complete the entire series of 100 color squares was measured by stop watch to the nearest fifth-second (200 ms).

5.2.2.4.2 Logical Relations   In this task, fifty adjectives were typewritten in a list on a test card. Subjects were required to look at each word and then say aloud a word having the *opposite* meaning of the word printed on the card. If the experimenter determined the response to be inappropriate or incorrrect, he said "No," and the subject was required to respond correctly before proceeding to the next word. Again, the measurement here was the time required to complete the list of 50 items.

5.2.3 Results

Hollingworth did not provide measurements for individual subjects, nor did he provide numbers for group averages. Averaged results were given in graphs, and results from individual subjects were given in prose form only. Response latencies in the color-naming task were in general higher for afternoon sessions than for morning ones, under all conditions. The effect on control and blank days, however, was appreciably less than on days when either a large dose of alcohol or a small one was administered. According to Hollingworth (1923, p. 229), "average results in this case are overdetermined by the contributions of Subject II, and in part by Subject V." Although control doses had no effect on performance, he noted that, "Small Alcohol doses slow up performance temporarily, and Large doses produce a more prolonged inferior performance, from which recovery is made by the end of the day" (p. 229).

The same general pattern of morning performance versus afternoon performance held for the entire group in the logical relations (opposites) task: performance was better in the morning than in the afternoon. Hollingworth noted that morning averages were irregular but not distinguishable from each other. Afternoon levels, however, tended to be more distinct from each other. Afternoon performance was inferior on control days as compared to blank days, and performance on small alcohol dose days was even further diminished. The most diminished afternoon performance was found on large alcohol dose days, with recovery not evident until the final trial.

5.2.4 Discussion

As in the experiment by Dodge and Benedict (1915), this study measured temporal durations for naming visual stimuli. One difference, however, was that scores were expressed in the present study as either the total time required to see and say 100 color-card stimuli or the total time required to read and give antonyms to a list of fifty adjectives; in Dodge and Benedict, the response latency for each stimulus reaction pair was measured separately. But in both studies, it is possible to compare the two conditions (sober and intoxicated) only for the whole set of stimuli; that is, subsets of the stimuli cannot be compared. In the study by Dodge and Benedict, because words differed in the exact location of an articulation sufficient to effect a circuit break, not all response latencies would be comparable. In the study by Hollingworth, it is possible that some colors would be more difficult to name (would require longer response latencies) than others; by the same token, some adjectives or their antonyms might have required a longer time to access lexically.

As Hollingworth pointed out, the processes assessed by these two paradigms differed. In Dodge and Benedict's study, it was a set of neuromuscular processes that were being investigated, among them the patellar reflex and reciprocal innervation of the finger. Hollingworth, however, maintained that more "mental" processes were investigated in his study. Both the color-naming and the logical relationships tasks did indeed tap deeper language processes than did the reading task in Dodge and Benedict. Both the color-naming task and the antonym task required semantic processing and lexical access, tasks that we would properly call "cognitive" today. As in the case of Dodge and Benedict, although responses were in the speech mode, the actual measurement was of the response latencies; here, as in the earlier work, it was not specifically the speech signal itself that was measured.

5.3 JETTER, 1938a

In this study, Jetter reported a large-scale clinical study of the relation between clinical diagnoses of acute alcoholic intoxication and chemical measurements (blood- and urine-alcohol) taken at the same time. At the time this article appeared, Walter W. Jetter was a resident pathologist at the Buffalo City Hospital (Buffalo, New York) and an instructor in biological chemistry at the University of Buffalo Medical School in Buffalo, New York.

5.3.1 Subjects and Methods

5.3.1.1 Subjects
Subjects for this study were 1159 consecutive patients admitted to the Buffalo City Hospital over a 3-year period with preadmission diagnoses of acute alcoholism. Of these, 1150 blood samples were obtained, and of these, 1000 subjects were shown chemically to be alcohol-positive, and 150 subjects alcohol-free. Of the 1000 subjects, 740 were diagnosed as clinically intoxicated, according to the criteria discussed below.

5.3.1.2 Methods
5.3.1.2.1 Chemical Indicators   Determination of blood- and urine-alcohol concentration was based on the ability of alcohol to decolorize potassium dichromate in acid solution (Heise, 1934). Blood samples were drawn upon admission, and, when possible, urine samples. BAC was expressed as a percentage of alcohol by weight per 100 cc of blood, urine-alcohol concentration as a percentage of alcohol by weight per 100 cc urine.

5.3.1.2.2 Diagnosis of Clinical Intoxication   A clinical diagnosis of acute alcohol intoxication in this study required absolutely that the patient exhibit gross gait abnormality or be unable to walk. Additionally, the patient had to exhibit at least two of the following criteria: (a) gross abnormality of speech or inability to speak, (b) flushed face, (c) dilated pupils, (d) alcoholic breath odor.

In order to diagnose gait abnormality, the patient was asked to walk across a room, from one end to the other. According to Jetter (1938a, p. 477), "if gross swaying, reeling or staggering were not present, the test was considered negative." In the case of speech abnormality, "the patient was required to answer simple questions only such as his name, residence, and so on. If definite slurring or incoherence was not present the test was considered to be negative" (p. 477).

5.3.2 Results

5.3.2.1 Correlation of Alcohol Concentrations and Clinical Intoxication

For the 1000 chemically blood-alcohol-positive patients, the most prevalent clinical criterion was breath odor, presenting in 90.3% of all cases. Gait abnormality, speech abnormality, and dilated pupils were present in 70%–75% of cases. Least prevalent among the diagnostic criteria was flushed face, which was present in only 60.6% of the cases. As mentioned above, the presence of abnormal gait was absolutely necessary to maintain the clinical diagnosis. Of the 750 cases presenting with gait abnormalities, there were 10 cases that could not be correlated with at least two of the other clinical criteria. Consequently, the number of diagnosed cases was 740.

A smaller number of samples ($N = 381$) of urine than blood were obtained upon admission. Of these, 372 were cases in which alcohol was found in both urine and blood; in nine cases, only a urine sample was obtained, and in all of these cases, alcohol was found. In a number of respects, the numbers for urine-alcohol-positive cases replicated those for blood-alcohol-positive cases. In both cases, the most prevalent positive clinical criterion was an odor of alcohol on the breath; of the 381 urine-alcohol-positive cases, 339 (88.8%) presented with alcoholic odor of breath. The order of the remaining four clinical criteria was likewise the same for blood-alcohol- and urine-alcohol-positive cases: in descending order, these were gait abnormality (75.3%), speech abnormality (70.1%), dilated pupils (68.0%), and flushed face (57.7%).

The curve for increasing acute clinical intoxication indicated that clinical intoxication rose as BAC increased, except for a slight decrease in clinical intoxication diagnoses at 0.40% BAC; at 0.35% BAC, 96.0% of the cases (71 of 74) were diagnosed as clinically intoxicated, and at 0.04%, 93.3%

(14 of 15). At BACs of 0.45 and 0.50%, 100% of the cases (5 of 5 and 2 of 2) were diagnosed as clinically intoxicated. Similar results were obtained for those cases providing urine samples, clinical intoxication rising as a function of urine-alcohol concentration.

5.3.2.2 Alcohol Concentrations and Specific Clinical Criteria

In this section, we consider the relationship between alcohol concentrations in blood and urine on the one hand and the five clinical criteria for intoxication (gait abnormality, speech abnormality, dilated pupils, flushed face, and alcoholic odor of breath) on the other. There was a close fit among the curves for clinical intoxication, gait abnormality, and speech abnormality, when these were plotted as a function of BAC. Alcoholic odor of breath was generally higher than any of these three, and the curves for flushed face and dilated pupils, although close to each other, appeared to have little relation to any of the other clinical criteria or to the diagnosis of clinical intoxication. In the specific case of perceived speech abnormality, positive tests occurred less than 20% of the time at 0.05% and 0.10% BAC. Incidence rose to close to 40% at 0.15% BAC, and at 0.20% BAC approximately doubled to 80%. Positive cases of 100% occurred at 0.45% BAC, with some fluctuation occurring beforehand, that is, between 0.30% and 0.45% BAC.

When plotted as functions of urine-alcohol concentration, the curves for the five clinical criteria were similar to those for BAC. The curve for positive gait abnormality followed very closely the curve for diagnosed clinical intoxication. In general, speech abnormality rose with urine-alcohol content, and as before, alcoholic odor showed the highest positive test prevalence among the five criteria. Flushed face and dilated pupils increased with increased alcohol concentration, but not monotonically, nor was there a close fit to the clinical intoxication curve. Finally, there were decreases in the positive test curves for a number of the clinical criteria at various points for urine-alcohol levels of 0.40% and above.

5.3.3 Discussion

Jetter (1938a) is the first study discussed here in which BAC was actually measured. However, in contrast to later studies, the results of chemical analysis were not taken to be the diagnostic criterion for intoxication. Rather, Jetter sought to correlate the results of chemical tests with those of clinical intoxication; it was, in fact, the clinical diagnosis, based on the observation of behavioral symptoms by trained observers, which was the more widely accepted criterion of intoxication. Clinical signs such as abnormal gait, slurred speech, flushed face, dilated pupils, and alcoholic odor of breath as indicative of intoxication had been widely known for some time.

This study thus established a correlation between chemical indicators of intoxication (blood and urine sampling) and clinical/behavioral indicators of intoxication. Because gait abnormality was an absolute criterion for the diagnosis of clincal intoxication, there was a good fit between the blood/ urine-alcohol curves and the curves for gait abnormality. Of interest, here, though, was the correlation of speech abnormality with both chemical indicators and gait abnormality. If the incidence of gait abnormality indicates various BACs, then the incidence of speech disturbances may do so as well. This was the first study discussed here to demonstrate a relationship between BACs and speech.

5.4 JETTER, 1938b

This experimental study followed up the clinical study reported in Jetter (1938a). In the earlier study, alcohol concentrations were known, but in the present study both the actual amount of alcohol ingested and BAC were known. In both studies, clinical criteria were used to assess acute alcoholic intoxication. When this article appeared, Walter W. Jetter was a resident pathologist at the Buffalo City Hospital (Buffalo, New York) and an instructor at the University of Buffalo Medical School in Buffalo, New York.

5.4.1 Subjects and Methods

5.4.1.1 Subjects
Subjects were 20 "young normal adults." All subjects were characterized as "either occasional drinkers or, in a few instances, total abstainers" (p. 487). The sex of subjects was not reported.

5.4.1.2 Dosage and Intervals
Dosage was an "approximately 10%" concentration of alcohol. Subjects were divided into four dosage groups; each group contained five subjects. Dosages were calculated as a specified amount of alcohol/kg body weight: Group 1:1.00 cc; Group 2:1.25 cc; Group 3:1.50 cc; and Group 4: 2.00 cc. Ingestion of the alcohol began in the morning either on an empty (fasting) stomach or after a light breakfast. Ingestion was completed 45 min after commencement.

5.4.1.3 Measurements
Two measurements were made: (a) BAC and (b) examination for acute alcoholic intoxication according to the criteria established in Jetter (1938a). Clinical criteria were (a) gait abnormality, (b) speech abnormality, (c) alco-

holic odor of breath, (d) flushed face, and (e) dilated pupils (see section 5.3.1.2).

A blood sample was taken 1 hr after completion of the first drink; intervals thereafter were 2, 3, 4, 6, 8, 12, and 24 hr after completion of the first drink. In all, eight blood samples were taken to examine BAC, according to the procedure outlined in Jetter (1938a, p. 476).

5.4.2 Results

5.4.2.1 Blood-Alcohol Curve

For all groups, BACs rose from termination of consumption until the 2-hr postconsumption measurement interval; at that point, all subjects in all groups showed peak blood-alcohol levels. Peak blood-alcohol levels, all occurring at 2 hr postconsumption, for each group (highest BAC in each group) were as follows: Group 1, 0.10%; Group 2, 0.13%; Group 3, 0.15%; and Group 4, 0.19%. From the peak at 2 hr postconsumption, blood-alcohol levels began to decline, fairly abruptly from 2–6 hr postconsumption and somewhat more gradually thereafter. By 8 hr postconsumption, all subjects in Group 1 were alcohol-free; by 12 hr postconsumption, all subjects in Group 2 were alcohol-free, although two subjects in this group were alcohol-free at 8 hr postconsumption. As might be expected, subjects in Groups 3 and 4 took longer to metabolize and eliminate. Subjects in Group 3 appeared to be alcohol-free by 12 hr postconsumption, but some subjects in Group 4 were not alcohol-free at that point. In any event, by the measurement interval at 24 hr postconsumption, all subjects were alcohol-free.

5.4.2.2 Clinical Intoxication

In addition to blood-alcohol measurements, several measures of clinical intoxication were also collected from the twenty subjects. Clinical criteria applied here were the same used in Jetter (1938a): gait abnormality, speech abnormality, flushed face, dilated pupils, and alcoholic odor of breath. Each criterion was judged to be either present or absent in an individual subject, and a diagnosis of clinical intoxication depended absolutely on the presence of gait abnormality plus two of the four remaining criteria. Table 5.4.1 shows the number of subjects from each group who exhibited each clinical criterion, as well as the number of subjects from each group who were diagnosed as clinically intoxicated.

5.4.3 Discussion

One question that arises from the data presented in Table 5.4.1 is when observations for determining clinical intoxication were made. Jetter did not indicate when the observations were made or whether all the observations

TABLE 5.4.1   Clinical Criteria and Clinical Intoxication[a]

Criterion/Intoxicated	Group 1 (1 cc/kg) N = 5	Group 2 (1.25 cc/kg) N = 5	Group 3 (1.5 cc/kg) N = 5	Group 4 (2 cc/kg) N = 5
Alcoholic odor	5	5	5	5
Flushed face	5	4	4	1
Dilated pupils	3	3	2	3
Speech abnormalities	2	3	1	5
Gait abnormalities	2	4	2	5
Intoxicated	2	4	2	5

[a] From Jetter (1938b)

were made either at the same time or at the same observation interval. Jetter also compared the number of cases of clinical intoxication at various BACs from this experimental group with cases at similar concentrations from the hospital group studied in Jetter (1938a). At all levels, a greater percentage of the (nonalcoholic) experimental subjects were determined to be clinically intoxicated than of the hospital group. Jetter attributed the differences in incidence of clinical intoxication to the different drinking habits of the two groups. Whereas the experimental subjects from Jetter (1938b) were occasional drinkers or nondrinkers, the hospital group consisted primarily of "chronic alcoholics, the majority having known alcoholic histories of long standing" (Jetter, 1938b, p. 489). The lower incidence of clinical intoxication at comparable blood-alcohol levels among the hospital group would thus be attributable to acquired tolerance of the intoxication effects of the alcohol. This is probably true, although neither Jetter (1938a) nor Jetter (1938b) mentioned how this determination was made. Jetter (1938a), in fact, mentioned that in the determination of speech abnormalities, only simple questions, such as name and address, were posed. How drinking histories or habits were ascertained for the hospital group was not reported.

5.5 ROMANO, MICHAEL, AND MERRITT, 1940

This work presented case studies of five patients suffering from cerebellar degeneration due to excessive use of alcohol. Two cases presented with speech anomalies. The work described in this article emanated from the Neurological Unit of Boston (Massachusetts) City Hospital, the Medical Clinic at Peter Bent Brigham Hospital (Boston, Massachusetts), and the Departments of Neurology and Medicine of the Harvard Medical School (Cambridge, Massachusetts).

This was a case study of five patients presenting with similar symptoms. All were males who were addicted to prolonged and excessive use of alcohol. Family histories appeared to be insignificant, and among the five, the symptoms were fairly uniform. In all five, there was progressive cerebellar ataxia involving principally the lower extremities. Furthermore, two presented with nystagmus, two with speech disturbances, and four with slight or moderate cerebellar ataxia of the upper extremities.

The first patient who presented with speech disturbances was a white male, age 36. He was admitted to the hospital complaining of unsteadiness of the legs, which had existed for approximately 2.5 years; additionally, "there had been a slight change in the patient's speech in the last few months" (p. 1232). Among other symptoms, a physical examination revealed that "speech was slightly dysarthric" (p. 1232). The second patient was a 53-year-old white male. Upon admission to the hospital, he also complained of gait unsteadiness, which had existed for 4 years. For 2 months he had been unable to walk unaided; additionally, "one and one-half years before admission he noted that his speech was becoming slightly thick" (p. 1234). This latter indication was borne out upon physical examination, when his speech was characterized as "thick and slurred" (p. 1234).

In contrast to subjects in the studies discussed up to this point, it appears that the subjects in Romano et al. were not intoxicated at the time of their examination. Thus, the speech disturbances observed in two of the subjects were not an effect of acute alcohol intoxication but rather of prolonged and excessive use of alcohol, which had caused chronic pathological cerebellar changes. This cerebellar degeneration could only be inferred, however, since all patients were alive when examined and autopsy information was therefore lacking. Nevertheless, symptoms in these five cases corresponded very closely with symptoms described in the literature, with cerebellar degeneration confirmed by autopsy.

In addition to the direct cause of chronic alcohol ingestion, Romano et al. also considered the problem of nutrition deficiency as a contributing factor in these instances of cerebellar degeneration. Four of the subjects were reported to have had a history of inadequate diet, but none of the patients exhibited signs of edema, pellagra, or peripheral neuritis. Nevertheless, Romano et al. suggested that either separate or combinatorial effects of excessive alcohol and malnutrition might be responsible for cerebellar degeneration.

This study is included here because of the connections it attempted to establish between alcohol and cerebellar disease, as well as between cerebellar disease and certain ataxic signs, including changes in speech. As discussed in Chapter 2, alcohol appears to affect a variety of subcomponents of the central nervous system, including the cerebellum. The effects on speech may stem from various specific loci, but the cerebellum appears an especially good candidate, because of its coordinating function over much of the motor control system. The acute effects of alcohol on speech are widely known, but the study by Romano et al. pointed out some of the chronic effects of alcohol on the cerebellum and thus on the motor control of speech.

5.6 HARTOCOLLIS AND JOHNSON, 1956

Hartocollis and Johnson proceeded from the hypothesis that fluency tests differing in the degree of restriction would be differentially affected by alcohol. The work described here emanated from the Department of Psychology at Michigan State University, in East Lansing, Michigan.

5.6.1 Methods

5.6.1.1 Subjects
Subjects for this study were 30 experimental subjects and 30 controls. All were males, ages 21–36, and college-educated to "guarantee adequate intellectual background." All were characterized as either casual or moderate drinkers; those characterized as either nondrinkers or heavy drinkers were not included in the study.

5.6.1.2 Alcoholic Preparation
The administered dosage of the experimental drink was calculated, using body weight, to produce a BAC of 0.10%. The beverage consisted of 20% absolute ethyl alcohol, 20% water, 60% grapefruit juice, and two drops of peppermint oil. As an example of the way the dosage was calculated, a subject weighing 150 lb was given a drink consisting of 56.8 cc of alcohol in a mixture totaling 284 cc. The control drink consisted of 40% water, 60% grapefruit juice, and two drops of peppermint oil.

5.6.1.3 Materials
Materials consisted of four verbal fluency tests differing in the restrictions placed on the words to be produced:

Test 1:   This test examined fluency under minimal restrictions. Subjects were required simply to name words for 3 min. The score was expressed as the number of words produced in that period of time.

Test 2:   In this test, subjects named words beginning with a certain letter. The letters used were S, P, M, and T, which had been shown to elicit similar numbers of responses. The score was expressed as the number of words produced in 3 min.

Test 3:   In this test, subjects named common classes of objects (birds, trees, vegetables, pieces of furniture). The score was expressed as the number of objects named in 2 min.

Test 4: This test examined fluency under maximal (for this study) restrictions. Subjects were required to name words with a specified meaning and also beginning with one of five specified letters. An example is "A place or building for athletic exercises: C D G H T." The score on this test was expressed as the number of correct words produced in 5 min.

Responses on all tests were oral and were recorded by the experimenter.

5.6.1.4 Procedure

Subjects were requested to fast for 2 hr preceding the experiment. The study was conducted in a small room with the subject seated on a couch. The experiment consisted of four phases: (a) a predrink testing period lasting approximately 21 min, (b) a drinking period of approximately 5 min, (c) a waiting period of approximately 25 min, and (d) a postdrink testing period of approximately 21 min.

During both the pre- and postdrink testing periods, each of Tests 1–3 was administered twice and Test 4 once. Both testing periods were balanced to take into account the alcohol curve after consumption of the alcoholic beverage. The order of the tests for both pre- and postdrink periods was thus: Tests 1, 2, 3, 4, 3, 2, 1. For the experiment, then, Tests 1–3 were each administered four times and Test 4 twice. For Tests 2 and 3, each administration required a different initial letter or a different object. For Test 4, different versions were administered pre-and postalcohol.

5.6.2 Results and Discussion

Table 5.6.1 shows the scores for both groups, before and after consumption of the beverage. Scores for the pairs of Tests 1 through 3 have been combined. Table 5.6.1 indicates general improvement in performance from the prealcohol condition to the postalcohol condition. Hartocollis and Johnson attributed this to a practice effect for both the experimental group and the control group. To eliminate this practice effect so that any differences between the

TABLE 5.6.1   Mean Scores of Experimental and Control Groups on Four Tests before and after Drink[a]

Test	Experimental Group		Control Group	
	Predrink	Postdrink	Predrink	Postdrink
1	201.93	211.56	211.33	233.93
2	91.93	91.93	86.23	98.76
3	48.06	50.33	46.40	46.87
4	21.80	20.96	22.80	23.80

[a] From Hartocollis and Johnson (1956). Copyright © 1956 by *Journal of Studies on Alcohol*, Rutgers University. Used by permission.

TABLE 5.6.2   Comparison of Experimental and Control Groups in Respect to Mean
Improvement on Four Tests[a]

Test	Experimental	Control	Difference	t
1	9.63	22.60	−12.97	2.15[b]
2	0.00	12.53	−12.53	3.92[c]
3	2.27	0.47	1.80	0.87
4	−0.83	1.00	−1.83	2.29[b]

[a] From Hartocollis and Johnson (1956). Copyright © 1956 by *Journal of Studies on Alcohol*,
Rutgers University. Used by permission.
[b] Significant at .05 level.
[c] Significant at .01 level.

experimental and the control group could be noted, Hartocollis and Johnson
compared the gains achieved by each group pre- to postalcohol and calculated the differences between them, as shown in Table 5.6.2.

From Table 5.6.2, it is clear that the improvements in performance from
the prealcohol to the postalcohol condition were greater for the control
group than for the experimental group in three of the four tests. Improvement
for the control group was better on Tests 1, 2, and 4 to a significant degree
as evaluated by a conventional t-test. On Test 4, however, improvement for
the experimental group was better than for the control group, although the
difference was not statistically significant. It is also possible to compare the
number of individual subjects in each group who improved or declined.
Such a comparison, with magnitude of changes ignored, is shown in Table
5.6.3. This analysis bears out results similar to the comparison of mean
improvement displayed in Table 5.6.2. Improvement was greater for control
subjects on Tests 1, 2, and 4, and for experimental subjects on Test 3.

TABLE 5.6.3   Comparison of Experimental and Control Groups in Respect to Number of
Subjects Who Improved[a]

Test	Experimental group (N = 30) Improved	Declined	Control group (N = 30) Improved	Declined	Chi-square
1	17	13	25	5	4.75[b]
2	18	12	25	5	6.42[b]
3	19	11	14	16	0.21
4	17	13	20	10	1.42

[a] From Hartocollis and Johnson (1956). Copyright © by *Journal of Studies on Alcohol*, Rutgers
University. Used by permission.
[b] Significant at .05 level.

Hartocollis and Johnson considered the question of what factors might account for the differences among performance improvements on Tests 1, 2, and 4 on the one hand and Test 3 on the other. They pointed out that a combination of effects might account for the difference. First, the tests themselves differed essentially in the degree of restriction of possible responses. Second, two effects of alcohol might be plausibly assumed: (a) a reduction of fluency, and (b) a reduction of conformity to standards of performance. The effects might combine to explain why results for Test 3 were different from those of Tests 1, 2, and 4.

On Test 1, performance was reduced by alcohol. The conformity effect would not be applicable in this case, because all responses were counted as being correct. On Test 2, performance was also reduced by alcohol. Similarly again, the conformity effect would not be applicable, because almost all responses would be counted as correct. On Test 4, performance was reduced by alcohol again. The conformity effect was irrelevant, because (ostensibly) there was only one correct answer.

The combination of effects in Test 3, however, would uncover the source of the different results. On this test, performance was in general reduced by alcohol, but at the same time, reduction in conformity would have a facilitative effect. The restrictions placed on responses in this test were flexible; standards were therefore lowered both in the quality of responses and in the possibility for repetition. Under the influence of alcohol, for instance, when naming "trees," such responses as "big tree," "family tree," "Christmas tree" were recorded and not scored as incorrect. Similarly, subjects in the postalcohol condition gave for "articles of furniture" such responses as "kitchen table," "dining table," and "study table"; again, responses such as these were accepted as correct.

Hartocollis and Johnson also pointed out the lack of variability in this study, in contrast to other studies, which had exhibited high variability in performance under alcohol. Finally, the authors pointed out two limitations to their study. First, in the experimental condition, the study was conducted only at an ostensible blood-alcohol level of 0.10%. Different blood-alcohol levels, achieved by larger or smaller doses, might produce different results. Second, they pointed out that the experimental conditions in a psychology laboratory might have been somewhat artificial. Differences in the results might be possible in other, less artificial environments.

In summary, Hartocollis and Johnson found that alcohol reduced fluency in the production of words. This was borne out by the results from Tests 1, 2, and 4. The general conclusion, however, could be overridden when a test allowed for a relaxation of standards of conformity or shifts in criteria, as shown in the results from Test 3. Hartocollis and Johnson suggested that this latter situation was probably similar to those to found in social situations.

5.7 FORNEY AND HUGHES, 1961

This study investigated the effects of alcohol on both verbal and arithmetic performance. It differed from other studies of the same type in that a distracting manipulation was introduced in the form of controlled delayed auditory feedback. At the time this work appeared, Robert B. Forney and Francis W. Hughes were affiliated with the Indiana University School of Medicine, in Indianapolis, Indiana.

5.7.1 Subjects and Methods

5.7.1.1 Subjects

Subjects were seven male and three female paid volunteers. All were either medical or graduate students. Subjects remained naive to the test procedure until 15 min prior to the beginning of the experiment.

5.7.1.2 Materials

The experiment consisted of six tests, from which 2 min of each were tape-recorded and scored later:

Test 1:   Verbal output: Subjects read a passage from *Aristotle's Selections* (Peters, 1957) as rapidly but distinctly as possible.

Test 2:   Forward count: Subjects counted from one forward as rapidly as possible for 2 min.

Test 3:   Reverse count: Subjects counted backwards from 500 as quickly as possible for 2 min.

Test 4:   Progressive count: Starting with one, subjects counted in multiples of four: 1, 5, 9, 13, 17, . . . for 2 min.

Test 5:   Addition: Subjects were given a mimeographed sheet of simple addition problems. These were read aloud by the subjects, who also supplied the answers.

Test 6:   Subtraction: Subjects were given a mimeographed sheet of simple subtraction problems. These were read aloud by the subjects, who also supplied the answers.

5.7.1.3 Procedure

All subjects were tested under two conditions: an alcohol condition and a nonalcohol condition. In the alcohol condition, subjects consumed a beverage composed of vodka mixed with a carbonated beverage. Quantities consumed contained 45 ml of 200-proof alcohol per 150-lb body weight. In eight of the ten subjects, this produced a BAC of approximately 100 mg%, but the remaining two subjects were required to consume additional alcohol to reach this level. BAC was determined 20 minutes after completion of consumption by measuring alveolar air using a Borkenstein Breathalyzer (Borkenstein & Smith, 1961; Monnier, 1956).

All tests were conducted in a soundproof room. Subjects spoke into a microphone connected to a tape recorder. The playback head on the recorder was monitored by an amplifier that fed into a set of headphones worn by the subject. This produced a 0.28-sec delay in audio feedback through the headphones. Sound levels were adjusted so that subjects could hear only the auditory feedback.

5.7.2 Results and Discussion

Mean BAC measured 20 min after completion of drinking was 97 mg% (SE = 3 mg%). Scoring was performed after the experimental procedure using a scoring form that recorded both errors and total output for each test. Additionally, errors were subdivided into the categories omissions, insertions, mispronunciations, "spasms (stammers)," prolongations, and "other." Performance appeared to be enhanced in the alcohol condition, although in most cases these differences were not significant. Significant changes occurred in the Reverse Counting task, in which the percentage of errors increased under alcohol, and in the Addition task.

Forney and Hughes noted that verbalization (as measured here) was not significantly impaired in subjects with BACs of approximately 100 mg% (0.10%). They proposed that although increased verbalization or decreased speech efficiency might follow alcohol ingestion, such measures could not be used to predict "shades of inebriation." They further noted that verbalization deficiencies followed the introduction of auditory feedback, but that this distracting factor was not enhanced by alcohol.

Finally, Forney and Hughes offered the following tentative conclusions (p. 192): (a) alcohol did not significantly increase scores in any of the tests; (b) verbalization was unaffected; and (c) ethanol tended to interfere with test performances in which mathematics were involved. The arithmetical tests in which such deficiencies became evident involved simple addition exercises and reverse counting.

5.8 KAWI, 1961

In this study, Kawi used slurred speech as a criterion threshold to measure other effects of alcohol. Here, Kawi expanded and slightly modified the concept of *sedation threshold* to mean the amount of alcohol required to produce slurred speech on two consecutive test periods; this was called the *slurred speech threshold*. Kawi thus investigated the use of the slurred speech threshold as "a relatively constant biological characteristic as a level at which studies of physiological and psychological phenomena can be carried out" (p. 8). When this article appeared, Ali A. Kawi was an Assistant Professor of Psychiatry at the State University of New York's Downstate Medical Center in Brooklyn, New York.

5.8.1 Subjects and Methods

5.8.1.1 Subjects

Subjects for this study were a group of 24 patients "presenting varying degrees of 'anxiety' " (p. 9) and were obtained from the psychiatric division of the Kings County Hospital Center in Brooklyn, New York. All were white males, between the ages of 16 and 36. The current admission was their first at a psychiatric hospital, and clinically, "they presented a picture of predominantly psychoneurotic or character disorder" (p. 9).

The following data were obtained for each subject: (a) basic information, including age, sex, race, degree of education, height, and weight; (b) an evaluation of the degree of anxiety using (i) clinical judgment, (ii) the figure-drawing test (Machover, 1949), and the Taylor Anxiety Scale (Taylor, 1951, 1953); (iii) the sedation thresholds for alcohol and amobarbital sodium. Additionally, information from psychological and psychomotor tests and from electroencephalographic (EEG) recordings was obtained; these are discussed in section 5.8.2.

5.8.1.2 Procedure

Three experimental conditions were employed in this study: a no drug condition, a drug condition under amobarbital sodium (a barbiturate), and an alcohol condition under ethanol. Four psychological and psychomotor tests were administered: (a) sentence completion, (b) two-hand coordination, (c) steadiness, and (d) tapping speed.

In the alcohol condition, alcohol was administered intravenously, with infusion effected by means of gravity. The slurred speech threshold was set to be the point at which a subject manifested slurred speech on two consecutive testing periods; slurred speech was tested for 20 sec of each minute.

5.8.2 Results

5.8.2.1 Correlations and Electroencephalography

The slurred speech thresholds for ethyl alcohol and for amobarbital sodium correlated positively and significantly: +0.58. Additionally, the correlations for the slurred speech threshold for ethyl alcohol and the measures of anxiety were as follows: Taylor Anxiety Scale, 0.40; clinical judgment, 0.69, and figure drawing, 0.29 (diffuse vs. inferred) and 0.13 (obsessive-compulsive vs. hysterical). In the no drug condition, all EEG recordings fell within the normal range. Kawi's general impression was that at the slurred speech threshold, there were no notable changes in brain potentials.

5.8.2.2 Projective and Psychomotor Tests

Performance on the two-hand coordination test showed significant deterioration under the effects of both amobarbital sodium and alcohol. Each of the two drugs produced separate effects of deterioration as compared to the no drug condition. Likewise, both drugs separately produced deterioration in performance on the tapping-speed test. In the steadiness test, however, alcohol alone appeared to improve performance over that in the no drug condition.

For the sentence completion task, two measures were made: content analysis and RT. In the analysis of content, Kawi found no noticeable differences between responses in the drug and the no drug conditions; no differences in the range and variety of responses could be attributed to the effects of alcohol. RT was measured as the time in seconds between the examiner's completion of reading the incomplete sentence and the commencement of the subject's response. There was a marked decrease in RT under the effects of alcohol. Under Kawi's analysis, this decrease could be accounted for by the effect of each of the two drugs when compared to the no drug condition. F values for effects on RT were order of tests, 0.62 (not significant); sequence of drug, 1.63 (not significant); drug effect, 20.94 ($p < 0.001$). F values for interactions were drug effect and order of test, 1.61 (not significant); effect and sequence of drugs, 4.26 ($p < 0.01$). Kawi attributed the significant interaction to learning and experience, whereby repetition of the test resulted in experience and "certain knowledge" that contributed to the "increase in spontaneity of responses" (p. 11).

5.8.3 Discussion

Three clinical phenomena were considered in the determination of the sedation threshold: slurred speech, bilateral nystagmus, and EEG changes. Nystagmus appeared to develop in most of the patients at a dose level higher than that desired for administration of the psychological and psychomotor tests. EEG changes, on the other hand, were only slight, and therefore insignificant. Thus, there remained the slurred speech threshold as representative of the sedation threshold for alcohol (and amobarbitol sodium).

Whereas other studies measured the effects of alcohol on speech, slurred speech was used in Kawi's study as a threshold at which other behavioral effects could be observed. Because speech is our main concern in this book, it is unfortunate that Kawi did not specify in more detail what constituted slurred speech for this study. The characterization slurred speech occurs throughout the medical literature, as well in applied situations (such as in incident reports by law enforcement officers), and yet it is very seldom given a technical or operational definition. As will be seen later on, there are measurable changes in the speech acoustic signal that indicate intoxication; however, slurred speech, although widespread, remains a fairly vague designation.

5.9 DUNKER AND SCHLOSSHAUER, 1964

At the time this chapter appeared, Erich Dunker was director of the Physiological Institute of the the University of Hamburg, in Hamburg, West Germany, and Burkhard Schlosshauer was Chief of the Ear, Nose, and Throat Clinic in Bremen, West Germany.

In order to examine the relationship between the vibration type of the vocal cords and the particular sound produced, Dunker and Schlosshauer (1964) used high-speed photography and stroboscopy. Specifically, they wished to find morphological changes in the vocal organs in the presence of altered voice perceptions, that is, hoarse voice.

Forty-six subjects, both male and female, were examined. Most were examined under various conditions up to eight times consecutively or on different days. The laryngeal sound was recorded in the pharynx using a Sonde microphone connected to a tape recorder. Among others, subjects examined included a professional singer (age 48 years), an amateur singer (age 44 years), a physician (age 24 years) with slight constitutional phonasthesia, and a male adult (age 79 years) with a tremulous voice but no apparent vibration irregularities.

Of particular interest to the present study is the case in which the experimenters asked "a university student to yell and sing with full voice when celebrating and consuming alcoholic beverages liberally" (p. 165). Dunker and Schlosshauer measured glottal width, speed and open quotient, frequency, and opening/closing time for this subject at three points in time: before alcohol, after alcohol and yelling, and after administration of a vasoconstrictor.

Examination of the various parameters revealed no significant differences for vibration values before and after alcohol. There was also a preservation of periodicity after the consumption of alcohol and yelling. However, amplitudes were different, and this difference was more pronounced subsequent to inhalation of a vasoconstrictor. In terms of width measurements, Dunker and Schlosshauer noted a distinct longitudinal wave, whereby the

> glottis first opens with a difference between right and left, in the center, thereafter frontally, and finally in the back. Frontally, the right vocal cord vibrates excessively widely and returns to the median line when the opposite vocal cord portion

is staying already in the median line. For the anterior parts of the vocal cords
there is even a phase difference between right and left. (p. 171)

Although there was normal complete closure of the vocal cords, there was
also increased formation of phlegm and weakness of the interarytenoid
muscle.

Dunker and Schlosshauer concluded that injury to the vocal apparatus
following alcohol and strain was minimal: changes affected only a single
vibration, and periodicity was preserved. There was a slight irregularity
insofar as there were alternating closing movements in the frontal and dorsal
glottal sections. With this minimal disturbance, however, it is difficult to
separate the effects of alcohol from the effects of undue strain on the voice
(i.e., yelling). Of all the cases of hoarseness examined by Dunker and Schlosshauer, the changes in vocal function following alcohol and yelling were
considered to be minimal.

CHAPTER 6

Research Review II: 1966–1982

6.0 OVERVIEW

Whereas the work reviewed in Chapter 5 was characterized as indicating a "medical/psychological" period of research on alcohol and speech, the research discussed in the present chapter can be called "psychiatric/speech-scientific." The holistic view of speech in the Chapter 5 studies, as evidenced by latencies as a measure of a speech response, is replaced by much more detailed analyses of the speech signal itself; this approach is manifested in a number of ways, including analyses of error patterns, of structural characteristics of speech, and of the use of speech in social communication.

One "holdover" from the previous period is Moskowitz and Roth (1971, discussed in section 6.4). Subjects in this study named objects presented as outline drawings in both an alcohol and a nonalcohol condition. Although this resembles Hollingworth's (1923) study described in Chapter 5, an additional variable introduced by Moskowitz and Roth was the determination of the relative frequency of the word that named each object. The major result from this study was that both word frequency and alcohol affect response latency in object naming.

Two studies discussed here, R. C. Smith et al. (1975, discussed in section 6.7) and Stitzer et al. (1981a, discussed in section 6.12), emanated from psychiatric research and dealt with alcohol effects on social aspects of verbal communication. R. C. Smith et al. (1975) examined formal aspects of social communication in social dyads in both alcohol and placebo sessions. A low dose of alcohol increased the amount of communication as well as the amount of overlap between the partners; there was also a decrease in the amount of acknowledgment that subjects offered their partners' statements. High doses of alcohol increased the amount of overlap, but at this dose, the amount of communication leveled off or decreased from the level of the low dose. In the same vein, Stitzer et al. (1981a) briefly reviewed social stimulus factors in drug effects, including the effects of alcohol on verbal communication. The studies by R. C. Smith et al. and Stitzer et al. do not exhaust the literature regarding the effects of alcohol (or certainly of drugs generally) on verbal behavior and social communication. They are included here as representative of a large body of research lying somewhat outside the main concern of this work, the effects of alcohol on the *speech signal*.

Two studies discussed here investigated perceptual judgments of speech produced under alcohol. Both studies used groups of listeners trained in speech or voice pathology to judge various aspects of the speech. In Andrews et al. (1977, discussed in section 6.8), listeners rated talkers in both an alcohol and nonalcohol condition on 114 perceptual scales reflecting the importance of various characteristics to spoken communication. Seven factors were identified as significant in the differential perception of sober and intoxicated speech. In Sobell et al. (1982, discussed in section 6.13), listeners judged speech produced before alcohol and in two alcohol conditions on five voice-quality dimensions: articulation, nasality, inflection, rate, and drunkenness. Three of these perceptual dimensions were found to be significantly affected by increasing alcohol levels.

One brief, wide-ranging article included for discussion in this chapter (Beam et al., 1978, discussed in section 6.9) reported speech, language, voice, and hearing impairments in alcoholic subjects. Assessments were made of oral sensation and perception, oral diadochokinesis, articulation and speech clarity, verbal-expressive ability, voice quality, and pure-tone hearing acuity.

The remaining studies discussed in this chapter dealt with various aspects of speech or language proper, in this case, speech errors, acoustics, and syntactic performance. Stein (1966, discussed in section 6.1) performed a structural linguistic analysis of speech recordings from 11 alcoholics; he found that at various linguistic levels, this speech appeared to fall within normal limits. Trojan and Kryspin-Exner (1968, discussed in section 6.2) examined the speech of three subjects producing isolated words before alcohol and at two levels of alcohol consumption. The researchers noted "general lingual dissolution," "phonetic disturbances," and "changes in vocal expression" (p. 219) as consequences of alcohol consumption. Phonetic disturbances included substitutions, omissions, and distortions of sounds. Zaimov (1969, discussed in section 6.3) examined speech disturbances brought about by alcohol consumption with a typology of speech errors, based on similarities in sound and meaning and on types and levels of the errors. Zaimov found that errors in speech increased as the amount of alcohol consumed increased.

Sobell and Sobell (1972, discussed in section 6.5) examined speech dysfluencies in alcoholics under acute alcoholization. A standard linguistic passage was read aloud and recorded before alcohol consumption, after a low dose of alcohol, and after a higher dose of alcohol. The recorded passages were then scored for speech errors using predetermined dysfluency criteria. The degree of intoxication was found to affect interjections, word omissions, revisions, suffix changes, and reading times, but was found not to affect repetitions, incomplete phrases, rhythm changes, and prefix changes. The study by Lester and Skousen (1974, discussed in section 6.6) combined substitution analysis and acoustic measurement techniques to examine the effects of alcohol on speech. Speech materials were recorded by talkers in both an alcohol and a nonalcohol condition. Substitution patterns included voiceless for voiced obstruents, alveolar fricatives for alveopalatal fricatives, and fricatives for affricates. Acoustic findings included lengthening of consonantal segments, suggesting that an important effect of alcohol is to increase durations.

Acoustic analysis formed just one component of Lester and Skousen's (1974) investigation of the phonology of intoxicated speech. Likewise, the study by Sobell et al. (1982) also included an acoustic component. Acoustic parameters were speaking rate, amplitude, and fundamental frequency. Results showed that duration for reading the entire passage was significantly longer (speaking rate was slower) in the high-alcohol condition than in the moderate-dose or no-alcohol conditions. Amplitude was higher in the no-alcohol condition than in either of the alcohol conditions, and no significant effects were found for fundamental frequency.

The only exclusively acoustic study during the period covered by this chapter was that of Fontan et al. (1978, discussed in section 6.10). Fontan et al. investigated the observation that, although alcoholics often present with difficulties in the intelligibility of their speech, their speech is not generally considered to be dysarthric in the usual sense. Fontan et al. tape-recorded a number of alcoholic subjects undergoing treatment and then submitted these recordings to spectrographic analysis. These instrumental analyses revealed system-wide alterations of a number of segments in the speech of these subjects; all classes of speech sounds were affected: consonants, vowels, and glides. Fontan et al. also considered the question of specific organic bases that might be responsible for these changes and suggested that the speech of the patients examined here showed some resemblances to the speech of patients with cerebellar syndromes.

Error–substitution and acoustic analyses can be considered to be structural analyses of speech, because they examine the units that make up the speech signal. Error and substitution analyses examine segment-sized units that form morphemes and words, and acoustic analyses investigate subsegmental elements of the speech signal. Another type of structural analysis was carried out by Collins (1980, discussed in section 6.11), in which the syntactic performance of alcoholic and nonalcoholic adults was examined. Spoken sentences were recorded and transcribed and then analyzed according to a standard procedure in terms of several grammatical characteristics. Results showed that alcoholics committed more syntactic and semantic errors than nonalcoholics and additionally showed a small deficit in the integrative aspect of expressive language.

Although the disciplinary eclecticism noted in the research discussed in Chapter 5 continued in the studies discussed in the present chapter, there was nevertheless a clear trend toward structural analyses of speech produced under alcohol, and this especially in segmental analyses (e.g., substitution analysis) and acoustic analyses of the speech signal.

6.1 STEIN, 1966

This study applied the analysis techniques of structural linguistics to the examination of the speech of 11 members of Alcoholics Anonymous. Speech was analyzed at a number of different levels. The author concluded that in general, the speech of these subjects fell within the "normal" range. This research was conducted while the author was a Research Fellow at the University of Buffalo (New York).

6.1.1 Subjects and Methods

Subjects for this study were seven male and four female alcoholics, all members of Alcoholics Anonymous who had been abstinent for from 4 months to 13 years. The author used rough economic criteria to determine that one subject was "upper-class," five "middle-class," and five "lower-class" (p. 107). Ethnically, three subjects were second-generation Polish-Americans, one each second generation Swiss-, Irish-, and German-American, and five third-generation or more Anglo-American.

Elicitation was by means of tape-recorded interviews, during which social histories of the subjects and a variety of speech behaviors were elicited. In addition to specific questions regarding such things as date and place of birth, elicitation included open-ended questions on general topics such as animals and pets, food and eating, and views about the future.

In all, 18 hr of recorded material were collected. A subset was selected for linguistic analysis, totaling 15 min, 34 sec, averaging about 1.5 min for each subject. The researcher also established for each talker a baseline for the talker's dialect according to sex, age, birthplace, social status, and ethnicity, according to a procedure described in Gleason (1961).

The linguistic analysis of the recorded materials was performed on four levels. First, phonetic and phonemic divergences from the talkers' baselines were noted; these included such details as appeared incongruous with the talkers' sex, age, social status, and ethnicity. The second level of analysis used a typewritten transcript of the speech sample upon which were noted stresses, pitches, and transitional phenomena. The third level analyzed tone-of-voice "or paralinguistic phenomena such as 'uh-huh,' 'uh-uh,' 'hm'" as well as inappropriate stress and pitch, and "drawl or clipping" (p. 108); analysis of this level also noted such phenomena as heavy aspiration, glottalization, and heavy friction. The fourth level analyzed voice quality characteristics such as "spreading of pitch range up or down, heavy rasp or openness, voicing or devoicing, sharp or smooth pitch transitions, forceful or relaxed articulation, jerky or smooth rhythm control, and increased or decreased tempo" (p. 108). Categories for analysis were based on those in Trager (1958).

6.1.2 Results

Results were reported in only the most general of terms. The basic finding was that the analysis revealed the speech of the subjects to fall within normal ranges. More specifically, the author compared the speech of these subjects to the speech of psychotic and severely neurotic patients, noting that in these cases, there was generally a clear divergence from baseline norms for talkers' profiles. In the case of the subjects in the present study, however, speech patterns "quite definitely belong on the normal rather than the deviant end of the continuum" (p. 108). Although there were individual anomalies, the general pattern was one of adjustment to patterns of communication of the subjects' peers. Stein concluded that the speech of abstinent alcoholics showed no more than normal variation, but whether this would also apply to nonabstinent alcoholic subjects was a question left open.

6.2 TROJAN AND KRYSPIN-EXNER, 1968

The purpose of this study was to test the hypothesis that speech sounds acquired "early" in childhood speech development (labial and dental nasals and plosives) are embedded in the extra-pyramidal motor system, and that speech sounds acquired "late" in development (velar nasals and plosives, all fricatives, and liquids) are localized in the cortical-bulbar motor system. Since this hypothesis could not be tested directly, Trojan and Kryspin-Exner employed two "disintegration processes" involving administration of alcohol and paraldehyde (a hypnotic) to induce changes in speech articulation and then to compare these results with the developmental and dysarthria literature. Although the effects of both alcohol and paraldehyde on speech were examined in this study, this discussion is limited to alcohol effects. Because the alcohol component of this work was reported mainly by Trojan, he alone will be cited in the following discussion. At the time this article appeared, F. Trojan was a university professor in Vienna, Austria, and K. Kryspin-Exner was a lecturer at the Clinic for Psychiatry and Nervous Diseases in Vienna, Austria.

6.2.1 Subjects and Methods

6.2.1.1 Subjects

This study used three volunteer subjects, all male; S1 was 26 years old, S2 36 years old, and S3 31 years old. None had speech defects or neurological disturbances at the time of testing.

6.2.1.2 Methods

Subjects were required to perform two tasks: (a) relate a self-experienced story, and (b) name (in German) a number of objects represented in color on cards. The words were chosen to provide approximately equal numbers of early and late acquired speech sounds, according to the authors. Subjects were tape-recorded under three conditions: (a) when sober, (b) after consumption of part of a total quantity of "heavy Austrian wine" (alcoholic content, approximately 13%), and (c) after consumption of the total amount. Obvious changes in articulation were subsequently analyzed spectrographically and compared with unchanged articulations. Table 6.2.1 gives the time of recording and the amount of alcohol consumed at the time of testing.

TABLE 6.2.1   Survey of the Point of Time of Recording and Amount of Alcohol Consumption[a]

	Subject					
	1		2		3	
Recording	PT[b]	Amount	PT	Amount	PT	Amount
a	18:45	—	19:38	—	19:50	—
b	19:50	1.0 L	20:35	0.75 L	20:55	1.0 L
c	20:15	1.38 L	21:10	1.0 L	21:25	1.38 L

[a] Note: A sufficient reabsorption period was allowed after respective consumption. From Trojan and Kryspin-Exner (1968). Copyright © 1968 by S. Karger AG, Basel. Used by permission.
[b] PT, point of time.

6.2.2 Results

Trojan noted three categories of change in articulation occurring after consumption of alcohol: (a) *general lingual dissolution,* comparable to the aphasic component in a combination of aphasia and *désintégration phonétique* (Alajouanine, Ombredane, & Durant, 1939); (b) *phonetic disturbances* (substitutions, omissions, and distortions), comparable to articulatory problems in dysarthria; and (c) *changes in vocal expression,* indicating brain stem participation, and which are lacking in pure dysarthria.

Trojan defined four categories of general lingual dissolution: (a) paragrammatical repetition of words and phrases; (b) other grammatical-syntactic errors (also errored sentence construction, anacolutha); (c) repetition of syllables; and (d) embolophrasia (meaningless speech). Trojan noted a definite increase in general lingual dissolution for all three subjects. The general course of this increase was from the sober condition to the small dose condition, but articulation appeared to be better in the large dose condition than in the small dose condition. Trojan offered two possible explanations for this: (a) "natural deviations in lingual functional proficiency," or (b) "compensatory efforts at correct lingual expression often found in a state of intoxication" (p. 220).

In the category phonetic disturbances or decay of sounds, Trojan reported the following speech sounds to be most in error: [l r s ʃ pf ts], further asserting that the affected sounds were late acquired ones. Trojan also noted isolated disturbances of [b ç x], as well as instances of vowel lengthening, similar to compensatory lengthening, for subject 3.

Changes in vocal expression were observed for all subjects. Most extreme changes in voice (and, according to Trojan, mood) were observed in S1, who exhibited:

> a higher pitch with increasing of the headvoice component of the mixed voice, gradually ascending bursts of laughter, and a euphoric-trophotropic intonation; in addition thereto, extensive relaxation of inhibitions, flatulence, and homosexual tendencies; further, a strong singultus (hiccup) (p. 222)

The situation for S1 is contrasted with that for S2, who "showed an increase in depth of pitch and the impression of good humor and peaceableness grew stronger" (p. 222). Finally, S3 "showed heightened aggression and symptoms of 'vox ergotropica (potent voice)' "; there was a further "tendency to diphthongize" (p. 222).

6.2.3 Discussion

Trojan suggested two separate levels for syllable formation and phonetic systems: a *vegetative-biophonetic* stage and a *cortical-phonologic* stage. According to him, the syllable was a unit of secondary function corresponding to mastication, a unit of primary function. In early work, Trojan (1955) had proposed that the earliest established sounds were those produced during voiced mastication, including nasals and labial and dental plosives. He further claimed that the plosives appear as clicks, from which the plosives are asserted to have originated. In this connection, Trojan cited Hayek, a Viennese anatomist, who postulated that earlier developing sounds were embedded in the extrapyramidal motor system, but that later developing sounds are embedded in the cortical-bulbar motor system. Trojan's contention was that alcohol and paraldehyde bring about decays of articulation comparable to *désintégration phonétique* (Alajouanine et al., 1939), and that in all these cases, the sounds that are acquired latest are the first affected, either by drugs or by brain lesions.

6.3 ZAIMOV, 1969

The analysis presented here was based on Wedensky's theory of parabiosis and Pavlov's theory of phase conditions. The basic regularity suggested by Zaimov was that in a pathophysiological nervous system, there is inhibition of regular neural paths and disinhibition of normally inhibited ones. The course of normal reactions is switched, and in language, this is manifested by confusion of linguistic units similar in sound or meaning. As such, speech disorders can then be a criterion for disturbances of consciousness. This work emanated from the Psychiatric Clinic of the Medical Faculty of Sofia in Bulgaria.

6.3.1 Subjects and Methods

Subjects were twenty volunteers who underwent an oral speech test (by reading text) and a writing test (by dictation) in three conditions. In the first condition, tests were administered first before any consumption of alcohol. An alcoholic beverage was prepared consisting of a 65% solution of alcohol made to taste like anise brandy. Subjects drank between 100 and 550 ml of this preparation in two alcohol conditions. In the first alcohol condition, subjects drank 50% of the prescribed quantity, and then in the second condition the remaining 50%. Fifteen of the subjects also underwent electroencephalographic (EEG) examination, and seven had blood-alcohol concentration (BAC) determined (specific method not stated).

Materials were either read or written from dictation. Using a preset passage allowed comparison of produced speech with the text, so that a clear determination of errors could be made. Zaimov (1969) did not mention the specific form of the stimuli, that is, whether they were paragraphs, sentences, or isolated words. Scoring employed a score sheet for speech errors that assigned these errors to cells in matrices. On the matrix for errors with an apparent relation to the text, one axis indicated the type of error (substitution, exchange, omission, repetition, contamination, repetition of a line, and skipping to a remote line) and the linguistic/orthographic level of the error (word, syllable, letter). Additionally, for the substitution category, one could indicate whether the substitution was related to the target by sound, by sense, or by both. The second axis indicated whether the error was anticipatory or perseverative, the total number of errors, and the number of corrected errors. On the matrix for errors without an apparent connection to the text, one axis listed the type of error (substitution, insertion, contamination) and the level of error (word, syllable, letter), whereas the second axis listed the total errors and the number of corrected errors. The scoring sheet for the written test was similar to the one for spoken responses, except that the categories 'Repetition of a line' and 'Skipping to a remote line' were left out and replaced with 'Mangling of words' . . . 'Substitution of lower case letters with upper case ones, and vice versa', and 'Error by using old orthography' (the test was administered in Bulgarian, which underwent orthographic reform in 1945) (p. 221, note). The typology allowed both a qualitative assessment and a quantitative assessment of speech errors.

6.3.2 Results

There was a general trend for the number of errors to increase as the amount of alcohol consumed increased. The relative prevalence of errors elicited in this experiment occurred in the following order: (a) anticipations and perseverations with apparent connection to the text, (b) errors without apparent connection to the text, (c) repetition of letters, syllables, and words, (d) repetition of a line or skipping to a remote line (in reading), (e) mangling of words (in writing), and (f) switching of lower- and upper-case letters (in writing).

6.3.3 Discussion

From these results, Zaimov (1969) concluded that error analysis of this type could be used to determine the level of impairment as well as the level of consciousness disturbance. A specific practical use, he said, would be in cases of automobile collisions, when samples of speech or writing could be gathered directly subsequent. Zaimov further claimed that in many cases, a measure of speech errors is more reliable than measurement of alcohol in the blood (blood samples were taken from 7 of the 20 subjects); it is not completely clear what objective standard Zaimov was using to compare this reliability. EEG was performed for fifteen of the subjects; changes were noticed at higher levels of intoxication, but Zaimov also noted that changes occurred much earlier in the speech analyses than in the EEGs. Finally, Zaimov noted that errors in both reading and writing increased at the level of 50-ml consumption, which, he said, contradicted the claim that small amounts of alcohol could increase mental functioning.

6.4 MOSKOWITZ AND ROTH, 1971

In this study, subjects produced the names of exhibited objects, which, according to Moskowitz and Roth (1971) is a "far more complex brain processing task" than a "relatively simple task in which the subject was required to make specified responses to two familiar stimuli presented in sequence" (p. 969). The performance measure was the response latency to the onset of speech. Moskowitz and Roth proceeded from a previous finding in the literature that the time to onset of naming an object is inversely proportional to the logarithm of frequency of appearance of an object's name in written language (Oldfield & Wingfield, 1965). Moskowitz and Roth, however, employed the additional variable of alcohol consumption. This work emanated from the Institute of Transportation and Traffic Engineering at the University of California at Los Angeles and from the California State College at Los Angeles.

6.4.1 Method

6.4.1.1 Subjects
Subjects were 12 male university graduate students, at least 21 years of age, with 20/20 vision (if necessary, corrected). They were self-described as "light," "social," or "party" drinkers. Male graduate students were used exclusively, to minimize sex and education level differences.

6.4.1.2 Alcoholic Preparation
The alcoholic preparation consisted of 1 oz of 80-proof vodka per 40 lb of body weight, mixed with an equal volume of orange juice, that is, 0.52 g alcohol/kg of body weight. The alcohol dose was calculated to raise BACs to between 0.06 and 0.08%. The control beverage consisted solely of orange juice equal in volume to the entire alcoholic preparation.

6.4.1.3 Materials
The stimulus materials were 30 outline drawings of objects selected on the basis of the frequency of their names in written English, according to the Thorndike-Lorge (1944) word count. The 30 test items were selected from six frequency groups (number per million words): Group 1 (0.1–0.9): gyroscope, seahorse, metronome, tuningfork, stethoscope; Group 2 (1–10):

octopus, horseshoe, anvil, dice, microscope; Group 3 (11–30): windmill, typewriter, screw, cigarette, anchor; Group 4 (31–50): hammer, drum, needle, glove, rabbit; Group 5 (51–10): basket, pie, key, clock, pipe; Group 6 (> 100): book, eye, chair, shoe, tree. Additionally, five practice items were presented, the names of which covered the range of frequencies: a skull, a penguin, a telephone, a bed, and a pencil.

6.4.1.4 Apparatus and Procedure

Subjects were seated in a sound-attenuated booth facing a window. A Hunter Cardmaster was placed on a table outside the booth in front of the window. A card was viewed when revealed by an opening shutter activated by an electronic timer. Placed directly in front of the subject was a microphone, which stopped the timer when spoken into. A clock recorded the elapsed time (from presentation of the object until the onset of speech) to the nearest 0.1 ms; for analysis, this was later rounded to the nearest millisecond.

Subjects were tested twice (once with alcohol and once without) between 11 A.M. and 1 P.M. on two successive days. Testing order was counterbalanced so that six of the subjects received alcohol on the first day and the remaining six on the second day. Subjects were instructed to fast for 4 hr preceding the experiment and not to consume drugs (including alcohol and caffeine) for the preceding 24 hr. Subjects were required to consume the alcoholic or control preparation within 10 min. The testing then began 30 min after completion of consumption. The 35 stimulus outline drawings (5 practice and 30 scored) were presented every 10 sec in random order, differing for each subject and treatment.

6.4.2 Results

Both alcohol and word frequency produced significant effects on response latency. Table 6.4.1 shows the results of a three-way analysis of variance (ANOVA) on the effects of alcohol, word frequency, and treatment order. For alcohol, the mean square difference was approximately 67.21; for word frequency, 179.71. Figure 6.4.1, which plots response latencies as a function of word frequency under both conditions, demonstrates that the logarithm of word frequency was approximately linearly related to the inverse of response latency under both conditions.

Figure 6.4.1 also illustrates the effect of alcohol on response latencies. In the control condition, the mean response latency was 705 ms, but after alcohol, it was 786 ms. The mean difference was therefore about 11.5%. Figure 6.4.1 also indicates a trend towards an alcohol effect that was increasingly larger the less frequently a word occurred, but this trend was not statistically significant, a result also borne out by the data in Table 6.4.1,

TABLE 6.4.1   Analysis of Variance[a]

Source	df	Mean squares	F
Order (A)	1	0.09001	—
Subjects within groups	10	51.4724	—
Alcohol (B)	1	67.21266	6.928*
A × B	1	219.97825	22.671**
B × subjects within groups	10	9.7029	—
Word frequency (C)	5	179.71161	66.041**
A × C	5	0.23210	0.08
C × subjects within groups	50	2.7212	—
B × C	5	2.61254	1.141
A × B × C	5	11.28856	4.928**
B × C × subjects within groups	50	2.2903	—

[a] From Moskowitz and Roth (1971). Copyright © 1971 by *Journal of Studies on Alcohol*, Rutgers University. Used by permission.
*$p < .05$
**$p < .001$

which show a nonsignificant interaction between alcohol and word frequency.

As indicated in Table 6.4.1, there was a significant interaction between alcohol and treatment order. This suggests a differential effect of alcohol on response latencies as a function of session order. Moskowitz and Roth analyzed the data for practice effects and found that latencies were shorter in the second session.

6.4.3 Discussion

Two major results emerged from this study: first, as shown in Figure 6.4.1, word frequency has a significant effect on response latency in object naming, and second, alcohol also affected response latency by increasing it independently of word frequency. According to Moskowitz and Roth, these findings supported the view that alcohol impedes the rate at which the brain processes information. They pointed out that usual reaction times (RT) for executing simple responses to stimuli are in the range of 150 to 200 ms, but that response latencies for naming objects (without alcohol) are typically in the 500 to 1400 ms range, indicating that in this task the brain is faced with greater complexity. They proposed that the object-naming task could be broken down into two separable components: (a) identifying the object, and (b) finding the name of the object in the word storage system (lexicon). Other evidence for this separation of identification and lexical access are "tip-of-the-tongue" phenomena, in which objects can be identified but not named, and certain types of aphasia, in which patients can provide correct

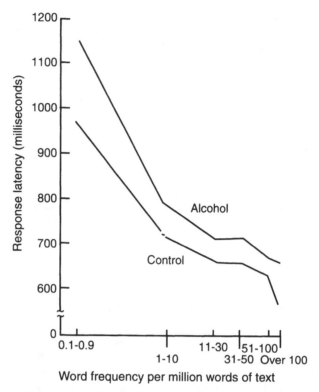

FIGURE 6.4.1   Response latencies as a function of word frequency under control and alcohol treatments. (From Moskowitz and Roth, 1971. Copyright © 1971 by Rutgers University. Used by permission.)

descriptions of objects but cannot without difficulty actually name the object spontaneously.

Moskowitz and Roth further pointed out that the evidence of variation in latencies as a function of word frequency speaks first for an increased central-processing demand for less frequent words, and second, the effects of alcohol involve central processing rather than simple sensorimotor connections or peripheral motor responses.

6.5 SOBELL AND SOBELL, 1972

In this study, Sobell and Sobell analyzed the effects of alcohol on speech using 13 operationally defined speech errors. This research was conducted while Linda C. Sobell was affiliated with the University of California at

Riverside and Mark B. Sobell with Patton State Hospital in Patton, California. At the time this article appeared, both authors were affiliated with the Orange County Department of Mental Health, Alcoholism Services, in Santa Ana, California.

6.5.2 Methods

6.5.2.1 Subjects

Subjects were 16 male patients self-admitted to Patton State Hospital (Patton, California) for alcohol treatment, who volunteered to participate in the study. All subjects had abstained from alcohol consumption for at least 3 weeks prior to the study and were not currently under medication. All spoke and read English fluently.

6.5.2.2 Apparatus and Testing Procedure

A tape recorder (Concord F-400) with automatic volume control was used to record subjects' readings in an acoustically isolated room. A voice-sensitive microphone was placed approximately 12 in. in front of the subject. The experimenter used stereo headphones both to monitor the readings and to score speech errors. The reading was a 613-word-long passage (McDavid & Muri, 1967), which was read aloud and recorded in three conditions in three separate sessions: mildly inebriated, moderately inebriated, and sober. Session orders were counterbalanced to allow for practice effects, and all sessions were separated by 48 hr.

In alcohol sessions, pairs of subjects at an experimental bar drank up to 16 1-oz preparations of 86-proof liquor (or its alcohol equivalent) in a 3-hr period. Testing occurred once when a subject was sober (48 hr before or after the two drinking sessions), once after the subject had consumed 5 oz of 86-proof liquor (or its alcohol equivalent), and once after consumption of 10 oz of 86-proof liquor (or its alcohol equivalent). In the two alcohol conditions, recordings were made immediately after the fifth or the tenth drink.

Although Sobell and Sobell pointed out that direct assessment of BAC would have been preferable, apparently this procedure was not possible. Instead, BAC was estimated from the quantity of alcohol consumed. In the mildly inebriated condition, given that most subjects consumed 5 oz of alcohol within an hour, Sobell and Sobell estimated the BAC at the time of recording to be approximately 0.10 g/100 ml (corrected from 0.10 g/ml appearing in the article text). Similarly, all subjects consumed the 10-oz dose of alcohol within the first 2 hr of the session, so that an estimate of 0.25 g/100 ml (corrected from 0.25 g/ml in the article text) BAC could be made for the time of recording.

6.5.2.3 Scoring Procedure

Scoring was performed by the senior author using the tape recordings made of the reading samples. Scoring was based on 13 types of speech errors, partly derived from an earlier study by W. Johnson et al. (1959). These errors were: (a) Interjections, including (i) Word, (ii) Phrase, (iii) Sound/Syllable; (b) Word Repetitions; (c) Phrase Repetitions; (d) Sound/Syllable Repetitions; (e) Revisions (single words); (f) Incomplete Phrases; (g) Broken Words, including (i) Rhythm Change, (ii) Suffix Change, (iii) Prefix Change; (h) Time to Read Passage; and (i) Word Omissions. W. Johnson et al. (1959) had originally suggested only seven categories of speech errors; new to the present study were the division of categories (a) and (g) into subcategories and categories (h) and (i). Sobell and Sobell defined (g, ii) "Broken Word—Suffix Change" and (g, iii) "Broken Word—Prefix Change" as "each word in the passage which was altered from its original context by omission, change, or addition of a suffix or prefix, respectively" (p. 864). Category (h) "Time to Read Passage" was defined as "the total number of seconds taken to read the passage aloud from beginning to end (including any pauses and hesitations)," and category (i) "Word Omissions" as, "each single word which was not verbalized although it appeared in the original passage. This does not include cases where another word or part of a word was substituted for the omitted word" (p. 864).

A given error could be assigned to only one category, even though, as Sobell and Sobell pointed out, the categories were not completely independent. A two-way ANOVA, with degree of inebriation as the independent measure and testing order as a repeated measure, was calculated for each of the thirteen categories.

6.5.3 Results

Table 6.5.1 presents mean scores for the thirteen scoring categories as a function of degree of intoxication. Degree of intoxication was found to affect (a) Word Interjections, (b) Phrase Interjections, (c) Syllable/Sound Interjections, (d) Word Omissions, (e) Revisions, (f) Broken Words–Suffix Change, and (g) Reading Time. On the other hand, the following were apparently not affected by alcohol (i.e., there were no statistically significant changes): (h) Word Repetitions, (i) Phrase Repetitions, (j) Sound/Syllable Repetitions, (k) Incomplete Phrases, (l) Broken Words—Rhythm Change, and (m) Broken Words—Prefix Change.

Experimental order significantly affected Revisions and Broken Words—Rhythm Change. According to Sobell and Sobell, these results were possibly due to a practice effect, because orders in which the intoxicated condition preceded the sober one produced more errors than in orders in which the

TABLE 6.5.1   Mean Time to Read Passage and Mean Number of Errors as a Function of
Degree of Intoxication for 16 Alcoholic Subjects (length of reading passage-613 words)[a]

Error category	Degree of intoxication		
	Sober	5 ounces	10 ounces
Mean time (sec) to read passage	233.50	243.62	312.06
Mean word interjections	5.81	7.31	10.56
Mean phrase interjections	0.31	0.38	3.08
Mean sound/syllable interjections	0.56	1.38	3.13
Mean word omissions	2.86	3.25	5.94
Mean revisions	3.48	3.38	6.50
Mean word repetitions	2.62	0.75	0.88
Mean Phrase repetitions	0.38	0.19	0.25
Mean sound/syllable repetitions	1.31	0.86	0.50
Mean broken words—suffix change	2.81	3.50	5.31
Mean broken words—prefix change	0.00	0.00	0.00
Mean broken words—rhythm change	0.69	1.44	1.50
Mean incomplete phrases	0.00	0.00	0.62

[a] From Sobell and Sobell (1972). Copyright © 1972 by the American Speech-Language-Hearing
Association. Used by permission.

conditions were reversed. There were two significant interaction terms:
Phrase Interjections with Order and Sound/Syllable Interjection with Order.

6.5.4 Discussion

The results of this experiment allow what the authors referred to as a "profile
of alcohol-induced disfluent speech of alcoholics" (p. 865). Sobell and Sobell
cautioned that (a) such a profile "can only be generalized to alcoholic
subjects" (p. 865), although "it is reasonable to assume that persons who
are not alcoholics will probably demonstrate the same general types of
speech changes when inebriated" (p. 866); and (b) because BACs were not
assessed directly, "the experiment reported here can only claim *ordinary*
[italics added] levels of intoxication" (p. 866). Given these caveats, then,
the profile would suggest that (at least) the following changes occur in the
speech of alcoholics from a sober state to more intoxicated ones: (a) reading
time increases significantly; (b) interjections (all three types) increase significantly; (c) word omissions increase; (d) broken word—suffix changes increase; (e) word revisions increase (word revisions are words that are read
incorrectly but corrected afterwards); (f) there are no changes in the three
types of repetition; (g) the categories Broken Word—Rhythm Change, Broken Word—Prefix Change, and Incomplete Phrases do not change in response to alcohol.

The authors proposed that the profile of alcohol-affected speech is roughly equivalent to slurred speech. They further pointed out that the effects of alcohol may be different in casual, conversational speech from the effects found here for read passages and proposed that future research investigate other types of speech. Finally, they suggested that speech changes, if found to be reliable and consistent across subjects, might serve as an observable measure of alcohol intoxication.

6.6 LESTER AND SKOUSEN, 1974

This study investigated alcohol-induced speech changes occurring at a stage when speech is still coherent. The techniques used were a combination of speech error analysis, acoustic analysis, and phonological analysis. At the time this article appeared, Leland Lester and Royal Skousen were affiliated with the linguistics department at the University of Texas in Austin, Texas.

6.6.1 Methods

Subjects were "all perfectly healthy normal people, who had English as their native language" (p. 238). The number of subjects was not reported, but the text implies more than one. The alcoholic preparation was 86-proof bourbon whiskey, administered in 1-oz doses every 20 min for approximately 5–7 hr. Materials consisted of a list of isolated words to be read aloud and a sample of spontaneous connected speech elicited in the context of a monologue by the subject or a conversation between the subject and the experimenter. The first speech sample was collected before administration of the first alcohol dose (i.e., in a sober condition). Subsequent samples were collected every 20 min immediately prior to the administration of the next dose of alcohol. Specific instrumentation was not noted in the published report, although R. Skousen has reported (personal communication, May 1995) that oscillographic tracings were used for measurements.

6.6.2 Results

Lester and Skousen (1974) first noted that "drunk speech appears to be drawn out" (p. 233), citing Kozhevnikov and Chistovich's (1965) observation that normal (unaffected by alcohol) slow speech shows lengthening mostly in vocalic segments. Lester and Skousen's results, however, showed lengthening mainly in consonantal segments. This lengthening occurred primarily in unstressed syllables, but syllables with primary stress showed little or no proportional increase in duration. This was observed, for example, in the word *locomotive*. Syllabification of *locomotive* would yield *lo-co-*

mo-tive, and stress assignment would assign primary stress to the third syllable, secondary stress to the first syllable and no stress to the second and final (fourth) syllables. As regards lengthening, the initial [l] of *lo-* and the initial [k] of -*co-* were both lengthened. Neither of the syllables containing these consonants bears primary stress, although *lo-* does bear secondary stress; in any case, -*co-* is clearly unstressed, and its consonant, [k], was lengthened to a considerable degree. Although Lester and Skousen did not rule out the lengthening of vocalic segments in alcohol-influenced speech, they did point out that this speech also contained lengthening phenomena not exhibited in normal (sober) slow speech.

Lester and Skousen further found a number of sound substitutions in the data. First, they observed final-obstruent devoicing, such as in the words *tease* [tis], *dog* [dɔk], and *judge* [dʒʌtʃ]. Second, they observed a merger of [s] (the initial sound in *sell*) with [ʃ] (the initial sound in *shell*), as in the words *yes* [yɛʃ] and *spin* [ʃpɪn]. Although Lester and Skousen referred to a "merger" of the two segments, all examples given showed an English /s/ being substituted for by an [ʃ]. Last, they observed the substitution of affricates by fricatives, such as in *church* [ʃʌrtʃ] and *judge* [ʒʌdʒ].

Lester and Skousen found that substitutions such as these did not generally occur until approximately the tenth reading, but that even after that point the substitution patterns were inconsistent. An example of this was the final obstruent in *tease,* which was correctly produced as a voiced fricative on the twelfth and thirteenth readings but was incorrectly devoiced on the tenth and eleventh readings (i.e., the two preceding readings), as well as on the fourteenth. Likewise, both *church* and *judge* contain both an initial and a final affricate; however, in both cases, only the initial affricate exhibited the fricative substitution pattern.

6.6.3 Discussion

The authors proposed that the observed substitutions were not to be interpreted as phonemic substitutions, because whether sober or intoxicated, speakers would have the same underlying phonological representations (psychological representations in Lester and Skousen's terms). For instance, they noted that in a sober pronunciation of *tease,* there is already some devoicing of the final obstruent, and the preceding vowel is longer than in the (nonsense) word [tis]. Furthermore, the voiceless portion of the final segment in *tease* is actually longer than the voiced portion, and the final segment in [tis] is over twice as long as the final segment in *tease.* In the rendition under alcohol, there was no change in the length of the vowel, but there was a phonetic change in the character of the final segment. The voiced portion of the final segment was shortened, and the voiceless portion (present even in a sober manifestation) was increased. The length of the final consonant

remained approximately the same as in the sober condition, and any perceptual change (devoicing) could be attributed to the earlier (approximately
100 ms) onset of the voiceless portion. That lengthening processes were
found in alcohol-affected speech that are not found in normal "slow speech"
suggested that alcohol effects are not simply a matter of slowing down
speaking rate; rather, there appeared to be changes unique to alcohol.

Lester and Skousen further noted that final obstruent devoicing is observed in child language and explained this within the framework of "Natural Phonology" (see Donegan & Stampe, 1979): the innate, inherent tendency is to devoice final segments; child language is also subject to this
tendency, and children learning English must learn to overcome it, as English
has both voiced and voiceless final segments. This learned behavior is com-
promised under the influence of alcohol.

Other characteristics of alcohol-affected speech, however, are not characteristic of child language, as Lester and Skousen (p. 237) pointed out. These
include the substitution of [s] by [ʃ] (also found by K. Johnson et al., 1990,
but not by Künzel et al., 1992) and the substitution of affricates by fricatives.
Finally, Lester and Skousen also pointed out that the speech of patients with
cerebellar disorders is often described as sounding "drunken." In this regard,
Lester and Skousen suggested that further investigation of this type of speech
might have implications for the study of alcohol-affected speech.

6.7 SMITH, PARKER, AND NOBLE, 1975

This study investigated alcohol effects on verbal communication within
social dyads. Whereas previous studies had concentrated on psychological
aspects of communication (e.g., content and affect), this study examined
formal aspects of speech. Previous studies had investigated formal properties
of communication in the context of other drugs, and it had been found
that these properties might be sensitive to the drugs' effects. For instance,
Lennard, Jarvik, and Abramson (1956) found that LSD increased the density of speech statements and rate of interruptions; Lennard, Epstein, and
Katzung (1967) showed that chlorpromazine increased initiation rates of
verbal communication and the proportion of communication directed to
others; and Reiss and Salzman (1973) showed that secobarbital increased
rates of speech and the occurrence of interruptions and overlaps.

This work emanated from the Department of Psychiatry and Human
Behavior at the University of California at Irvine. When the article appeared,
Robert C. Smith was affiliated with the Department of Psychiatry at the
University of Chicago (Chicago, Illinois).

6.7.1 Methods

Subjects for this study were 18 male–female couples, ages 21–30 years.
These couples had been acquainted for several months and were either

spouses or close friends. Excluded were abstainers, heavy drinkers, and heavy users of other psychoactive drugs. Subjects were instructed to fast for at least 3 hr before each experimental session. The task for each session involved a period of free discussion.

Each couple participated in an alcohol (low-dose) and a placebo session according to a balanced crossover design. The two sessions, each of which lasted approximately 2 hr, were separated by approximately 2 weeks. Subjects were informed that they might receive either no drug or a different drug from their partner, but in fact both members of the couple, in each session, received either alcohol or a placebo. In addition, six couples participated in a third session involving a higher alcohol dose (high-dose).

The alcohol preparation consisted of 80-proof vodka in a peppermint-flavored carrier. The placebo preparation was the masking carrier without alcohol. The alcohol preparation was administered on a volume by weight basis, or milliliter absolute alcohol per kilogram body weight. Doses differed for men and women in the low-dose condition; doses in the high-dose condition were higher than in the low-dose condition, but were the same for men and women. Specific doses per session were as follows: Low dose: Men: 1.0 ml/kg, Women: 0.83 ml/kg; High dose: Men: 1.50 ml/kg, Women: 1.50 ml/kg. To prevent precipitous decreases in BAC in latter parts of the test sessions, alcohol preparations were administered in two doses, the first dose approximately 1 hr prior to measuring a prediscussion BAC (from breath), and the second immediately after measuring the prediscussion BAC. A second BAC was measured postdiscussion.

Verbal information was coded for the second 10 min of each interaction based on typed transcripts. Coding employed two broad categories: (a) Volume, Length, and Patterning of Communication and (b) Acknowledgment in Communication, both based on categories developed by Mishler and Waxler (1968) for their study of psychiatrically disturbed families. The more detailed coding categories subsumed by the broad categories were as follows:

1. Volume, length and patterning of communication were as follows:
   a. Words (total number of words produced by each talker)
   b. Acts (total number of "acts" [see Mishler & Waxler, 1968] produced by each talker)
   c. Initiations (number of times each talker initiated a statement that elicited response)
   d. Overlap and interruptions in speech (number of instances in which partners spoke simultaneously plus number of interruptions)
2. Acknowledgment in communication
   a. Stimulus fragment (number of acts serving as stimuli for partners' communication that were fragments rather than complete acts)

b. Complete or partial acknowledgment (number of responses showing complete or partial acknowledgment of stimulus)
c. Recognition (number of responses recognizing previous speaker's having said something without specific response to intent or content)
d. Nonacknowledgment (number of responses coded for degree of acknowledgment but not showing acknowledgment or recognition of partner's stimulus)
e. Response fragments (number of responses that were fragments)
f. Too little information
g. Not ascertainable because of poor transcription
h. Codable responses (sum of responses coded as Complete/Partial acknowledgment or response fragments)

6.7.2 Results

Mean BACs (in mg/100 ml) for both alcohol conditions, pre- and postdiscussion, were as follows: prediscussion low-dose mean = 55 (SD = 13), prediscussion high-dose mean = 76 (SD = 11), postdiscussion low-dose mean = 65 (SD = 14), postdiscussion high-dose mean = 101 (SD = 22). There was no difference in BACs between the male and female subjects. Correlations between BACs and various other factors were generally absent. BACs were not related to changes in verbal communication, and there were no significant correlations between individual BACs and changes in verbal communication between the placebo and alcohol sessions. Furthermore, there was no correlation between individual BACs and speech characteristics in the alcohol session alone.

The most consistent effect of alcohol was an increase in the amount of interrupting and overlapping speech. There was more overlap in the low-dose condition than in the placebo condition, as well as more overlap in the high-dose condition than the low-dose. There was a significant increase in the number of acts and a similar trend in number of words in the low-dose condition. A highly significant increase in the number of initiations was noted, and this was not simply a matter of increasing the amount of communication or of shortening the length of responses, as there was no significant correlation between change in the number of words or number of acts and the change in number of initiations. Furthermore, there was no significant shortening of the length of each statement, that is, no significant decrease in the number of acts per statement or words per act.

The tendency to increase the amount of communication from the placebo to the low-dose condition appeared to be reversed for the high-dose session, so that total words, total acts, and number of initiations all decreased from their low-dose levels and approached placebo-level measures. The decrease in words from the low-dose condition to the high-dose condition was significant, but the difference in words between the high-dose and the placebo conditions was nonsignificant.

This study offered limited support for the authors' hypothesis that alcohol would decrease acknowledgment and responsiveness. In the low-dose condition, there was a small but consistent trend for decreased acknowledgment. Among the specific measures were a significant decrease in the proportion of responses showing complete or partial acknowledgment and a decrease in acknowledgment to stimuli that could definitely be acknowledged. Furthermore, there was a trend toward increasing the proportion of vague responses that could not be acknowledged, a small but nonsignificant increase in the proportion of nonacknowledging responses, and a small but nonsignificant decrease in the index of *positive acknowledgment* (the proportion of responses showing either acknowledgment or recognition).

Overall, the authors found evidence that alcohol did affect some formal aspects of verbal communication and that "alcohol appeared to make social communication more disorganized and intoxicated subjects seemed less likely to follow conventional rules of etiquette in their speech" (p. 1397). In the low-dose condition, overlapping and interruption were more frequent, and responses tended to show less acknowledgment. Most significantly, the amount of communication and initiations increased with alcohol.

6.8 ANDREWS, COX, AND SMITH, 1977

This work addressed the question of whether there are perceptible differences in speech resulting from alcohol when listeners do not identify the talkers as intoxicated. Listeners judged the speech of talkers in both sober and intoxicated conditions using a perceptual response inventory. When this article appeared, Moya L. Andrews was an Assistant Professor of Speech and Hearing Sciences at Indiana University, W. Miles Cox, a postdoctoral scholar in the Department of Psychology at Indiana University, and Raymond G. Smith a Professor of Speech Communication at Indiana University (Bloomington, Indiana).

6.8.1 Subjects and Methods

Stimulus voices were those of three young adult male graduate students, determined to be normal speakers, who read aloud a short passage adapted from Montagu (1958), chosen for its articulatory complexity and tendency to elicit speech errors:

> During eighteen-ninety to eighteen-ninety-seven, a young Dutch physician,
> Peter Brinker, journeyed to Java searching for the missing link. Brinker discovered

at Jesselton in central Java, a skull fragment, a thighbone, a lower jawbone fragment and three teeth. These looked strikingly manlike, though the skullcap looked quite primitive. An upright striding creature probably possessed this femur. The apelike superior skull surface and manlike femur suggested this descriptive label: erect ape man. (Andrews et al., 1977, p. 140)

Each voice was recorded in two conditions, sober and, 2 weeks later, intoxicated. In the intoxicated condition, 20 min prior to recording, each talker consumed three alcohol doses, each containing 1.5 oz of 80-proof vodka mixed with 3 oz of fruit juice and ice. Speakers reported feeling "considerably inebriated" at the time of recording. Voices were recorded and played back on a cassette tape recorder. Presentation was through two extended-range speakers.

Listeners were 27 students from advanced classes in voice and speech. The response measure was a perceptual inventory developed to study the perception of stuttered speech (Andrews & Smith, 1976). In the development of the instrument, 800 subjects rated the importance of 500 qualities to spoken communication. From these, 114 terms were then identified, representing 31 positive and 29 negative factors.

Each of the 114 scales was administered to each of the listeners three times: (a) subjects were asked to estimate the importance of the characteristic to any message; (b) subjects were asked to estimate the amount of the characteristic in either the sober or intoxicated recording of the passage; and (c) 2 days later, subjects were asked to estimate the amount of the characteristic in the alternate condition.

6.8.2 Results and Discussion

As listed in Table 6.8.1, seven factors were found to be significant in the differential perception of sober and intoxicated speech; these were Efficient, Reasonable, Self-Confident, Scholarly, Artistic, Theatrical, and Untrained.

TABLE 6.8.1   Means and Significance Levels of Differences between Perceptions of Sober and Intoxicated Speakers $(N = 27)$[a]

Factor	Sober	Intoxicated	t	p
Efficient	4.98	4.38	2.10	0.05
Reasonable	6.98	6.34	2.12	0.05
Self-confident	5.83	4.58	3.84	0.001
Scholarly	5.62	5.18	2.33	0.05
Artistic	2.50	2.06	2.29	0.05
Theatrical	2.06	1.40	2.34	0.05
Untrained	3.87	4.60	2.90	0.01

[a] From Andrews, Cox, and Smith (1977). Copyright © 1971 by Central States Communication Association. Used by permission.

Each factor included a number of different scales that helped to define and delimit it.

The factor *efficient* was measured best by the scales *skillful, efficient,* and *right.* The significance of this factor indicated a perception of lowering of economy and precision of speech resulting from alcohol intake. The factor *reasonable* was best represented by the scale *reasonable* and somewhat less so by *rational.* Results for voices in both the sober and intoxicated conditions rated above the midpoint for reasonableness, but voices in the sober condition were rated higher. The factor *self-confidence* was measured by *able, self-confident, self-assured, confident,* and *relaxed*; the latter two scales, however, showed high contamination. Alcohol appeared to affect this factor more than any other, and the difference for this factor between the two conditions was significant beyond the 0.001 level; this suggested a high degree of listener ability to detect changes in self-confidence after consumption of alcohol.

The factor *scholarly* was measured by *scholarly, skilled, intelligent,* and *expert,* with the best measure deriving from *scholarly* and *intelligent.* Voices in both conditions were rated above average on this scale, but the mean rating for sober recordings was considerably higher than for intoxicated ones. The factor *artistic* was measured by *admirable, adventurous, artistic, beautiful, bold,* and *colorful*; best were *artistic, beautiful, bold.* Voices in both conditions were rated extremely low in both conditions, but intoxicated voices were rated lower than sober ones. The factor *theatrical* was best measured by the scale *theatrical.* Ratings for both conditions were rated near the lower end of the scale, but worse so for the intoxicated condition.

Of the 29 negative factors, *untrained* showed the only significant contrast. This was best measured by the scales *inexperienced, self-conscious, tense, unsure,* and *untrained.* The mean rating for the intoxicated condition was significantly above the rating for the sober condition.

Finally, an overall index was derived from clusters of related scales, averaged and normalized. The midpoint of this overall scale was 1.125; the index for the sober condition was 0.99, for the intoxicated 0.88, and the difference was significant beyond the 0.01 level. Andrews et al. reported that listeners, upon being informed of the nature of the experiment, were surprised to learn that some of the voices were recorded after talkers had consumed alcohol. On this basis, Andrews et al. proposed that characteristics of intoxicated speech were not apparent from read passages.

The research reported in Andrews et al. is an early examination of the perception of alcohol-affected speech. Subsequent research (e.g., Klingholz et al., 1988; Künzel et al., 1992; Pisoni & Martin, 1989) also had perception components, but in those experiments, listeners were asked to determine (a) which of a pair of sentences was produced under alcohol, or (b) whether or not a sentence presented in isolation was produced under alcohol. The scaling technique used in Andrews et al. is not directly comparable to these other types of tasks, but it does provide evidence that alcohol does indeed induce changes in speech that are perceptible to listeners.

6.9 BEAM, GANT, & MECHAM, 1978

The purpose of this study was to determine whether communication deviations might be definable in the alcoholic population. When this article appeared, Sandi L. Beam was affiliated with the Division of Speech Pathology and Audiology at the University of Utah in Salt Lake City, Utah; Ralph W. Gant was affiliated with the Utah Division of Alcohol and Drugs and the Utah Division of Rehabilitation Services, Utah State Board of Education; and Merlin J. Mecham was affiliated with the Division of Speech Pathology and Audiology at the University of Utah.

6.9.1 Subjects and Methods

Subjects for this study were nine male (age range 30–60 years, mean 45.7 years) and six female (age range 26–50 years, mean 44.8 years) alcoholics. All had been diagnosed as alcoholics, but there were no other medical diagnoses, and none had received any speech or audiological diagnostic or intervention therapies in the past. All were from the lower and middle socioeconomic classes. Twelve subjects were native speakers of English, and four had learned English as a second language (accent was irrelevant in this study). All had at least average intelligence and education, and none were taking any medication that might impair their speech at the time of testing.

The study consisted of a number of tests to assess communication abilities. First, subjects were given an oral stereognosis test requiring them to identify four forms (e.g., a circle and a triangle) placed in their mouths. Second, oral diadochokinesis measured tongue-lip-palate mobilities during rapid successive movements. On this test, rates of fewer than eleven movements per 5 sec were deemed inadequate. Third, speech clarity was evaluated with a short articulation test. Fourth, the Carrow Elicited Language Inventory (Carrow-Woolfolk, 1974) was used to indicate short-term memory abilities for sentences, word-searching or substitutions, semantic distortions, and syntactic breakdowns. Fifth, subjects were given a pure-tone audiometric examination for thresholds between 250 and 8000 Hz. Last, in order to assess the voice characteristics of pitch, loudness, rate, quality, and resonance, the W. Johnson et al. (1963) criteria were applied to a 15-min speech sample; these were evaluated twice by the same clinician, using a five-point scale ranging from acceptable to severe impairment.

6.9.2 Results

On the oral stereognosis test, eleven of the fifteen subjects were unable to identify more than 50% of the objects (normal subjects identify 90%). Oral diadochokinesis showed that eleven subjects had overall rates of movement below that of normal adults. Fourteen subjects displayed at least one aspect of unacceptable voice quality. Of these, seven had noticeable interferences, and another seven had marked disorders. Two males in the latter group were diagnosed as spastic dysphonic. Twelve of the subjects presented with losses of hearing acuity: two mild, eight moderate, and two severe.

Misarticulation was moderate for individual words and acceptable for the age and linguistic backgrounds of the subjects. There were, however, problems with conversational speech, characterized by Beam et al. as "slurred or muffled"; factors contributing to the impression were inappropriate rate, intonation, articulation, and syntax. In the test of language abilities, eleven subjects displayed verbal-expressive breakdowns, and eight subjects showed a slowing in verbal information processing or verbal receptive facility; this was indicated by diminished ability to understand or process instructions. The Carrow Elicited Language Inventory indicated a moderate impairment for short-term memory for sentences and verbal reproduction, as indicated by inability to complete a sentence or reproduce tenses and articles correctly.

6.9.3 Discussion

This pilot study pointed out the persistence of speech anomalies in chronic alcoholics. Subjects in this study were diagnosed alcoholics, but all but one had been abstinent for between 3 weeks and 13 months (mean, 15.3 weeks; median and mode, 8.6 weeks). Although subjects appeared to fall within normal limits on the articulation test (with isolated words), the researchers did note anomalies (slurred or muffled speech) in conversational speech. Thus, the disturbances observed here are comparable either to those studies that elicited spontaneous conversational speech or, perhaps less convincingly, to those that required reading aloud of written passages. In the latter case, dysfluencies may not be directly comparable, because one of the categories in the present study was syntax, which would not be apparent in read passages.

This study was relatively wide ranging in terms of the types of measures made. However, the results of this study need to be considered within the context of other studies examining the same population (alcoholics), and such investigations are a decided minority in the literature on alcohol and speech. An early study, Romano et al. (1940) examined five patients, but descriptions of speech were unfortunately lacking in detail. Stein (1966) noted that the speech patterns of eleven recovering alcoholics did not deviate significantly from expected patterns for non-alcoholics; again, however, no details were available in the published report. Two studies examined acoustic patterns of the speech of alcoholic subjects: Fontan et al. (1978) and Niedzielska et al. (1994), but Beam et al. (1978) did not perform acoustic analyses. The study reported in Sobell and Sobell (1972) used alcoholic subjects, but they were also acutely intoxicated before measurements were made. Perhaps the best match for comparison of results is the study by Collins (1980), who compared syntactic performance in alcoholic and nonalcoholic adults. In this case, Collins found better performance on the standard measures among the nonalcoholic subjects. These results are consistent with those of Beam et al., who found diminished performance among the alcoholic subjects on the Carrow Elicited Language Inventory.

6.10 FONTAN, BOUANNA, PIQUET, AND WGEUX, 1978

This study was an instrumental investigation of the speech of hospitalized recovering alcoholics who, although evidencing some speech problems, did not present as dysarthric in the usual sense. The analysis revealed some consistent changes in speech affecting a wide range of segment types, including vowels, consonants, and glides. Fontan et al. considered the question of the precise relationship between the observed speech anomalies and the organic impairments brought on by alcoholism. At the time this work appeared, M. Fontan, J. M. Piquet, and F. Wgeux were affiliated with the Psychiatric Clinic at the Regional Hospital Center in Lille, France, while G. Bouanna was an Assistant of Phonetics at the University of Lille III.

6.10.1 Methods

Subjects were 38 alcoholic males, ages 21–58 years (mean = 40 years). Of these 38, 35 were being hospitalized for detoxification at the time of the study; three additional subjects had been abstinent for a number of years. Elicitation consisted of nondirected, spontaneous interviews lasting from 10 to 15 min. These took place in a quiet room, in which subjects were tape-recorded using a Sony Stereo tape recorder TC 630 . A microphone was placed approximately 30 cm away from the subject. Spectrographic analysis was performed using a Kay Sonograph, using a 300-Hz band-pass filter permitting analysis between 85 and 8000 Hz.

6.10.2 Results

6.10.2.1 Subjective Tape Analysis

Two of the tapes were not used because of strong dialectal pronunciations. In the remaining tapes, three types of articulatory anomalies were found.

In the first type, entire groups of words, including entire sentences, were unintelligible, even after repeated examination. The second type did not involve impairment of intelligibility at the discourse level, but there were syllable-level distortions necessitating repeated listenings. A third type involved a "general impression of haziness and masking"(p. 534), but careful listening was necessary for the investigators to perceive distortions. In fact, instrumental analysis was often necessary to clarify that the speech was in fact modified.

All of the subjects exhibited anomalous speech at least once, and there did not appear to be any relationship between these anomalies and extent or duration of addiction or sobriety. Anomalous speech was noted even for those subjects who had abstained for a relatively long period, although the investigators did notice a tendency for speech anomalies to be more frequent at the beginning of treatment.

6.10.2.2 Acoustic Analysis

Three tapes with background noise were eliminated from analysis. Passages from the remaining were selected according to three criteria: (a) speech had to be auditorily perceptible but could not impair intelligibility and had to be susceptible to segmentation; (b) as far as the corpus permitted, every sequence of phonemes was examined; (c) wherever possible, the researchers tried to find similar sounds in similar phonetic sequences at different places in the discourse and with different speakers.

Most anomalies appeared to be consistent with an articulatory laxing (French: *relâchement articulatoire)*, that is, an enlargement of the vocal tract, most consistently realized as excessive labialization. Elsewhere, however, there was evidence of articulatory reinforcement (French: *renforcement articulatoire)*. The entire phonetic system was affected by these anomalies, showing changes in vowels, consonants, and semivowels.

Two major changes were observed for vowels: (a) compacting and (b) inappropriate lengthening. The authors noted that compacting of vowels resulted from enlargement of the vocal tract, which could be attributed to excessive labialization. They noted that vowel spectra could be characterized as either *compact* (with formants relatively close together), as in the vowels [a ɔ œ ɑ̃ ɔ̃)] , or *diffuse* (with formants relatively far apart), as in the vowels [ɛ e o u y i ɛ̃)]. In the spectrograms, vowel compacting appeared as a lowering of F2 by approximately 300 Hz for round vowels and 700 Hz for spread vowels.

The second anomalous vowel articulation, inappropriate lengthening, was characterized by Fontan et al. as a reinforcement rather than as a laxing. They first noted that accented syllables in the normal sense are rare, because, although French words are generally accented on the final syllable, this accent is lost in favor of a phrasal accent. Accentuation of a vowel can be realized by an increase in either intensity or duration. However, they noted that in connected speech, intensity, rather than duration, is the usual way of realizing accent, and duration is employed only in special circumstances such as poetry. They further asserted that it is easier to lengthen a vowel with a low frequency (FØ) than one with a high frequency. The spectrograms revealed that some subjects, in contrast to normal spoken French, lengthened unaccented vowels, lengthened final vowels excessively, and lengthened spread vowels more than rounded vowels.

The spectrographic analysis also revealed changes in consonants. Although there were no changes in place of articulation, the following were noted: (a) change of voiceless to voiced, (b) change of stops to fricatives, (c) vocalization of the labiodental [v], and (d) aspiration of stops. The first three were considered to be weakening, the fourth strengthening. The change of voiceless segments to voiced segments was revealed spectrographically for stops by an absence of a white portion prior to the burst in low frequencies and by the lack of a return to zero on the sonority intensity curve. In fricatives, the spectrogram showed a more intense darkening in low frequencies and a very slight lowering of the sonority intensity curve. Both stops and fricatives were affected: no instances of the voiceless stops [p t k] could be isolated in the spectrograms, and among the fricatives, changes from [s] to [z] and from [ʃ] to [ʒ] were observed. Additionally, it was observed that the voicing of [b d g] actually increased.

Another weakening process, observed in all but five of the patients studied, was the change of stops to fricatives. In these cases, stop characteristics were absent spectrographically; that is, there was no white span (indicating occlusive silence), there was no burst, and there was a continuous dark area at high frequencies. All consonants thus appeared spectrographically as fricatives. Because no articulations, including stops, achieved complete closure, there was an emission of air corresponding to a fricative; these fricatives were at the same place of articulation and of the same voicing as the apparently targeted stop.

The third consonantal weakening was the vocalization of the voiced labiodental fricative [v]. Spectrographically, normal productions of this segment would appear as two areas of darkening, one at low frequencies indicating voicing and the other at midfrequencies (around 4000 Hz), corresponding to fricative noise. In the spectrograms from this study, however, it took on the appearance of a vowel; that is, there was a wide darkened band at low frequencies (up to approximately 1500 Hz). Actually, one of these vocalized [v]s could be considered a glide [w], with a somewhat more anterior place of articulation, corresponding to the excessive labialization noted above. For productions of [w], there was a marked loss of consonantal characteristics, so that these in turn appeared vowel-like.

One apparent strengthening process affected the consonants, the aspiration of voiceless stops. Spectrographically, this appeared as a dark area following the stop burst; concomitantly, there was a peak in the sonority curve, corresponding to a puff of air, following the usual trough for the consonant. This articulation could be considered reinforcing insofar as aspiration can be characteristic of voicelessness. All but four subjects exhibited this aspiration, and only voiceless stops were affected. Fontan et al. noted that the actual frequency of the phenomenon may not have been reflected in the task used in this study.

Twelve of the spectrograms proved difficult to segment, although some phonemes could be recognized, especially, the fricatives [s z ʃ] and the following vowels. The traces exhibited a constant vocalization, indicated by a concentration of energy in the lower frequencies, which Fontan et al. attributed to the excessive labialization noted earlier. Both voiced and voiceless stops appeared not to be present, as indicated by lack of a silent portion and plosive spike. The majority of segments were ill-formed or missing, evidence of extreme articulatory laxing.

Three types of anomalies could thus be distinguished in this study: (a) those amenable to analysis using the spectrograph, (b) those that resisted instrumental analysis, and (c) those that affected intelligibility. The first type was quite frequent; the latter two, although considered to be more serious deviations, were widely dispersed and intermittent within the corpus.

6.10.3 Discussion: Possible Etiologies

Fontan et al. further considered possible etiologies for the phonetic changes found in this study. They first distinguished, within alcoholism, transitory dysarthrias during acute episodes and dysarthrias indicative of constitutional changes. Two disparate types of cases were cited. In one case, one of the subjects was recorded during a period of acute, extreme intoxication, exhibiting impairment of coordination and equilibrium. The audiotape revealed sections of stammering and unintelligibility, as well as a number of hesitations. Many of the spectrograms, however, were quite interpretable: there was evidence of articulatory laxing for which the subject, apparently aware of his condition, was trying to compensate through inappropriate lengthening or aspirated stops. Three other cases concerned subjects whose long-term chronic alcoholism had apparently resulted in mental deterioration (e.g., confusion). Nevertheless, they did not sound dysarthric, nor did their spectrograms reveal the types of changes in alcoholized speech noted previously.

Fontan et al. cited a number of studies (Chevrie-Muller, Dordain, & Gremy, 1970; Chevrie-Muller & Grappin-Gilette, 1971; Dordain, Degos, & Dordain, 1971; Dordain & Dordain, 1972; Gremy, Chevrie-Muller, & Garde, 1967) incorporating oscillographic analyses of dysarthric speech in cases of bulbar/pseudobulbar and cerebellar syndromes. Bulbar syndromes resulted in articulatory insufficiency and a change in voice timbre. Cerebellar syndromes involved motor deficiencies, resulting in articulatory insufficiency and a "rough, slack, irregular, explosive, and scanning" voice (p. 539).

A comparison of the oscillographic and spectrographic results was also conducted. One similarity found in the two analytical methods was voicing of voiceless consonants in bulbar syndromes. Because oscillographic evidence would not indicate labialization and the resulting vowel compacting, there would be no basis for comparison between the present findings and those from either of the dysarthrias on this point. The main difference was in the fricatives, which were unaffected in the alcoholics but affected in the dysarthrics. The similarities, especially between the alcoholics and the bulbar palsy patients, pointed to articulatory laxing or insufficiency. Additionally, there was compensatory strengthening in all three cases. A definite conclusion was not possible on the basis of these comparisons, although evidence did seem to point to a neurological basis; nevertheless, a functional component, for example, a simple lack of attention, could not be necessarily excluded.

Finally, Fontan et al. considered the relative advantages and disadvantages of the type of spectrographic study undertaken here. The main disadvantage is that an acoustic analysis is just that, an analysis of the speech signal itself; it provides no direct view of the pathologies that might underlie or cause the changes such as the ones observed in this study. Other clinical methods would help, such as those that could uncover laryngeal pathologies, for example, electromyography or stroboscopy. On the other hand, spectrography is capable of uncovering very small differences in the speech signal, as well as purely functional articulatory anomalies. Furthermore, spectrography is a relatively simple, noninvasive technique for investigating at least one aspect of the effects of alcohol and alcoholism on speech.

Fontan et al. represents an early application of instrumental acoustic analysis to the study of alcohol and speech. A number of phenomena found in this study are reported elsewhere in the literature. For example, the phenomenon of *compacting*, that is, lowering of F2, is also reported in Pisoni et al. (1986) and in Behne and Rivera (1990), and vowel lengthening is reported by Künzel et al. (1992). Overall devoicing is also reported in Pisoni et al. (1986).

In spite of results that are consistent with other research, however, the usefulness of the report by Fontan et al. is diminished by at least two factors. First, no explicit measurement criteria or analysis techniques were provided, nor were specific measurements. Second, there was no explicit comparison of the results reported here with acoustic characteristics of speech produced by nonalcoholic talkers. These two factors together make it difficult to assess the true magnitude of the changes noted here, as they relate to normal speech, to speech produced under acute intoxication, and to speech produced under nervous system disorders.

6.11 COLLINS, 1980

This study investigated adult syntax with a statistical comparison of the syntactic performance of nonalcoholic and alcoholic adults. This work was based on the author's doctoral dissertation, and at the time this article appeared, he was affiliated with the John Jay College of Criminal Justice, City University of New York (New York, New York).

6.11.1 Method

Subjects were 39 males and females medically diagnosed as alcoholics who were members of resident alcoholism treatment programs. Subjects ranged from 22–55 years old and had been alcoholics for 2.0–30.0 years (mean: 13.88 years, median: 12.25 years, SD: 6.49 years). An additional 39 male and female nonalcoholics, matched for age, IQ, and years of education, served as controls. All subjects were white, native-born, American-educated speakers of American English. Subjects consumed no stimulants or depressants for 12 hr preceding the study. Subjects were first screened for sociolinguistic parameters, freedom from speech defects, and hearing acuity (puretone audiometric screening at 20-dB thresholds). IQ scores were obtained using the Quick Test (Ammons & Ammons, 1962).

For recording, a Sony TC-110 cassette recorder equipped with a Sony ECM-965 microphone were used. For audiometric screening, a Maico Model 19 was used. Samples of language were gathered using stimulus pictures from the Thematic Apperception Test (Murray, 1943); sampling of spontaneous speech continued until a minimum of 50 sentences or sentence attempts was obtained. Audio recordings were made of all elicitations., which were transcribed by the author and verified as to their accuracy by experts in linguistics and speech pathology.

The measurement of language development was the Developmental Sentence Scoring (DSS; Lee, 1974), used and normalized with children. Norms established for children were of course not applicable to adults; however, measures were used here to make comparisons between the alcoholic and nonalcoholic subjects. The DSS provides a numerical index of sentence complexity on the basis of eight grammatical items, as well as a measure of the degree of sentence completeness (sentence point). This determination is made by comparing the spontaneous language sample obtained with a sequence of developmental norms. The grammatical categories used in scoring are (a) indefinite pronouns; (b) personal pronouns; (c) main verbs;

(d) secondary verbs; (e) negatives; (f) conjunctions; (g) interrogative reversals; (h) *wh*-questions; and finally a "sentence point category": complete sentences received a "1," incomplete sentences a "0." Scores for each of the first eight grammatical categories could range from 1 through 8. Also obtained was a DSS score, the mean of the above nine categories.

A total of 3900 sentences or sentence attempts were analyzed. Mean scores were calculated for both the alcoholic and nonalcoholic groups in each of the grammatical categories, the sentence point score, and the DSS score. A correlated *t*-test determined significance of differences found between the two groups, and a coefficient of correlation was computed.

6.11.2 Results

In general, the language performance of alcoholics was similar or inferior to that of nonalcoholics. Performance of the nonalcoholics was better than that of the alcoholics in seven of the ten categories examined, although alcoholics outperformed nonalcoholics in the remaining three (negatives, conjunctions, and *wh*-questions). Of the differences found in performance for the ten categories, however, only three were significant. Nonalcoholics performed significantly better in two categories: sentence-point and DSS score; alcoholics scored higher in the category *wh*-questions. Other differences were not significant.

6.11.3 Discussion

Collins (1980) noted that although gross patterns of syntactic performance were similar for both the alcoholic and nonalcoholic group, a further general tendency was that nonalcoholics outperformed alcoholics. In terms of the developmental scoring used here, the syntax of the nonalcoholics could be characterized as more advanced and complete. Collins further noted that the significant difference in performance in the sentence-point category was largely attributable to three types of errors committed by the alcoholic group: (a) subject-verb agreement, (b) sentence fragments, and (c) semantic errors (non sequiturs, etc.). Collins attributed the superior performance in the wh-question category to a possible integrative language deficit. According to this line of reasoning, a *wh*-question "seeks information with minimal linguistic output on the part of the speaker" (p. 287). The alternative to a *wh*-question, a yes–no question, "must be used in combination with an information-laden structure that minimizes the need for a complex response" (p. 287).

6.12 STITZER, GRIFFITHS, BIGELOW, AND LIEBSON, 1981a

This study, a chapter from *Behavioral Pharmacology of Human Drug Dependence,* reviewed existing data supporting the interaction of drugs and social stimuli. Although a number of drugs and a number of behaviors were examined, discussion here is limited to alcohol and to verbal behavior. When this article appeared, the authors were affiliated with the Departments of Psychiatry at the Baltimore (Maryland) City Hospitals and the Johns Hopkins University School of Medicine in Baltimore, Maryland.

Stitzer et al. (1981a) proposed that two general classes of studies have been carried out to study drug and social behavior interactions, differing primarily in the subject populations studied and the methodologies used. The first type of study originates from work in drug abuse research. Subjects in these studies have a history of abuse, and experiments are generally conducted in inpatient research facilities. In these studies, drugs are typically self-administered to a maximum allowable dose. The categories of social behavior are defined in advanced, with operational scoring performed by institutional staff. Comparisons are generally made with observations gained during periods when the drugs are not available. In these studies, finally, there is no experimental control of the independent variable, that is, drug intake.

A second type of study originates in clinical psychopharmacology. In typical cases, such studies examine the effects of acute doses of drugs on normal volunteers or psychiatric patients. Study is generally of groups of two to four subjects seated together in an experimental situation. Verbal behavior is a typical dependent variable. The drug is administered to one member or multiple members of the group. Doses are generally acute, and the dose may be an independent variable. Observational techniques in these studies are both quantitative and qualitative and may involve automated equipment with voice-activated relays in the case of studies of verbal behavior.

Stitzer et al. pointed out that alcohol has been the most widely studied drug for its effect on verbal behavior (others have included barbiturate sedatives, stimulants, opiates, phenothiazine tranquilizers, benzodiazepine tranquilizers, marijuana, and hallucinogens). Two studies were cited that suggested an enhancement of social conversation by acute doses of alcohol. In R. C. Smith et al. (1975; see section 6.7 above), it was found that the effects of a dose of alcohol administered to both members of a social couple induced small increases in the amount of speech and increases in initiation and overlap. Pliner and Cappell (1974) found that when a 0.5 g/kg dose was administered to groups of volunteers, observational ratings on an "amusement index" showed higher scores for a group given alcohol than for one receiving a placebo.

Further confirmation of conversation facilitation was to be found in Stitzer, Griffiths, Bigelow, and Liebson (1981b). In this study, the amount of verbalization was recorded by throat- mounted microphones connected to voice-operated relays. Same-sex subject pairs met in 1-hr sessions daily for 5 days. One of the members of the pair received either test doses of alcohol or a placebo, while the other member of the pair received only the placebo. Doses in the amount of 1 to 6 oz of 95-proof alcohol consumed one-half hour prior to each session appeared to enhance the amount of vocalization for the partner receiving the alcohol, whereas the vocalization of the partner receiving the placebo remained for the most part unaffected. Additionally, the effect appeared to be dose-related.

Stitzer et al. found that evidence such as that above supported the proposal that alcohol in acute doses enhances verbal behavior among nonalcoholic volunteers. They found, however, no consistent results from studies of nonalcoholic volunteers allowed to self-administer alcohol chronically. For instance, McGuire, Stein, and Mendelson (1966) reported that (an unspecified dose of) alcohol increased socialization in three members of a four-person group. On the other hand, other investigators found no such effect.

Finally, Stitzer et al. (1981a) noted that among inpatient alcoholic subjects, chronic self-administration does appear to facilitate social behavior. Social behavior appears to remain intact with heavy drinking by alcoholics and drops off only after extremely high doses.

6.13 SOBELL, SOBELL, AND COLEMAN, 1982

Sobell et al. (1982) pointed out that only three studies examining the effect of alcohol on speech had been conducted up to this time: Zaimov (1969), Sobell and Sobell (1972), and Andrews et al. (1977). Collective results from these studies demonstrated that moderate to high doses of alcohol could cause dysfluency in both alcoholic and nonalcoholic subjects. In the present study, Sobell, Sobell, and Coleman compared the speech of nonalcoholic subjects who read a standardized paragraph across three conditions: (a) sober, (b) after a relatively small dose of alcohol, and (c) after a relatively large dose of alcohol. To make these comparisons, both human perceptual judgments and acoustic analysis were used. In addition, an ancillary study was conducted to examine vocal quality deviation and thereby to assess possible relationships between observed dysfluency and psychomotor impairment. The research for this article was conducted while Linda C. Sobell and Robert F. Coleman were affiliated with Vanderbilt University and the Dede Wallace Center Alcohol Programs in Nashville, Tennessee. When the article appeared, Linda C. Sobell and Mark B. Sobell were affiliated with the Clinical Institute of the Addiction Research Foundation in Toronto, Ontario, Canada, and with the University of Toronto, while Robert F. Coleman was affiliated with Eastern Virginia Medical School in Norfolk, Virginia.

6.13.1 Subjects and Methods

Subjects were 16 male undergraduate students ranging in age from 18–22 years (mean = 20 years). They were judged to be normal speakers who were moderate or social alcohol drinkers without drinking problems, as assessed by the Drinking Practices Questionnaire (Cahalan et al., 1969), the brief Michigan Alcoholism Screening Test (MAST) (Pokorny et al., 1972), and the CAGE questionnaire (Mayfield et al., 1974). No subject had a medical condition that contraindicated participation in the study. Subjects agreed to abstain from food and drink for 4 hr prior to the experiment.

The standardized passage read by the subjects was from Montagu (1958), which had also been used in the study reported as Andrews et al. (1977). Speech samples were recorded in a sound-treated room on a Revox A-77 stereo tape recorder, using a Bruel & Kjaer microphone placed 6 to 8 in. in front of the subject. Spliced samples were re-recorded onto an identical machine. The samples were elicited in a single session under three conditions. In the first condition, subjects had 0.00% BACs (no alcohol), as measured by an Alco-Analyzer gas chromatograph (Model 1000). In the second condition, subjects read the same passage after consuming a dose of 190-proof grain alcohol mixed with 4 parts of chilled tonic water. This dose was prepared according to a formula of 0.345 g 190-proof alcohol per kg body weight and was designed to raise BACs to a peak of 0.05%. The dose was administered approximately in thirds over a 10-min period. Ten minutes after completion of consumption of this dose (moderate dose), subjects gargled, rinsed, and read the passage for the second sample. Immediately subsequent to completion of the reading the gas chromatograph was used to assess BACs.

After this breath analysis, subjects consumed a dose of alcohol identical to the first; the combination of the first (moderate) dose and this dose (high dose) was designed to raise BACs to a peak of 0.10%. As with the first dose, subjects repeated the wait, gargle, rinse sequence and then read the passage for the third time. Again, immediately after completion of the reading, BACs were assessed with the gas chromatograph.

Three tapes were prepared for listening. Ordering of subjects and conditions were partially counterbalanced across the three tapes. Listeners were nine graduate students, trained in speech pathology but naive to the nature of the experiment. The scores from two judges were reported by Sobell et al. to be "extremely aberrant" and were excluded from analysis; the remaining seven scores were averaged to produce a single score for each sample. The judges rated the speech samples using the following categories: (a) articulation, (b) nasality, (c) inflection, (d) speaking rate, and (e) drunkenness. Evaluation entailed placing a point along a 15-mm line, labeled only at its endpoints as "very good" and "poor." Before the actual evaluation, judges heard a tape providing examples of the first four rating dimensions. No training was provided for evaluation of the fifth dimension, "drunkenness," and judges were asked to rate this category according to any previous experience with intoxicated speech.

The acoustic analysis of the speech samples was conducted according to the following parameters: (a) fundamental frequency, (b) amplitude, and

(c) speaking rate. Fundamental frequency was measured using a Fundamental Frequency Indicator (see Baken, 1987; Hollien, 1990). Speaking rate was measured as the total time for reading the passage, including pauses and errors. Amplitude was analyzed as the average of amplitude peaks across the reading sample.

6.13.2 Results

Although the prescribed dose of 0.345-g 95% alcohol per kg of body weight had been designed to raise BACs to a peak of 0.05% in the moderate condition and 0.10% in the high condition, Sobell et al. reported that most subjects did not achieve the desired peak BACs. Some possible causes of this included individual variability, short duration of peak BAC, and differential adipose tissue density.

In the high-dose condition, further examination revealed considerable between-subject variability, but interestingly (and unexpectedly), subjects fell into two well-defined groups. Half (eight) of the subjects had BACs ≥ 0.079% (not 0.79% as reported in the text of the article), and the other eight subjects had considerably lower BACs. Details are given in Table 6.13.1. On the basis of this dichotomy, actual peak BAC was employed as a between-subjects factor in further analyses.

As shown in Table 6.13.2, a significant effect of alcohol dose for speaking rate and amplitude were found. There were no other significant effects. For speaking rate, the authors found that a significantly longer time was required to read the passage in the high-dose condition than in the moderate-dose or no-alcohol conditions. No further significant differences were observed between the moderate-dose and no-alcohol conditions. Amplitude was found to be significantly higher in the no-alcohol condition than in either the

TABLE 6.13.1 Comparison of Alcohol Dose and Actual Peak Blood-Alcohol Levels for All Subjects and for Subjects Grouped as Having Attained Levels < 0.079% and ≥ 0.079%[a, b]

| | Alcohol dose administered | | | |
| | Moderate (expected BAL = 0.050%) | | High (expected BAL = 0.100%) | |
Group	Mean	Range	Mean	Range
All subjects (*n* = 16)	0.026	0.016–0.051	0.078	0.045–0.117
Peak BAL ≥ 0.079% (*n* = 8)	0.028	0.016–0.051	0.098	0.079–0.117
Peak BAL < 0.079% (*n* = 8)	0.023	0.018–0.027	0.058	0.045–0.073

[a] From Sobell, Sobell, and Coleman (1982). Copyright © 1982 by S. Karger AG, Basel. Used by permission.
[b] All blood-alcohol level (BAL) values are in grams of alcohol per 100 ml of blood volume.

TABLE 6.13.2   Mean Scores for Rate and Amplitude as a Function of Alcohol Dose for 16 Nonalcoholic Subjects[a]

	Alcohol dose[b]		
	No alcohol	Moderate	High
Rate (sec)	31.19 (a)	31.88 (b)	34.19 (c)
Amplitude (dB)	73.59 (d)	72.83 (e)	73.19 (f)

[a] From Sobell, Sobell, and Coleman (1982). Copyright © 1982 by S. Karger AG, Basel. Used by permission.

[b] $p < 0.01$ by Newman-Keuls test for (c) vs. (b), (c) vs. (a), (d) vs. (e); and $p < 0.05$ for (d) vs. (f).

moderate- or high-dose conditions, and no significant difference was revealed between the moderate- and high-dose conditions. Again, no significant effects were found for fundamental frequency.

In the analysis of vocal quality dimensions, significant main effects for alcohol dose were found for articulation, speaking rate, and drunkenness, and no significant main or interaction effects for the remaining dimensions nasality or inflection. To the human judges, subjects sounded more drunk, less articulate, and slower in the high-dose condition than in either the moderate-dose or no-alcohol conditions.

6.13.3 Discussion

The results of this study demonstrated that consumption of alcohol affects vocal quality and that furthermore, these effects are dose-related. Of the three acoustic parameters, two were affected by alcohol. Of the five vocal quality dimensions, three were affected, as BAC increased.

The high-dose condition was found to be the most important factor in changes in vocal quality and acoustic dimensions, with one exception. Although most parameters showed a significant difference between the high-dose condition, on the one hand, and moderate-dose/no-alcohol conditions, on the other, a significant effect for amplitude was found between the no-alcohol condition and the moderate-dose condition; in this case, amplitudes were significantly higher in the no-alcohol condition.

Sobell et al. pointed out that the significantly longer reading time in the high-dose condition was consistent with earlier findings, in particular, the findings of Sobell and Sobell (1972). Although speaking rate was affected by the high-dose and amplitude by the moderate dose, no effect for either dose was found for fundamental frequency. Sobell et al. offered some possible explanations for this. It might have been that the ability to self-monitor pitch remained unaffected by alcohol, or the sampling method may not have been sensitive enough to small perturbations in frequency (*jitter*).

Among the vocal quality dimensions, speaking rate, articulation, and drunkenness were significantly affected by the high alcohol dose, but nasality and inflection remained unaffected by either dose. Sobell et al. pointed out that nasality is often difficult to judge, especially by human listeners, and also, since FØ was unaffected (see above), the related perceptual measurement, inflection, might also be expected to remain unaffected. Finally, Sobell et al. pointed out the "curious finding" that the alcohol dose (in this case, either high or moderate) appeared to be the primary determinant of speech dysfluency, rather than the actual peak BAL. This might be attributable to high between-subjects variability found in this study.

CHAPTER 7

Research Review III: 1985–1996

7.0 OVERVIEW

In the previous two chapters, we discussed 22 articles on alcohol and speech appearing from 1915 to 1982, a span of almost 70 years. In this chapter, we discuss more than that number appearing since 1985. Except for the literature on social and verbal interaction, the review of the research literature on alcohol and speech in these three chapters is very nearly exhaustive, so that as much research was reported from 1985 to 1996 as had been in the seven decades prior.

What might account for this sudden proliferation of research on alcohol and speech? One answer is that the impression of sudden and widespread interest in this type of research is only illusory. Of the 25 works discussed in this chapter, 15 come from just two laboratories, one in Wiesbaden, Germany (5 works), and the other in Bloomington, Indiana (10 works). Furthermore, between these two research groups, all of their reports in the literature represent just two laboratory experiments and one case study.

However, if massive growth of interest is in fact illusory, it is nevertheless true that growth of the literature itself is not, and this can be attributed to the approach to research on alcohol and speech taken by investigators since 1985. Just two approaches inform almost all of the research reported in this chapter: acoustic-phonetic and, to a somewhat lesser extent, phoniatric-logopedic. Of the independent research published since 1985, the only work not within one of these two realms is Higgins and Stitzer (1988), which reported on the amount of speech produced by subjects in isolation (without a social context) under the acute effects of alcohol. All of the remaining research approached the topic through analyses of the effects of alcohol either on the acoustic signal or on the vocal organs used to generate speech. And, it is most certainly the acoustic analyses and the wide-spread availability of computer instrumentation that are responsible for the large growth in the literature.

Research from both the Wiesbaden group and the Bloomington group are first and foremost acoustic studies, whether involving analysis of speech or analysis of voice. If one reads between the lines in almost any of the research from either of these two groups, there is a discrepancy between the amount of data collected and the amount of data analyzed and reported. Even given the possibility of negative results, it remains a fact that speech is an extremely rich acoustic signal, with a multitude of variables and parameters susceptible to measurement. Furthermore, even with the aid of powerful, fast computer technology, instrumental methods in speech analysis are still extremely labor- and time-intensive techniques, requiring enormous amounts of analysis time from highly skilled scientists. Considering one or all of the reports from the Wiesbaden and Bloomington groups, it is clear that not all of the recorded speech materials have yet been analyzed, not all of the subjects have been accounted for, and, most importantly, not all of the possible measurements have been made. This last fact is an important one for future research, for with high-quality tape recording or better yet, direct digital storage, raw speech data are well preserved, and as new analysis techniques are developed, they can be applied to existing speech data. Maintenance of digital records such as these permits new results and replication using exactly the same speech samples. For example, the last report discussed in this chapter (Cummings et al., 1996) applies new analysis techniques to data collected over 10 years before for the first report discussed (Pisoni et al., 1985). Research findings reported in the literature since 1985 thus represent only the tip of the iceberg of possible results; even if no other human subjects participate in any other experiments, refined and improved acoustic analysis could generate important new results into the 21st century.

Reports from the Bloomington group are of two types. In the early 1980s, research was undertaken at Indiana University under contract with General Motors Research Laboratories to investigate the feasibility of an ignition interlock system for automobiles based on speech-analysis techniques, preventing ignition if on-board equipment determined from the speech signal that a potential driver was intoxicated. To that end, a study was conducted to find reliable acoustic cues or markers in the speech signal indicating intoxication. Then, in 1989, after the grounding of the U.S. tankship *Exxon Valdez,* the Bloomington researchers were retained by the National Transportation Safety Board to analyze tape-recorded radio transmissions to determine if the ship's captain was intoxicated around the time of the grounding.

Research from the Indiana University/General Motors study are Pisoni et al. (1985, 1986), Pisoni and Martin (1989), Behne and Rivera (1990), and Behne et al. (1991). These studies found that both experienced and naive listeners were able to determine at above-chance levels (a) which of two presented sentences was produced under alcohol and (b) whether or not a single sentence presented in isolation was produced under alcohol. Consistent speech errors produced under alcohol included vowel and consonant lengthening, consonant deletion, deaffrication, distortion of the phoneme /s/, devoicing, and velarization. Acoustic measurement of intoxication included increased word and sentence durations, increased duration of stop closure, incomplete stop closure in affricates, postvocalic devoicing, lowered F2 and F3, reduction in the ratio of intervowel-to-word duration, higher mean amplitude and fundamental frequency, and increased variability in amplitude and fundamental frequency. Another more recent report, using the same acoustic analysis techniques developed in the earlier Bloomington studies, is Dunlap et al. (1995). Dunlap et al. found reliable increases in total sentence durations from prealchohol to postalcohol recordings. Finally, a new analysis of the General Motors data is reported in Cummings et al. (1996). Using inverse filtering, the glottal waveform can be analyzed alone, without vocal tract characteristics. Cummings et al. found reliable differences in jitter and shimmer measurements between speech produced with and without alcohol.

Publications from the Bloomington group discussed in this chapter regarding the *Exxon Valdez* are K. Johnson et al. (1989, 1990) and Pisoni et al. (1991). Tape recordings from the *Exxon Valdez* were available from a number of time intervals around the time of the grounding. In analyzing the captain's speech, the Bloomington researchers found changes around the time of the grounding consistent with previous laboratory findings, including changes on a least three levels: gross effects, segmental effects, and suprasegmental effects. Gross effects included error revisions, in which Captain Hazelwood produced an error and then corrected himself. Segmental effects included a number of misarticulations of liquid and sibilant consonants and word-final devoicing. Finally, suprasegmental effects included reduced speaking rate and change in pitch range.

Forensic aspects of this research were in fact the driving force behind the research program of the Wiesbaden group, whose members were affiliated with various law enforcement agencies in Germany. The research was multidisciplinary, with acoustic-phonetic, perceptual, and phoniatric-logopedic components. Reports from this research project include four addresses: Künzel (1990, 1992), Braun (1991), Eysholdt (1992), and one monograph: Künzel et al. (1992). In the acoustic-phonetic area, findings included changes in nasality, segmental lengthening, incomplete articulations, changes in fundamental frequency, reduction in speaking rate, and increases in the number and duration of pauses. The perceptual findings replicated the results of the Bloomington group: untrained listeners could determine above chance whether a sentence presented in isolation was produced under intoxication or not. The phoniatric-logopedic analysis investigated changes in the voice as well as direct observation of the pharynx using endoscopy and stroboscopy. No morphological changes in the larynx were found, but there was a decrease in vocal-fold amplitudes and mucosal waves . Changes in voice included slight dysphonia and increases in fundamental frequency range and maximum phonation time. Thus, alcohol was shown to produce changes in both phonation and articulation.

A third group of researchers, affiliated with the University of Florida and the Veterans Administration Medical Center, both in Gainesville, Florida, are represented here by Hollien and Martin (1996). This study continues the type of analysis exemplified by the Bloomington and Wiesbaden groups, that is, a combination of instrumental and perceptual analyses. Results from the Gainesville group included (a) correlation of subject behavior with physiological measures of intoxication, (b) changes in FØ and increases in misarticulations, and (c) increases in task-completion time on passage reading and diadochokinetic tasks. Perhaps most importantly, however, this research addresses several important methodological problems of research on alcohol and speech.

With the exception of Higgins and Stitzer (1988), the remaining research discussed in this chapter followed one or another of the research lines undertaken by the Bloomington, Wiesbaden, and Gainesville groups. Klingholz et al. (1988) examined recognition of intoxication based on automated acoustic analysis of the speech signal. Signal-to-noise ratio (SNR) distributions, fundamental frequency distributions, and long-term average power spectra could discriminate between sober and intoxicated conditions with error rates less than 5%, and a combination of SNR and fundamental frequency produced correct discrimination in all cases. The ratio of F1/F2 showed wide variance in its ability to discriminate, and changes appeared only at higher levels of intoxication. In his doctoral dissertation and a subsequent article, Swartz (1988, 1992) examined the effects of alcohol on voice onset time (VOT) and determined that this was in fact resistant to the effects of alcohol.

The report from the National Transportation Safety Board (NTSB) (1990) included analyses of the *Exxon Valdez* tapes from two independent research groups, Linda Sobell and Mark Sobell in Toronto (whose research was discussed in Chapter 6) and Pisoni and his colleagues in Bloomington, Indiana. In the same vein, Brenner and Cash (1991), investigators with the NTSB, reviewed the relevant research on alcohol and speech and its application to the *Exxon Valdez* case. Four main effects of alcohol on speech played a role in the safety board's determination that Captain Hazelwood was intoxicated: decrease in speaking rate, speech errors, misarticulations, and changes in vocal quality.

More recently, Niedzielska et al. (1994) performed acoustic analyses of the speech of control subjects and two groups of alcohol-dependent subjects (short- and long-term). Analysis of mean and maximum jitter values, harmonic structure, periodicity-to-aperiodicity ratios in vowels, and intonation variability revealed differences between the control group and both of the alcoholic groups. Furthermore, differences between the two alcoholic groups indicated only functional changes in the more short-term alcoholics but organic changes in the more long-term alcoholics.

K. Johnson et al. (1993) conducted electropalatographic and electroglottographic investigations of four talkers at five alcohol concentrations. Using these physiological techniques, they found that changes in speech and voice were sporadic rather than all-encompassing and proposed a model incorporating random noise and selective attention to account for the pattern of results. Watanabe et al. (1994) investigated the effects of alcohol using both acoustic analysis and fiberscopic examination of the hypopharyngeal and laryngeal mucosa. Acoustic results were consistent with previous findings from the Bloomington and Wiesbaden groups, including lowered fundamental frequency, increase in frequency range of phonation, decrease in mean airflow, and changes in vowels. However, contrary to the findings of Künzel et al. (1992), Watanabe et al. did find changes in the vocal folds, including capillary dilation, edema, and vocal-fold injection.

The research conducted during the period beginning around 1985 was thus narrowed from the eclectic research of previous periods and centered on acoustic and phonetic analysis of the speech signal. However, as an examination of the relevant literature will show, within acoustics and phonetics there is an amazingly wide range of analysis procedures and measurements, so that the large amount of research conducted on alcohol and speech summarized in this chapter can only be expected to continue.

7.1 PISONI, HATHAWAY, AND YUCHTMAN, 1985

This research report and the publication in section 7.2 (Pisoni et al., 1986) are essentially the same. Both emanated from a research program conducted under a contract between General Motors Research Laboratories (Warren, Michigan) and Indiana University; the research was conducted in the Psychophysiology and Speech Research Laboratories in the Department of Psychology at Indiana University (Bloomington, Indiana, USA). Pisoni et al. (1985) is the final report to the GM Research Laboratories, and Pisoni et al. (1986) is the published version of that report. Although the published version (1986) is more widely available (the 1985 version is essentially an internal document), the 1985 report is more complete, and so we discuss this research here. Other reports from the same research project are Pisoni and Martin (1989), Behne and Rivera (1990), and Behne et al. (1991).

As originally conceived, the project had the following major goals: (a) to determine if reliable and consistent changes could be observed in an acoustic analysis of speech obtained under laboratory conditions in which the talkers were intoxicated to known BACs, and (b) to determine if human listeners could reliably discriminate and identify intoxicated speech. The laboratory conditions design feature mentioned in (a) was especially important, because, as the researchers noted, only one previous experiment (Sobell et al., 1982) had previously investigated the effects of alcohol on speech under laboratory conditions, but this study had not controlled for or specified actual alcohol concentration. Pisoni et al. reported two perceptual experiments, a phonetic transcription study, and two sets of acoustic analyses.

7.1.1 Perceptual Studies and Phonetic Transcription

7.1.1.1 Preparation of Materials

Materials for recording included both auditory and visual stimuli. The auditory stimuli were 204 monosyllabic words and 66 sentences prerecorded in citation format by a male talker in the following manner. The stimuli were recorded in a sound-attenuated IAC (Industrial Acoustics Company; New York, New York) booth with an Electro-Voice (Model D054) microphone fed to an Ampex AG-500 tape recorder. Stimuli were low-pass filtered at 4.8 kHz and digitized at a 10-kHz sampling rate through a 12-bit A/D converter. The stimuli were edited into separate stimulus files using a digital waveform editor running on a PDP 11/34 computer (Digital Equipment Corp.). Four stimulus tapes were constructed by outputting the digital waveforms through a 12-bit D/A converter, low-pass filtering at 4.8 kHz, and recording them on audiotape at 7.5 ips.

Two of the test tapes thus constructed contained first the isolated words with 1 sec of silence between words. These were followed by all of the stimulus sentences recorded with 3 sec of silence between sentences. A different random ordering of both words and sentences was used for each of the two tapes. The two remaining tapes were made in a similar manner, except that all of the sentences preceded all of the isolated words.

The visual stimuli consisted of 38 isolated spondees (disyllabic words consisting of two stressed syllables, e.g., *inkwell, sundown*), 15 complete sentences, and 3 passages of meaningful connected text (i.e., paragraph length or longer). The spondees and sentences were presented to talkers on a cathode-ray tube (CRT) display; the passages were typewritten separately on white paper.

7.1.1.2 Recording of Talkers

A set of recordings was made for all five studies reported here and formed a digital database. Talkers were nine male students, recruited through a newspaper advertisement and paid for their participation. All nine were at least 21 years old and native speakers of English with no history of speech, language, or hearing problems. Screening for these subjects included the Michigan Alcoholism Screening Test (Selzer, Vinokur, & Van Rooijen, 1975), the MacAndrew Scale (MacAndrew, 1965), the socialization subscale of the California Psychological Inventory (Gough, 1969), and an alcohol consumption questionnaire. Subjects were limited to those determined to be moderate social drinkers at a low risk for alcoholism. Subjects were requested to abstain from consumption of food and drink for at least 4 hr prior to commencement of the experiment. Talker characteristics for the four subjects used in this study are summarized in Table 7.1.1, which includes ages; blood-alcohol concentrations (BACs) at the beginning (Initial BAC) and end (Final BAC) of recording; scores on the Michigan Alcoholism Screening Test (MAST), socialization subscale, and MacAndrew Scale; and self-reported total alcohol intake during the 30 days prior to the experiment (converted to ounces of 200-proof alcohol).

Each talker participated in two recording sessions, once without and once with alcohol. Sessions were counterbalanced, with half the talkers intoxicated and the other half of the talkers sober in the first session. In the control condition, talkers were tested with a Smith and Wesson Breathalyzer (Model 900A) to ensure there was no alcohol in their systems. For alcohol recording sessions, talkers were first weighed and given a breath test. The alcohol preparation consisted of one part 80-proof vodka to three parts orange juice for a dose of 1-g alcohol/kg body weight, designed to raise BAC to 0.10% over a period of 45 min. During this time period, approximately one-third of the preparation was consumed in each of three 15-min

TABLE 7.1.1 Talkers' Ages, Blood-Alcohol Concentrations (BACs) at the Beginning and End of Recording, Test Scores,[a] and Self-Reported Total Alcohol Intake[b, c]

Talker	Age	Initial BAC	Final BAC	MAST	SOC	MAC	Alcohol intake
1	26	.10%	.10%	2	35	22	6.15
2	21	.17%	.10%	5	30	27	16.8
3	21	.15%	.10%	6	36	24	8.94
4	22	.16%	.10%	3	39	23	3.53

[a] MAST, Michigan Alcoholism Screening Test; SOC, socialization scale; MAC, MacAndrew scale.
[b] Self-reported alcohol intake during the previous 30 days (converted to number of ounces of 200-proof alcohol).
[c] From Pisoni, Hathaway, and Yuchtman (1985). Used by permission.

periods. After consumption of the entire dosage, subjects rinsed their mouths, and BAC was measured. If BAC was less than 0.10%, the same dose was repeated. Audio recordings were then made when BAC was at least 0.10%. Subjects were naive to the actual purpose of the experiment and were informed only that the study was to examine the effects of alcohol on memory and on shadowing and reading.

Audio recordings were collected in a sound-attenuated booth. Talkers wore a matched and calibrated pair of TDH-38 headphones with an EV C090 LO-2 microphone attached to a boom, 4 in. in front of the mouth. Recordings were made on an Ampex AG-500 tape recorder. Recording levels were adjusted for each subject at the beginning of the first session and then held constant across both sessions.

In the shadowing task, half of the sober talkers and half the intoxicated talkers heard and repeated the sentences first. The remaining talkers heard and repeated isolated words first. Talkers were instructed to listen carefully to each stimulus sentence or word and then to repeat it quickly aloud (i.e., to shadow) as soon as possible. After the shadowing task, spondees and sentences were presented on a CRT controlled by a computer. The orders sentences:words or words:sentences were maintained from the shadowing task. Presentation rate in this task was controlled by the subjects, who pressed a button for presentation of the next item. In the passage-reading task, subjects were instructed to read each passage aloud at a normal rate.

Subjects who had received alcohol took a final BAC test after completion of all recordings and were then transported home in a prepaid taxi.

7.1.1.3 Perceptual Experiments

Two perceptual experiments were conducted: listeners in the first experiment (Perceptual Experiment I) were six Speech Research Laboratory staff members. Listeners in the second experiment (Perceptual Experiment II) were 21 undergraduate students from an introductory psychology course. Listeners in Perceptual Experiment I participated as part of their regular laboratory duties, whereas listeners in Perceptual Experiment II participated in order to fulfill a curriculum requirement.

Stimulus materials for both experiments were 34 of the shadowed sentences obtained in both conditions. Each sentence contained one or two "key words," which contained a range of phonemes with special emphasis on fricative clusters. The recorded sentences from all four talkers were low-pass filtered at 9.6 kHz and digitized at a 20-kHz sampling rate through a 12-bit A/D converter. Speech samples from Talkers 1 and 2 were also low-pass filtered at 4.8 kHz and digitized at a 20-kHz sampling rate.

The thirty-four sentences were extracted for each talker in both conditions. Two tests (A and B) of matched pairs of sentences were formed by digitally splicing together a sentence produced in the sober condition with its corresponding production in the intoxicated condition from the same talker. One second of silence separated the sentences in each pair. The sentences in Test A were randomly ordered, and the sentences in Test B were in the opposite order.

In Perceptual Experiment I, listeners heard taped renditions of sentences produced by Talkers 3 and 4 from Set A. Sentences were blocked by talker and recorded in random order with 4 sec of silence between each of the sentence pairs. For Perceptual Experiment II, two audiotapes were made with sentences from all four talkers. One of the tapes contained randomized pairs of sentences separated by 4 sec of silence and blocked by talker. The second tape for Perceptual Experiment II contained randomized pairs of sentences separated by 4 sec of silence and blocked by talker. The two tapes in Perceptual Experiment II each contained a different talker order. Stimuli from Talkers 1 and 2 were the recordings with a frequency cutoff at 4.9 kHz; for Talkers 3 and 4 the cutoff was 9.8 kHz.

The procedure used in the perceptual tests was an A–B forced-choice task. Subjects listened to each pair of sentences and had to decide which of the pair was produced when the talker was intoxicated. Subjects were told that only one sentence of each pair was spoken under this condition. Responses were recorded by circling either A or B for each pair of sentences on an answer sheet. All listeners in Perceptual Experiment I heard the same tape; in Perceptual Experiment II, half of the listeners heard one tape, and half the other. In addition to their A–B responses, subjects were also asked to provide a confidence rating for each pair of sentences indicating their degree of certainty in the response. For each response, subjects were asked to rate their confidence on a scale of 1 to 5: 1 indicated that subjects were "just guessing," 2 "not sure," 3 "probably right," 4 "sure," and 5 "very sure."

7.1.1.4 Phonetic Transcriptions

Two listeners trained in phonetic transcription made independent narrow transcriptions of the key words in the sentences from all four talkers under both conditions using one of the tapes also used in Perceptual Experiment II. The transcribers were unaware of which of each pair of sentences was produced under intoxication, and each of the transcribers heard and transcribed the tape twice. Disagreements after the first listening were noted for special attention at the second listening, but discrepancies were otherwise not resolved.

7.1.1.5 Perceptual Experiments and Phonetic Transcriptions: Results

Individual percent correct scores for the six listeners from Perceptual Experiment I were 92.6, 88.2, 66.2, 77.9, 77.9, and 91.2%. All listeners performed above chance, and the mean proportion of correct responses was

82.4% (SD = 10.2%). Mean proportion correct responses for Talker 3 was
82.8% (SD = 18.1%) and for Talker 4, 81.9% (SD = 19.0%). The correlation between confidence ratings and accuracy of responses was high. As indicated in Table 7.1.2, confidence rose as accuracy rose.

Results from Perceptual Experiment II were similar to those from the first perceptual experiment, although overall, listeners in Perceptual Experiment II were less accurate than those in Perceptual Experiment I. The mean proportion of correct responses across all 21 listeners was 73.8% (SD = 06.5%). Table 7.1.3 gives individual mean percent correct responses for each of the listeners. Mean percentage of correct responses for the four talkers were as follows: Talker 1, 72.3% (SD = 6.5%); Talker 2, 70.0% (SD = 21.3%); Talker 3, 80.3% (SD = 14.9%); Talker 4, 72.7% (SD = 15.9%). Similar to results from Perceptual Experiment I, listeners' confidence ratings correlated highly with their response accuracy. As Table 7.1.4 indicates, the more confident a listener was in responding, the more likely the response was correct. Both experienced and naive listeners could thus identify, above chance, a sentence produced while the talker was intoxicated in an A-B paired-comparison task.

For phonetic transcription, interjudge reliability was calculated as the percentage agreement between the two transcribers on the key words for all speakers in both conditions after the second listening. In this task, the transcribers agreed on 296 of the 304 key words, or about 97.3% of the time. In descending order of frequency, the following were the speech errors or changes in speech recorded by the transcribers in the sentences produced under intoxication (devoicing and palatalization, occurred with equal frequency): (a) vowel lengthening, (b) deletions and partial articulations, (c) deaffrication, (d) s-distortions, (e) consonant lengthening, (f) devoicing, (g) palatalization. Table 7.1.5 shows the number of each type of error occurring in both conditions. As can be seen, there was a clear increase in number of speech errors in the intoxicated condition over the sober condition.

TABLE 7.1.2   Percent Correct by Rating Category (First Perceptual Experiment)[a]

Rating category	Number correct	Number of times used	Percent correct	Standard deviation (%)
1	18	37	35.9	21.7
2	55	86	64.0	22.8
3	109	126	83.6	12.4
4	78	81	93.8	08.0
5	76	78	98.2	03.1

[a] From Pisoni, Hathaway, and Yuchtman (1985). Used by permission.

TABLE 7.1.3 Performance of Listeners
(Second Perceptual Experiment)[a]

Listener number	Mean percent correct
1	64.0
2	73.5
3	69.9
4	77.9
5	85.3
6	74.3
7	69.9
8	77.2
9	73.5
10	73.5
11	80.1
12	67.6
13	64.0
14	71.3
15	74.3
16	82.4
17	70.6
18	83.1
19	69.9
20	83.8
21	64.0
Mean	73.8%
SD	06.5%

[a] From Pisoni, Hathaway, and Yuchtman (1985).
Used by permission.

Vowel lengthening was the most common speech change, occurring 14 times in the intoxicated condition. Second most prevalent was consonant deletion or partial articulation. Most frequently deleted or partially articulated were the liquids [l r], followed by [n] and [ŋ], and finally [d] (two occurrences). There were six occurrences of deaffrication in the intoxicated

TABLE 7.1.4 Percent Correct by Rating Category (Second Perceptual Experiment)[a]

Rating category	Number correct	Number of times used	Percent correct	Standard deviation (%)
1	245	434	58.4	18.0
2	430	637	66.1	09.1
3	684	914	75.4	10.8
4	476	563	86.5	08.9
5	273	308	92.8	11.5

[a] From Pisoni, Hathaway, and Yuchtman (1985). Used by permission.

TABLE 7.1.5   Total Transcribed Errors in Key Words[a]

Error	Sober	Intoxicated
Vowel lengthening	1	14
Deletions and partial articulations	0	13
Deaffrication	1	6
[s]-distortions	0	4
Consonant lengthening	0	2
Devoicing	0	1
Palatalization	0	1

[a] From Pisoni, Hathaway, and Yuchtman (1985).

condition, three affecting the voiced affricate and three the voiceless. One occurrence of apparent deaffrication of [ts] (in the word *it's*) was noted in the sober condition. Distortion of [s] was observed four times; in two cases the production was palatalized (approaching [ʃ]), and in two cases it was dentalized. Consonant lengthening affected [ŋ] once word finally and [s] once in a cluster. Additionally, the voiced affricate was devoiced once, and the liquid [l] was velarized once.

7.1.2 Acoustic Analyses

In addition to the perceptual and transcription studies, acoustic analyses were performed on the recordings. These analyses were of two types; first, a sentence-level analysis of global measures of duration, energy, and voicing; and second, a segmental analysis examining the acoustic correlates of several classes of sounds in the frequency and temporal domains.

7.1.2.1 Materials, Digital Signal Processing, and
Analysis Parameters

Materials for the acoustic analyses were the same 34 sentences used in the perceptual and transcription studies. The key words in those 34 sentences were used in the segment-level acoustic analysis. In preparation for acoustic analysis, all sentences underwent digital signal processing. All sentences were low-pass filtered (9.6 kHz cutoff) and digitized at 20,000 samples per second. Each digitized sentence was stored in a separate computer file for further processing. A preliminary analysis was performed using digital signal processing algorithms incorporated in Interactive Laboratory System (ILS) software. Linear prediction analysis (autocorrelation method) was performed using a window length of 25.6 ms with a shift (frame) of 12.8 ms between consecutive windows. Prior to computation, each window was filtered (Hamming window) and preemphasized. The analysis yielded 21 analysis coefficients used to calculate formant frequencies, bandwidths, amplitudes, and overall power level. Finally, a pitch extraction algorithm was used to determine the voicing of a segment, and, in the case of voiced segments, to estimate the fundamental frequency of that segment.

In the sentence-level analysis, acoustic parameters were calculated for each of the 34 sentences as wholes, to determine global, long-term properties. The acoustic parameters used were of four main types (p. 16):

1. Temporal measures
   a. overall sentence duration
   b. total duration of voiceless segments of the sentence
   c. total duration of voiced segments
   d. duration of glottal fry (segments that were labeled as voiceless due to extremely low FØ, i.e., below 60 Hz)
   e. total duration of silent intervals (levels below 40 dB)
   f. voiced-to-voiceless ratio (i.e., the sum of duration in [c] and [d] above, divided by the total duration of [b] and [e])
2. Voicing decision parameters (calculated separately for voiced and voiceless segments)
   g. first reflection coefficient
   h. value of zero crossing
   i. amplitude of cepstral peak
   j. amplitude of absolute and normalized residuals
   k. voicing decision statistic (a value representing a weighted combination of parameters [g] and [h])
3. Power parameters
   l. peak power for a given sentence
   m. first four moments of mean rms values (mean, standard deviation, skewness, and kurtosis)
4. Pitch measures (calculated for voiced segments)
   n. first four moments of FØ

The segmental acoustic analysis investigated the effects of alcohol on specific classes of speech sounds. First, each of the 38 key words was divided into a sequence of labeled phonetic segments. The label assigned to each segment was one of the following: (a) voiced strident fricatives [z ʒ], (b) voiceless strident fricatives [s ʃ], (c) voiced weak fricatives [v ð], (d) voiceless weak fricatives [f θ], (e) voiced affricates [dʒ], (f) voiceless affricates [tʃ], (g) stops, (h) closure preceding voiced stops, (i) closure preceding voiceless stops, (j) nasals, (k) vocalic (vowels, glides, and liquids). Segmentation was performed by visual inspection of the speech waveform using a digitally controlled waveform editor with cursor controls (Forshee & Nusbaum, 1984). In addition to displaying a waveform, the program also simultaneously displayed spectral information and power and voicing parameters to assist in locating segment boundaries. After segmentation and labeling of segments, the key words were analyzed, stored, and labeled. The analysis program calculated the acoustic parameters listed above for the sentence-level analysis, as well as the following spectral measures: (a) the slope of the mean power spectrum of the segment; (b) the half-power frequency (the point above and below which half of the energy was concentrated); (c) normalized distance measures between the onset, middle, and offset of the segment. Finally, for all segment categories and some segments in specific environments, mean values and variances of the acoustic parameters were calculated.

7.1.2.2 Acoustic Analyses: Results

7.1.2.2.1 Sentence-Level Acoustic Analysis   The most consistent difference in sentences between conditions was an overall change in durations. For all four talkers, mean sentence durations were longer in the intoxicated condition than in the sober condition. The magnitude of this increase in duration ranged from 75 ms (Talker 4) to 153 ms (Talker 2). Furthermore, the majority of sentences were lengthened in the alcohol condition rather than shortened; depending on the talker, from approximately 70% (Talker 2) to 97% (Talker 1) of the sentences showed increased duration. The acoustic analysis further revealed that increased sentence duration was due largely to increased durations for voiceless segments as opposed to voiced segments. A comparison of the number of voiced frames and the number of voiceless frames in the sentences produced in both conditions revealed that increases in the number of voiceless frames were greater than increases in the number of voiced frames.

The acoustic analysis revealed no consistent changes in those acoustic parameters corresponding to voicing activation. However, as Figure 7.1.1 shows, fundamental frequency was somewhat more variable (i.e., standard deviations were larger) in the intoxicated condition than in the sober condition.

7.1.2.2.2 Segment-Level Analysis   It might be supposed that changes in individual segments would be reflected in modifications to the spectra of those segments. In fact, however, the segmental analysis revealed no spectral differences for stops, fricatives, nasals, or vowels that could be attributed to alcohol consumption. Observed changes involved temporal, rather than spectral, properties, reflecting the durational differences noted above in the sentence-level analysis.

The production of a stop consonant characteristically requires that airflow be briefly but completely blocked behind the relevant articulators. The acoustic consequence of this closure is silence, and on a waveform display, the closure will appear as a span of no energy, that is, a more or less straight line. Examination of the waveforms for the initial [g] in the word *girl* revealed

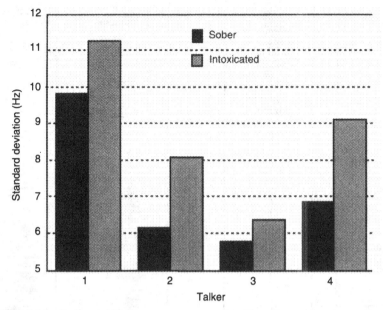

FIGURE 7.1.1   Pitch variability across sentences produced by talkers while sober and intoxicated. (From Pisoni, Hathaway, and Yuchtman, 1985. Used by permission.)

that closure durations for all talkers except Talker 2 were longer in the intoxicated condition than in the sober condition. For Talker 2, glottal pulsation continued through what should have been the closure, and in fact, complete closure was not achieved. The result of incomplete closure was a fricative-like segment. Figure 7.1.2 shows the relevant waveforms for the initial stop in *girl* in both conditions for Talker 4. A similar situation obtained for the initial [g] in the word *grapes* and for the initial [d] in *dishes*. The remaining English voiced stop, the labial [b], presented only minor changes in closure duration.

Like stops, affricates involve completely blocked airflow. However, whereas stops are released abruptly, affricates are released into a relatively prolonged fricative-like portion. The second consonant in the word *pajamas* is a voiced affricate, and Figure 7.1.3 shows waveforms of the affricate [dʒ] as produced by Talker 1 in both conditions. Here it is evident that Talker 1 failed to achieve complete closure for the stop portion of the affricate, resulting in "leakage" of noise where there should have been a (short) span of silence. A further example involved the phrase *garbage cans,* which contains a sequence of an affricate followed by a stop: the final segment in *garbage* is a voiced affricate, and the initial segment in the word *cans* is a voiceless stop. Figure 7.1.4 shows that in the intoxicated condition,

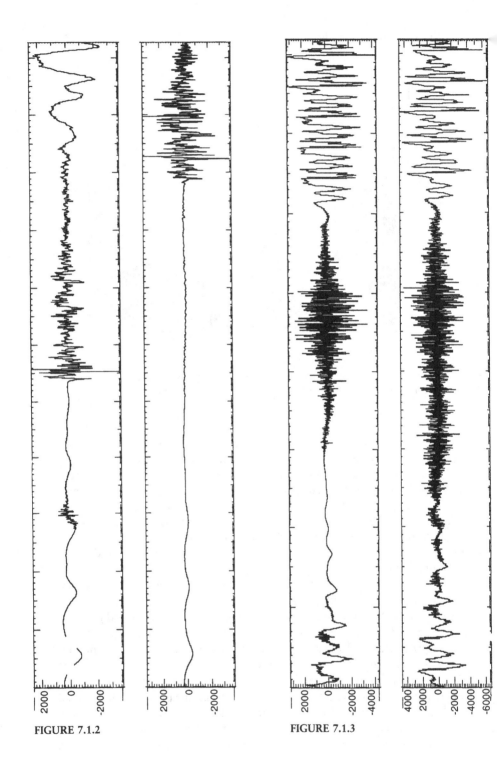

FIGURE 7.1.2

FIGURE 7.1.3

182

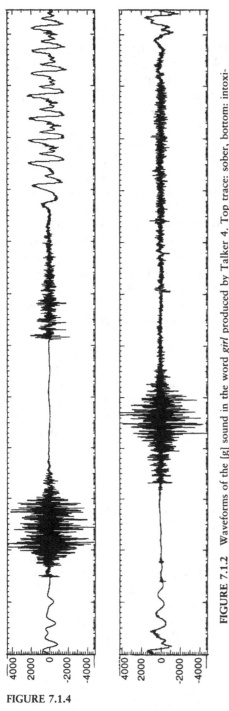

FIGURE 7.1.2 Waveforms of the [g] sound in the word *girl* produced by Talker 4. Top trace: sober, bottom: intoxicated condition.

FIGURE 7.1.3 Waveforms of the [dʒ] sound in the word *pajamas* produced by Talker 1. Top trace: sober, bottom: intoxicated condition.

FIGURE 7.1.4 Waveforms of the [dʒk] sounds in the end of the word *garbage* and the beginning of *cans* produced by Talker 4. Top trace: sober, bottom: intoxicated condition.

FIGURE 7.1.4

Talker 4 achieved complete closure for neither the affricate nor the stop. Failure to achieve complete closure under intoxication during production of an affricate was most evident for the voiced affricate, but two talkers (2 and 4) showed the same effect for the final voiceless affricate. Finally, alveolar [ts] is analyzed variously as an affricate (a single phonological segment) or as a cluster of stop followed by fricative (two phonological segments). Nevertheless, for the word *it's*, some of the talkers showed the same effect under intoxication as with the alveopalatal affricates described above.

A further segmental change under intoxication occurred in sequences of a vowel followed by the voiced alveolar fricative (as in the word *he's*). The usual progression of articulatory events for this sequence is that as the amplitude of the vowel decreases, constriction for the fricative consonant begins, accompanied by glottal pulsation. At the point of maximum constriction (but not complete closure), frication noise is produced, accompanied by intermittent voicing. Under alcohol, however, talkers exhibited two types of deviation from this: (a) either the onset of constriction began well within the vowel (rather than toward the end of it), or (b) a voiceless interval followed the vowel, so that a voiceless, rather than a voiced, fricative was produced.

The final segmental alteration revealed by the acoustic analysis involved the result of releasing exceedingly high pressure in the production of the voiceless bilabial stop. This articulation resulted in a "popping" sound characterized by a low-frequency, high-amplitude waveform. Although this phenomenon occurred for the word *play*, in no case did it occur in the word *splay*. This was attributed this to an analysis that the [p] is voiceless in *play* but voiced in *splay*.

7.1.3 Discussion

Pisoni et al. noted a seeming paradox in the results from this study. Although the results of the perceptual studies indicated that listeners could reliably discriminate between speech produced with and without alcohol, the frequency of salient speech errors (e.g., lengthening, deaffrication) in the alcohol condition was fairly low. They noted that some additional cues, perhaps less salient, must be contributing to correct perceptual discrimination. These additional cues might be found in the acoustic record, which was also examined in this study. The most consistent acoustic change was a significant increase in sentence durations, that is, a slowing of speaking rate under alcohol. In addition, control of abrupt closure and opening of the vocal tract were also affected by alcohol.

Pisoni et al. concluded that "alcohol intoxication affects the acoustic-phonetic properties of speech in a systematic and consistent manner" (p. 21). These changes occured at both the sentence level and at the segmental level. Reduced rates of articulation were observed, as well as increased pitch variability. Impairments of fine articulation were found in the production of voiced stops, affricates, and stop clusters. In addition to these production characteristics, this study also found that listeners could "reliably discriminate and identify sentences produced by an intoxicated talker in matched samples of speech from the same talker" (p. 22). From these, Pisoni et al. concluded that acoustic changes in speech might possibly "serve as an index of sensory-motor impairment due to the depressant central nervous system effects of alcohol" (p. 22).

Finally, Pisoni et al. suggested a number of future directions for research on alcohol and speech, including (a) a demographic broadening of the talker samples, to include subjects of differing ages and gender; (b) evaluation at other BACs; (c) addition of further acoustic measurements, including measurements of sonorant segments (vowels, etc.) and intonation and stress patterns; (d) broadening the perceptual study to include (i) different types of listeners, such as "trained" listeners (e.g., law enforcement officers) and (ii) different perceptual tasks, such as absolute identification tasks (in contrast to the A–B paired-discrimination task described here); and (e) investigation into the possibility of employing automated digital signal processing techniques to develop algorithms for the identification of intoxicated talkers from speech samples.

7.2 PISONI, YUCHTMAN, AND HATHAWAY, 1986

This work is the published version of Pisoni et al. (1985). With minor differences, the two reports are essentially the same.

7.3 HIGGINS AND STITZER, 1988

This work examined the effects of alcohol on the amount of talking produced under various doses of alcohol. Previous research had established that rates of social conversation increased both when alcohol was administered acutely to nonalcoholics and when it was self-administered by alcoholics. Comparable increases in conversation had been observed under the acute administration of opiates, d-amphetamine, and secobarbital (Babor, Meyer, Mirin, McNamee, & Davies, 1976; Griffiths, Stitzer, Corker, Bigelow, & Liebson, 1977; Stitzer et al., 1981b; Stitzer, McCaul, Bigelow, & Liebson, 1984); on the other hand, marijuana appeared to have decreased conversation (Babor, Rossi, Sagotsky, & Meyer, 1974a, 1974b; Babor, Medelson, Gallant, & Kuehnle, 1978; Babor, Mendelson, Uhly, & Kuehnle, 1978; Higgins & Stitzer, 1986). The present study differed from other studies of verbal output in that subjects produced monologues with no conversation partner present. At the time this article appeared, Stephen T. Higgins was affiliated with the Human Behavioral Pharmacology Laboratory, Departments of Psychiatry and Psychology at the University of Vermont in Burlington, Vermont. Maxine L. Stitzer was affiliated with the Behavioral Pharmacology Research Unit in the Department of Psychiatry and Behavorial Sciences at The Johns Hopkins University School of Medicine, in Baltimore, Maryland.

7.3.1 Subjects and Methods

7.3.1.1 Subjects

Subjects for this study were six volunteers (five male, one female). All drank alcohol socially. Their average age was 23.8 years ($SD = 5.6$ years); average body weight was 165 lb ($SD = 16.9$ lb); and self-reported average alcohol consumption was 7.2 drinks per week ($SD = 8.5$ drinks). Subjects were requested to abstain from ingesting illicit drugs during the experiment and to refrain from consuming alcohol for 12 hr prior to the experiment and caffeine or food for 2 hr before. BACs were estimated using an Intoxilyzer (CMI Corp.) breath-alcohol analysis system before each session. Urine specimens were also collected periodically to ensure compliance with the request to abstain from illicit drugs. No positive results were recorded either for presession BACs or from urine analysis.

7.3.1.2 Apparatus, Procedure, and Data Analysis

The experiment was conducted in a sound-attenuated chamber. Subjects were seated facing a console. Vocalizations were detected with a nondirectional microphone (Sony model ECM electret) clipped to the subjects' clothing. The microphone was connected to a voice-operated relay and a PDP-8 computer (Digital Equipment Corp.). The nominal attack time for the voice-operated relay was less than 50 ms, and release time was 800 ms. Closures of 1 sec or longer of the voice-operated relay (VOR) were considered to be speech utterances, and all recorded utterances were then totaled to produce the measure of total seconds of speech. A white light was illuminated during the entire session, and a blue feedback light illuminated whenever the voice-operated relay was closed. A circular-lights device was located in a separate room. This apparatus was a wall-mounted panel with 16 button lights arranged in a circle with a diameter of 56 cm. Located in the center of the panel were a session start button and a point counter.

Four ethanol doses were administered to all subjects. These preparations consisted of 0 g, 22 g, 45 g, or 67 g of ethanol mixed with water to achieve 8 oz of liquid; this water/ethanol preparation was then mixed with 8 oz of orange juice. The ethanol preparations were consumed in 15 min. Subjects were exposed to each dose of alcohol at least three times in a mixed block design. Both experimenters and subjects were aware that the experiment involved consumption of alcohol but did not know the exact dose of each administered preparation.

The task for subjects was to produce speech monologues. Subjects were told that the white session light would be illuminated during the entire session, but that the blue light would be illuminated only when they were talking. Subjects could speak on any topic, and in any amount that they wished; however, they were told that they had to speak at least occasionally to indicate that they were awake. Only naturalistic speech was acceptable: subjects could not, for example, sing or whistle. In case subjects produced unacceptable vocalizations (e.g., singing), they were reinstructed to produce naturalistic speech. Baseline sessions were conducted daily until the amount of vocalization stabilized; this usually required four or five sessions. After establishment of baseline measures, alcohol treatment was introduced, and experimental sessions were conducted 3 days a week. Talking sessions began 30 min after completion of consumption of the alcohol or placebo prepara-tion and lasted 40 min; to assess within-session variation, the amount of speech was recorded separately for 0–10, 11–20, 21–30, and 31–40 min of each of the sessions.

The circular-lights task involved three 60-sec trials: before consumption of the preparation, before the talking session (30 min after completion of consumption), and after the talking session (70 min after completion of consumption). Points were accumulated by pressing buttons as rapidly as possible in response to random-sequenced illumination. Pressing a button activated a feedback tone, increased the point counter by one, and activated the next light. Subjects were instructed to accrue as many points as possible.

A number of self-report instruments were administered postsession, and subjects were instructed to answer based on how they felt during the experi-ment. The instruments were the following:

1. A 49-item (true/false) questionnaire based on the Addiction Research Center Inventory (ARCI; W. R. Martin, Sloan, Sapira, & Jasinski, 1971), consisting of five empirically derived subscales to measure sedative effects, euphoric effects, dysphoric and psychotomimetic effects, and amphetamine-like effects.

2. The 21-item (true/false) alcohol scale of the ARCI (Haertzen, 1966).

3. The Profile of Mood States (POMS), a 65-item five-point adjective rating scale factor analyzed into eight mood clusters: anxiety, depression, anger, vigor, fatigue, confusion, friendliness, and a total mood score.

4. A 100-mm visual-analogue line to rate the degree of drug-produced high, ranging from 0 (not at all) to 100 (highest I've ever been).

5. Five items for rating the degree of drug effect, sleepiness, drunkenness, relaxation, and alertness, ranging from 1 (mild) to 4 (extreme). In addition,

a 5-point scale for rating the degree of drug liking, ranging from 0 (not at all) to 4 (very much).

BACs were estimated from breath analysis prior to drinking, immediately prior to the talking session, and immediately following the talking session. Daily data for each of the subjects were averaged across repeated observations for each of the dose conditions, with three or four observations for each subject under each dose condition. Means for individual subjects were used in a two-way repeated measures analysis of variance (ANOVA) to assess effects on talking; the two factors were alcohol dose and within-session time (i.e., 0–10, 11–20, 21–30, and 31–40 min). The same analysis was used for both BACs and the circular-lights measures; one factor was alcohol dose; the second was minutes after completion of drinking. A repeated-measures (dose condition) one-way ANOVA was used in the analysis of the self-reported measures. Effects were considered significant at the p < 0.05 level and below.

7.3.2 Results

Average BACs increased as a function of alcohol dose from immediately prior to the talking session (30 min after completion of drinking) to immediately after the talking session (70 min after completion of drinking); effect of alcohol on average BACs was statistically significant. Table 7.3.1 shows average BACs for each of the dose conditions at 30 min and 70 min after completion of drinking. Additionally, there was a significant interaction of dose and time.

Figure 7.3.1 shows average seconds of speech produced (i.e., seconds of VOR switch closure) as a function of time periods within the talking session. In general, subjects produced more speech in the first half of the talking session than in the second half under all dose conditions. Additionally, a significant effect of dose on total amount of speech was found. Table 7.3.2 shows the average total seconds of speech in each of the four dose conditions. At 878 sec of speech, there was significantly more talking in the 67-g dose

TABLE 7.3.1   Average Blood-Alcohol Concentrations[a]

	30 min (%)	70 min (%)
Placebo	0	0
22 g	0.01	0.01
45 g	0.05	0.04
67 g	0.07	0.08

[a] From Higgins and Stitzer (1988).

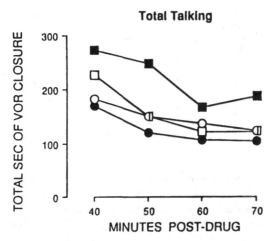

FIGURE 7.3.1   Average effects of placebo, 22 g, 45 g, and 67 g of alcohol on total seconds of speech (voice-operated relay switch closure) are shown in 10-min bins across the 40-min talking sessions. The bins represent total seconds of speech during 0–10 min, 11–20 min, 21–30 min, and 31–40 min of the talking session. Data points are means for six subjects. Filled squares = 67-g ethanol, open squares = 45-g ethanol, filled circles = 22-g ethanol, open circles = placebo. (From Higgins and Stitzer, 1988. Copyright © 1988 by Springer-Verlag. Used by permission.)

condition than in the other three doses; this was true for five of the six subjects. None of the other dose conditions differed significantly from each other on this measure. There was a significant interaction of dose and time, attributable to the decrease in speech produced during the 60-min bin in the 67-g dose condition. The 45-g dose produced a nonsignificant increasing trend during the first 10 min of the talking session, but this effect disappeared during the final 30 min. Average amount of speech produced for the 22-g dose was below the level in the placebo condition, but this difference was not significant.

TABLE 7.3.2   Average Total Seconds of Speech in a 40-Min Period[a]

Dose	Average total seconds of speech
Placebo	597.4
22 g	502.1
45 g	625.7
67 g	878

[a] From Higgins and Stitzer (1988).

TABLE 7.3.3 Average Scores on Circular-Lights
Task[a]

Dose	Predrug	30 min	70 min
Placebo	93.3	93.6	92.3
22 g	94.6	93.7	90.6
45 g	92.6	87.1	85.8
67 g	92.7	85.6	79.0

[a] From Higgins and Stitzer (1988).

Table 7.3.3 gives average scores on the circular-lights task. There were no significant differences across doses before administration of the ethanol preparation. Across all doses, there was a decrease in average scores from 30 min after completion of the drinking trial to 70 min after completion of the trial. The effects of alcohol on this measure were small but quite reliable across subjects. Decreased response rates from the 30- to 70-min interval in the 67-g dose condition were significantly lower than those in the placebo and 22-g conditions, but they were not significantly different from scores in the 45-g dose condition. The decreased scores in the 22-g and 45-g dose conditions were not significantly different from those in the placebo condition. For this task, there was no significant interaction of dose and time.

Of the postsession self-report measures, the following increased as a function of alcohol dose: high, drug effect, and drunkenness. There was a trend for drug liking to increase, but this was not statistically significant, and the following were also not significantly affected by alcohol: sleeping, relaxed, alert, and energetic. On the ARCI alcohol scale, there was a significant increase as a function of alcohol dose. Among the ARCI short-form subscales, only amphetamine significantly increased; although there were trends among the remaining four subscales, these were not statistically significant. Finally, on the POMS, only the confusion cluster increased significantly as a function of alcohol; the remaining clusters showed no significant effects of alcohol.

Alcohol thus induced a significant dose-dependent increase in the total amount of speech produced. Because speech was produced in isolation, Higgins and Stitzer concluded that a social context was not necessary for alcohol to produce increases in speech. However, alcohol also appeared to decrease response rates on the circular-lights task, so that the increase in speech under alcohol could not be attributed to an increase in overall activity levels.

7.4. KLINGHOLZ, PENNING, AND LIEBHARDT, 1988

This study examined the possibility of recognition of alcohol intoxication using automated acoustic analysis techniques. Klingholz et al. (1988) acknowledged previous work on alcohol and speech, mentioning the following studies: Andrews et al. (1977); Lester and Skousen (1974); Natale, Kanzler, Jaffe, and Jaffe (1980); Pisoni, et al. (1986); Sobell and Sobell (1972); Sobell et al. (1982); Trojan and Kryspin-Exner (1968); and Zaimov (1969). The authors suggested that all of these suffered from at least one of the following shortcomings in methodology: (a) BACs were not measured objectively; (b) BACs were so high, and thus intoxication effects so apparent, that acoustic analyses were superfluous; (c) there was only a very small number of subjects; (d) analyses were performed only qualitatively, either by auditory evaluation (listening) or by visual inspection of spectrograms. Klingholz et al., on the other hand, sought to achieve objective recognition of intoxication by automatic acoustic analysis, with BACs at a low to medium level and treated as a continuous independent variable. Klingholz et al. further pointed out the lack of automatic computer methods for measuring the effects of intoxication on errors, semantics, and phonemes. They suggested that changes in features of speech, rather than the features themselves, would provide the basis for recognizing intoxicated speech, and that the influence of alcohol would be most readily found in dynamic patterns of speech articulation rather than static ones. Because of individual variation, identification of intoxicated speech would rely on speaker-dependent references.

Implementation of such identification capabilities was by statistical analysis of both laryngeal and articulatory features in the speech signal. In the laryngeal domain, measurements were made of fundamental frequency (FØ) and SNR, whereas measurements of formant frequency were used to characterize articulation. In addition to the acoustic analyses, Klingholz et al. also conducted perception tests like those carried out earlier by Pisoni et al. (1985) to determine if acoustic changes corresponded to perceptual impressions. Establishing a relationship would be especially useful in real-world situations in which auditory witnesses would be required to estimate intoxication. At the time this work appeared, all three authors were affiliated with the Department of Otorhinolaryngology and Institute for Forensic Medicine at the University of Munich, Munich, Germany.

7.4.1 Methods

7.4.1.1 Subjects and Alcohol Preparation

Subjects for this study were 16 males, ranging in age from 25–35 years (mean = 28.7 years). All were nonalcoholic native speakers of German with no voice or speech disorders. Eleven were examined under both intoxicated and nonintoxicated conditions, and the remaining five served as nonintoxicated controls to examine the effects of prolonged use of the voice. The eleven alcoholized subjects were allocated target BACs ranging from 0.05–0.15% in 0.01% increments. The alcohol preparation consisted of beer concentrated at 40 g alcohol per liter; subjects were required to consume the entire preparation in 90 min. Target BACs were estimated using Widmark's (1932) formula equating BAC with grams of alcohol divided by a reduction factor (which accounts for the proportion of body weight attributable to contained water) times the body weight in kilograms. Blood samples were taken 20 min after cessation of consumption, and BACs were determined using a Perkin-Elmer F40 gas chromatograph. Prescribed BACs were not achieved exactly, and Table 7.4.1 shows actual achieved BACs. Recording took place immediately after blood sampling. After this recording, three of the subjects were administered further alcohol treatment.

7.4.1.2 Materials and Recording
Subjects read the beginning of a fairy tale and produced at least 2.5 min of speech; speech was produced once before administration of alcohol and then again immediately after blood samples were taken. The text was phonetically balanced and consisted of 40 sentences, or 520 words. Speech samples were tape-recorded in an acoustically isolated room.

7.4.1.3 Signal Processing
The recordings were digitized by a 12-bit A/D converter at a rate of 12.5 kHz. The 2.5 min spans of speech material were divided into five 30-sec portions for statistical analysis. Spectral analysis utilized an 80-ms time window with a 20-ms shift.

Fundamental frequency (FØ) was determined by using the product spectrum according to a procedure described by Schroeder (1968), allowing recognition of FØ in signals with a low SNR. Measurements of FØ were made only for frames containing voicing, as predetermined by selecting

TABLE 7.4.1   Target and Actual Achieved
Blood-Alcohol Concentrations[a]

Target BAC (in %)	Achieved BAC (in %)
0.05	0.67
0.06	0.77
0.07	0.80
0.08	0.87
0.09	0.88
0.10	0.93
0.11	0.97
0.12	0.101
0.13	0.124
0.14	0.137
0.15	0.159

[a] BAC, blood-alcohol concentration. From Kling-holz et al. (1988).

frames with low-frequency energy, and the pitch contour was smoothed. Because of the lack of sustained vowels in the speech samples, and because noise characteristics were unknown, the SNR could not be estimated using long time windows (e.g., Hiraoka et al., 1984), speech wave averaging (e.g., Yumoto, Kitzoe, Veta, Tanaka, & Tanabe, 1982), or an approximation of the noise spectrum (Kasuya, Otawa, Mashima, & Ebihara, 1986; Kitajima, 1981). Instead, because harmonics are defined by their frequency location, amplitude, and shape, harmonics were reconstructed to calculate harmonic energy.

First- and second-formant frequencies (F1, F2) were determined by a 14th-order linear predictive coding (LPC) model during voiced intervals, and time contours were smoothed. Time derivatives were determined by a differentiation (first backward difference in the contours, time interval 20 ms). The long-term average spectrum (LTAS) was determined using the Bergland fast Fourier transform (FFT). The waveform was used to determine estimated distributions of FØ, F1/F2, SNR, and time derivatives of FØ, F1, and F2.

7.4.1.4 Classification

Estimated distributions were classified using an n-dimensional Euclidean distance technique. Distributions of the same variable from the same subject were normalized as "profiles." If such a profile is regarded as an n-dimensional vector, where the frequencies in the classes represent the vector components, each profile represents a point in an n-dimensional space. Reference and test profiles set up point clusters in this space, and geometric distances between these points can be calculated as Euclidean distances between the vectors. Reference vectors were designated DT_r, whereas test vectors or relative distances, DR_r, were expressed as multiples of the mean distance between the reference vectors, where $DT_r = 1$.

7.4.1.5 Perceptual Judgments

A perceptual study was conducted using the first 30 sec of the text from all of the subjects in both the pre- and postalcohol conditions. These stimuli were used in two tasks: (a) an identification task, in which the recordings were presented in random order, and listeners were required to identify the sample as produced under alcohol or not; and (b) a discrimination task, in which pairs of sober/intoxicated (or intoxicated/sober) samples were presented in random order, and listeners were required to choose the utterance produced under intoxication. Twelve speech therapists served as listeners and received no prior training on the task. Listeners were further required, upon classification of a speech sample as produced under intoxication, to select one or more of six criteria as the basis for their decision. These criteria were (a) speech fluency (e.g., rate, pauses); (b) speech quality (e.g., monotonous, slurred); (c) speech errors (e.g., omissions, repetitions); (d) voice quality (e.g., roughness, breathiness); (e) voice instability (e.g., bitonality, voice breaks); and (f) voice effort.

7.4.2 Results

The SNR profile in the intoxicated condition differed from the sober profile. The peak amplitude was lowered or the peak shifted to a lower SNR. Thus, harmonic speech energy was lowered from the sober to the intoxicated condition. The intoxicated profile for FØ displayed an expansion and reduction in amplitude of the peak or peaks from the sober condition, indicating an increase in FØ variability in the alcohol condition. The F1/F2 profiles showed narrowing of the peak from the nonalcohol to the alcohol condition but no shifting of the peak toward 1. The LTAS profiles showed an increase in the occurrence of higher frequency spectral components from the nonalcohol to the alcohol condition. Table 7.4.2 shows differences between the sober condition and the intoxicated and control conditions for the acoustic parameters FØ, SNR, F1/F2, and LTAS. Differences between conditions for these variables were significant; differences between the nonalcohol and alcohol conditions for the time derivatives of FØ, F1, and F2 were not significant.

To assess the effects of BAC, Spearman's rhos were calculated, using test distance (DT_r) as a dependent variable, between BAC and DT_r of FØ, SNR, F1/F2, and LTAS profiles. There was no significant correlation between BAC and SNR, F1/F2, or LTAS. There was, however, a significant positive correlation between BAC and the FØ profile, as well as between BAC and the combined profiles for FØ and SNR. Three of the subjects continued drinking after the remaining eight had stopped. Two showed greater differ-

TABLE 7.4.2 Reference Distances, Test Distances, and Their S. D. for F_o, SNR, F_1/F_2, and LTAS Profiles in the Cases of Intoxication and Long-Term Voice Error[a,b]

Profile	DR_r	DT_r intoxication	$p1^c$	DT_r voice effort	$p1^c$	$p2^c$
F_o	1.0 ± 0.11	2.54 ± 0.68	0.001	1.58 ± 0.21	0.010	0.005
SNR	1.0 ± 0.04	2.05 ± 0.34	0.001	1.34 ± 0.24	0.010	0.005
F_1/F_2	1.0 ± 0.07	2.13 ± 0.82	0.001	1.31 ± 0.82	0.100	0.025
LTAS	1.0 ± 0.02	2.83 ± 1.65	0.001	1.98 ± 0.91	0.025	0.100

[a] From Klingholz, Penning, and Liebhardt (1988). Copyright © 1988 by American Institute of Physics. Used by permission.

[b] DR_r, reference distances; DT_r, test distances; SNR, signal-to-noise ratio; LTAS, long-term average spectra.

[c] Significance levels (Wilcoxon test) $p1$ and $p2$ evaluate the comparison to sober, respectively, to intoxicated condition.

ences from the nonalcohol condition at the high BAC than at the low BAC; one of the subjects, however, exhibited measurements closer to the nonalcohol condition at the higher BAC than at the lower BAC. Test differences for the five control subjects (i.e., all voice recordings made but no alcohol consumed) were less than for the intoxicated subjects, and these differences were significant.

The two perception tests yielded results as follows. In the identification task, the percent correct was 54.0%, that is, only 4% above the chance level of 50%, indicating no significant perception of intoxication. In the discrimination task using paired samples, percent correct discrimination was 61.1%. There was an increase of correct discrimination with increasing BAC, ranging from 54.2% at BAC < 0.1% to 82.0% for BAC > 0.1%. Results for subjective characteristics on which intoxicated judgments were based were: speech errors, 19.8%; speech fluency, 21.4%, speech quality, 19.5%; voice quality, 14.0%; voice instability, 4.7%; and voice effort, 20.6%.

7.4.3 Discussion

Alcohol-induced changes in speech were observed in both the laryngeal and the articulatory domains. Laryngeal differences were consistently found in changes in FØ, whereas articulatory changes (as in F1/F2 ratio and time derivatives of FØ, F1, and F2) were evident generally when BACs were higher.

A main concern in this research was possible forensic applications of the recognition techniques described here, specifically whether automated acoustic analysis of the speech signal could be used to determine whether or not a talker was intoxicated. The conclusion of Klingholz et al. was that such application would be questionable. First, because of variability in individual sensitivity to alcohol, even statistically significant measurements of change would not necessarily apply in every case. A resulting concern was that intoxicated persons might be misidentified as sober. Second, because of other factors contributing to voice changes (e.g., laryngeal disorders, neurological disease), a sober subject might be incorrectly identified as intoxicated. Third, automated acoustic analyses are expensive, and subjects might be uncooperative. In any case, the authors concluded that it would be absolutely necessary to have available long signal samples from both reference (nonalcohol) and test (alcohol) states.

7.5 SWARTZ, 1988

This work is the author's doctoral dissertation from Michigan State University (East Lansing, Michigan), in the Department of Audiology and Speech

Sciences. It examined VOT variability and how it might change as a function of physiological changes induced by alcohol. Eight male and eight female subjects recorded a number of tokens of [t] and [d] in phonetically identical contexts. Results indicated no significant differences in VOT variability as a function either of time or of alcohol. In addition, based on the durational measurements carried out here, the author found that three of the temporal features identified six different VOT types; as this does not impinge directly on our present concerns, it will not be discussed below. A published version of the major results of this study (except for the differentiation of the six different types of VOT) can be found in Swartz (1992).

VOT refers to "the interval between the articulatory release of the stop and the onset of vocal cord vibrations" (Kent & Read, 1992, p. 108). VOT can be expressed as a single number, that is, a measurement of time. It can thus be measured continuously, but in general, it is perceived categorically and is an important cue to the voicing of a consonant. VOTs can generally be classified as negative (the onset of voicing precedes the stop release), zero (the onset of voicing is simultaneous with the stop release), short-lag, or long-lag. Negative, zero, and short-lag VOTs thus contribute to the perception of voicing in stops, whereas long-lag VOTs indicate voicelessness. Figure 7.5.1 shows spectrograms for the English words *tie* and *die,* with VOTs marked as A and B respectively. As shown in this figure, VOT for the voiceless stop is approximately 160 ms, whereas the VOT for the voiced stop is much shorter, approximately 100 ms.

7.5.1 Subjects and Methods

Subjects were eight men and eight women between 21 and 26 years of age, all native speakers of General American English (the dialect of the midwestern and western United States of America). At the time of the study, none of the subjects had any speech or hearing problems. None were smokers, diabetics, prescription drug users, or known or admitted alcoholics. All were occasional drinkers of alcohol. Subjects received course credit for their participation.

Stimulus materials were ten seven-syllable-long sentences, five containing [t] in a crucial sequence and five containing [d] in that sequence. This sequence consisted of the voiceless interdental fricative [Θ], followed by the alveolar stop (either voiced or voiceless), and then the sequence [ul]. Subjects made recordings at four sessions, each held on a different day. Subjects consumed no alcohol before the first session or before two of the remaining three sessions; sessions under alcohol treatment were counterbalanced among the second, third, and fourth sessions. Sentences were randomly ordered in four different lists, and lists were counterbalanced among the four sessions for each subject. Each list was read twice in each session, producing a total of 20 sentences (20 stop tokens, or 10 for each stop) in each session.

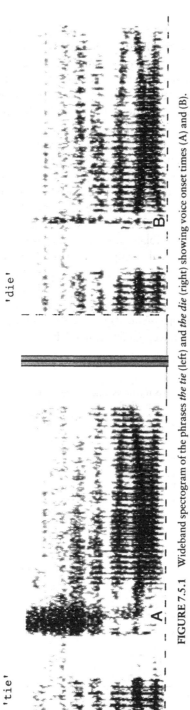

'tie' 'die'

FIGURE 7.5.1 Wideband spectogram of the phrases *the tie* (left) and *the die* (right) showing voice onset times (A) and (B).

The alcohol preparation employed was beer, administered in a dose of approximately 12 oz per 0.75 hr. Dosages were determined by reference to a chart provided by the police showing the number of 12-oz beers required for a person of a given weight to achieve a given level of intoxication. A 15- to 20-min deprivation period followed consumption in order to clear mouth alcohol. Approximately 1.5 hr after beginning of consumption, blood-alcohol concentration (BAC) was determined by means of a portable breath-alcohol testing device operated by a trained police officer. A BAC between 0.075 and 0.100% was required before recordings were made in the alcohol condition. Subjects with alcohol levels below or above the required window were tested subsequent to absorption or elimination. Table 7.5.1 gives the time required to reach the target BAC, the amount of beer in ounces consumed, and the recorded BAC for each of the subjects at the time of recording in the alcohol condition. In the sober condition, subjects were also tested with the breath analyzer to ensure absence of alcohol.

Speech material was digitally recorded at a sampling rate of 5 kHz, using a Macintosh SE computer with MacSpeech Lab 2.0 software; this software also permitted subsequent oscillographic and spectrographic display and acoustic analysis. Subjects' heads were fixed to maintain a constant microphone-to-mouth distance, which ranged between 3 and 6 in. Recording

TABLE 7.5.1   Time Required for Intoxicated Treatment, Alcohol Consumed, and Portable Breathalyzer Test (PBT) Level for Each Subject[a]

Subject	Time required for intoxication (hours:minutes)	Alcohol consumed (oz)	PBT level (%)
A	1:49	56	0.092
B	1:48	52	0.088
C	1:36	40	0.078
D	1:42	59	0.077
E	1:33	45	0.086
F	1:36	48	0.099
G	1:18	43	0.097
H	1:41	57	0.076
I	2:46	43	0.090
J	2:06	59	0.092
K	4:27	53	0.096
L	2:14	48	0.090
M	1:55	60	0.075
N	3:09	48	0.084
O	1:45	53	0.075
P	2:01	71	0.092
Mean	2:05	52.19	0.087

[a] From Swartz (1988). Copyright © 1988 by Bradford L. Swartz. Used by permission.

levels were adjusted for each subject and monitored and controlled using a VU-meter.

Waveform displays of the recording were produced, and VOT was measured by placing a cursor at the point of stop release (a spike) and a second cursor at the onset of voicing (periodicity); the time indicated between cursors was recorded as the VOT. In group and intrasubject measurements, only positive (≥ 0) VOTs were used (p. 62; see Klatt, 1975).

Both individual and group data were subjected to statistical analysis. Independent variables were subject, subject sex, treatments, sentence number, and sentence replication group; BAC was used as a covariate when comparing the four treatments, and the dependent variables were the VOTs for the two stops. The data analyzed included standard deviations for each subject, as a measure of changes in variability, rather than only variance about a mean; logarithmic transformations were used on standard deviations in order to ensure normality of samples. Reliability was estimated by an intraobserver test–retest procedure for all of the 1280 tokens of [d] or [t] (640 tokens of each). This procedure showed a mean difference of 1.46 ms, corresponding to a consistency of measure of less than one-third of an FØ cycle for females (assuming an average FØ of 225 Hz) and less than one-fifth of a cycle for males (assuming an average FØ of 110 Hz). For all ANOVAs, the 0.05 confidence level was used.

7.5.2 Results

As expected from previous research on VOT, there was a wide range of VOTs both within and across subjects, and this resulted in large standard deviations. Because of this variability, and in order to determine intrasubject consistency or inconsistency both over time and with the introduction of alcohol, analysis was performed on logarithmic transformations of the standard deviations. Table 7.5.2 presents logarithmic transformations of the standard deviations for each of the 16 subjects, for both stops, in all four conditions. The alcohol condition is uniformly listed as Condition 4 for analysis and presentation purposes, even though this condition was counterbalanced in order across subjects. Additionally, p-values are given in the rightmost column. As Table 7.5.2 shows, very seldom was there a significant difference in condition standard deviations. Only subjects A and C showed significant differences in variability across conditions. Subjects F, G, and K showed significant differences in variability across conditions for the voiced [d], but as seen from Table 7.5.2, these differences were not between the alcohol and nonalcohol conditions. Table 7.5.2 also shows standard deviations for the group of male subjects and the group of female subjects; here again, for both groups there was no signifcant difference in variability for either of the two stops across conditions. Thus, no significant differences

TABLE 7.5.2. Subject Log Transformations of Standard Deviations of [d] and [t] Voice Onset Times Across Four Treatments, and Respective p Values[a]

Subject/sex	Phoneme	Treatment				
		1	2	3	4	p
A male	d	1.66	2.43	1.74	2.31	.011*
	t	2.42	2.66	1.35	1.96	.013*
B female	d	2.15	3.43	1.97	1.83	.285
	t	2.70	2.66	1.97	2.68	.267
C female	d	1.83	2.52	1.21	2.05	.001*
	t	2.21	2.37	2.76	2.92	.018*
D male	d	2.42	1.96	2.36	1.96	.837
	t	2.85	2.72	2.33	2.51	.216
E female	d	2.17	2.16	2.00	1.77	.844
	t	2.86	2.69	2.95	2.94	.982
F female	d	1.98	1.36	2.06	2.17	.029*
	t	2.61	1.95	2.32	2.49	.398
G female	d	1.76	1.87	1.56	1.08	.041*
	t	2.82	1.76	2.14	2.15	.084
H male	d	1.69	1.68	1.68	2.03	.554
	t	1.95	2.50	1.84	1.54	.308
I male	d	2.09	2.15	2.01	1.96	.864
	t	2.52	2.36	2.65	2.85	.763
J female	d	1.97	1.84	1.97	1.59	.693
	t	2.34	2.18	2.22	2.11	.930
K male	d	1.78	1.64	1.94	0.00	.001*
	t	1.73	2.08	2.10	1.99	.794
L female	d	2.26	1.83	2.14	2.22	.103
	t	2.49	2.65	2.68	2.64	.961
M male	d	2.27	2.15	2.14	1.21	.621
	t	2.80	1.77	2.38	2.58	.431
N female	d	1.34	1.29	1.62	1.33	.906
	t	2.31	1.87	1.76	2.27	.171
O male	d	2.02	1.99	1.93	2.51	.457
	t	2.30	2.39	2.86	2.41	.068
P male	d	1.70	1.03	2.32	2.08	.327
	t	2.56	2.47	2.59	2.48	.918
males	d	1.95	1.88	2.01	1.76	.657
	t	2.39	2.37	2.26	2.29	.851
females	d	1.93	1.91	1.82	1.75	.606
	t	2.54	2.27	2.35	2.52	.220

[a] From Swartz (1988). Copyright © 1988 by Bradford L. Swartz. Used by permission.
* $p < 0.05$.

in the variability of VOTs were found within subjects between the alcohol and nonalcohol conditions or over time for each subject.

Besides comparing VOT standard deviations, Swartz also compared VOT means and performed several ANOVAs. Table 7.5.3 shows mean VOTs

TABLE 7.5.3   Means and Standard Deviations of
[d] Voice Onset Times across Treatments, Sexes,
and Sentence Numbers[a]

Variable	Mean	Standard deviation
Population	15.04	8.76
Treatment 1	15.39	8.84
Treatment 2	15.05	8.99
Treatment 3	14.51	7.89
Treatment 4	15.21	9.30
Males	12.88	8.81
Females	17.21	8.16
Sentence 1	15.81	8.65
Sentence 2	13.91	7.77
Sentence 3	16.13	9.21
Sentence 4	14.28	9.48
Sentence 5	15.07	8.50

[a] From Swartz (1988). Copyright © 1988 by Bradford L. Swartz. Used by permission.

and standard deviations for [d] for the four treatments, the two sexes, and
the five sentences, whereas Table 7.5.4 shows the same for [t]. ANOVAs
of VOTs across sentence replications, sex, treatments, and sentence numbers
are given for [d] in Table 7.5.5 and for [t] in Table 7.5.6. As Tables 7.5.5
and 7.5.6 show, for [d] VOTs, there was a significant difference only for

TABLE 7.5.4   Means and Standard Deviations of
[t] Voice Onset Times across Treatments, Sexes,
and Sentence Numbers[a]

Variable	Mean	Standard deviation
Population	73.79	18.03
Treatment 1	76.06	18.67
Treatment 2	71.39	17.04
Treatment 3	72.26	18.37
Treatment 4	75.45	17.74
Males	65.96	14.53
Females	82.62	16.85
Sentence 1	75.01	20.86
Sentence 2	69.93	17.90
Sentence 3	77.02	17.35
Sentence 4	74.41	17.87
Sentence 5	72.59	15.21

[a] From Swartz (1988). Copyright © 1988 by Bradford L. Swartz. Used by permission.

TABLE 7.5.5   Analysis of Variance for [d] Voice Onset Times across Sentence Group Replications, Sex, Treatments, and Sentence Number[a]

Source	SS[b]	DF[b]	MS[b]	F	p
Replication	19.95	1	19.95	.27	.605
Sex	2997.23	1	2997.23	40.29	.000*
Treatment	69.32	3	23.11	.31	.818
Sentence number	465.32	4	116.33	1.56	.183
Sex × Treatment	202.03	3	67.34	.91	.438
Sex × Sentence number	72.17	4	18.04	.24	.914
Within cells	41660.87	560	74.39		

[a] From Swartz (1988). Copyright © 1988 by Bradford L. Swartz. Used by permission.
[b] SS, sum of squares; DF, degrees of freedom; MS, mean squares.
* $p < 0.05$.

sex, whereas for [t] there were significant differences for sex, treatment, and sentence number. In no case, for either stop, was there a significant interaction of variables.

A direct assessment of the effects of alcohol on VOT was made by statistically weighting the three nonalcohol treatments and combining them into a single group, which was then compared to the single alcohol condition by t-test. No significant difference was found for either the [d] or the [t] VOTs. A variation of this analysis used level of intoxication as a covariate. For [d], this analysis revealed significance between sexes and between treatments, with a significant covariate regression effect. Although this might appear to indicate a difference between the alcohol and nonalcohol conditions, a comparison of sex and treatment means revealed that the alcohol condition was not significantly different from the three nonalcohol conditions, such that variance attributable to intoxication level was equally attrib-

TABLE 7.5.6   Analysis of Variance for [t] VOTs, Across Sentence Group Replications, Sex, Treatments, and Sentence Number[a]

Source	SS[b]	DF[b]	MS[b]	F	p
Replication	640.00	1	640.00	2.53	.122
Sex	49914.23	1	49914.23	197.70	.000*
Treatment	2562.28	3	854.09	3.38	.018*
Sentence number	3669.73	4	917.43	3.63	.006*
Sex × Treatment	1089.86	3	363.29	1.44	.230
Sex × Sentence number	811.12	4	202.78	.80	.523
Within cells	141384.25	560	252.47		

[a] From Swartz (1988). Copyright © 1988 by Bradford L. Swartz. Used by permission.
[b] SS, sum of squares; DF, degrees of freedom; MS, mean of squares.
* $p < 0.05$.

utable to sex or treatment variances. For both [d] and [t], intoxication level
was determined not to underlie any of the variances.

7.5.3 Discussion

A number of conclusions can be drawn from this study. Most importantly,
alcohol did not appear to affect VOT. Second, although two subjects showed

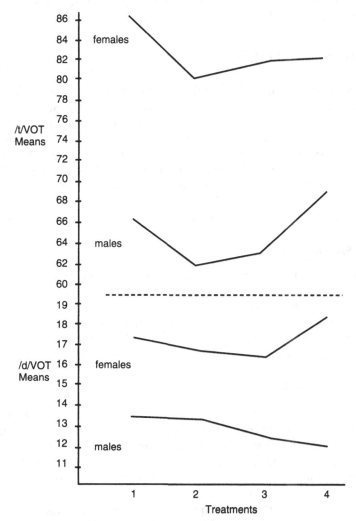

FIGURE 7.5.2 Male and female [d] and [t] voice onset time (VOT) means across treatments.
From Swartz, 1988. Copyright © 1988 by Bradford L. Swartz. Used by permission.

differences in variability for both stops over time, and three showed differences for [d], there did not appear to be a general difference in the variability of VOT over time. One significant difference, however, was in the VOT means between males and females. Figure 7.5.2 shows means for both stops for females and males across the four treatments (three sober, one intoxicated). As Figure 7.5.2 shows, there was a clear separation between the male and female means. In general, for both stops, females tended to use a significantly longer VOT than males. Finally, it should be noted that this study examined not only VOT means, but also standard deviations as a measure of variability.

7.6 PISONI AND MARTIN, 1989

This study reported on the research project undertaken by General Motors Research Laboratories and Indiana University to investigate the effects of alcohol on speech, reporting on two perceptual experiments and two analyses of speech production: phonetic transcription and acoustic analysis. This article reiterated a number of results reported in Pisoni et al. (1985), and the discussion below concentrates on a perceptual experiment using an absolute identification task. When this article appeared, David B. Pisoni and Christopher S. Martin were affiliated with the Speech Research Laboratory in the Department of Psychology at Indiana University (Bloomington, Indiana).

7.6.1 Speech Materials

Talker descriptions, materials, and procedures, including talker preparation and recording, were as reported in Pisoni et al. (1985; see section 7.1). Male university students served as talkers and recorded speech materials both before and after alcohol. Alcohol doses were calculated to raise subjects' BACs to at least 0.10%. Table 7.6.1 shows BACs for each of the eight subjects used in the present study, at the beginning of the recording session.

7.6.2 Perceptual Experiment

Results from the perceptual experiments reported in Pisoni et al. (1985) indicated that naive listeners could reliably identify speech produced under alcohol when a direct paired-comparison procedure was used. Pisoni and Martin suggested, however, that an absolute-identification task might better replicate conditions under which recognition of alcoholized speech would be performed in clinical and law enforcement settings. The perceptual experiment discussed here therefore required subjects to decide whether a single presented sentence was produced before or after alcohol consumption.

Materials for this experiment consisted of 24 of the 34 sentences used in the perceptual experiment described in Pisoni et al. (1985) and included

TABLE 7.6.1 Talkers' Blood-Alcohol
Concentrations (BAC) at the Beginning of the
Recording Session[a]

Talker	BAC (%)
1	0.10
2	0.17
3	0.15
4	0.16
5	0.15
6	0.13
7	0.19
8	0.13

[a] From Pisoni and Martin (1989). Copyright © 1989
by Williams & Wilkins. Used by permission.

recordings from all eight talkers listed in Table 7.6.1 in both the sober and
intoxicated conditions. Each of the talkers contributed 12 sentences from
each of the conditions. Two files were compiled for presentation, differing
in that each speaker-sentence combination appeared on one file in the sober
condition and on the other file in the intoxicated condition. Successive
sentences were separated by 5 sec of silence.

Two groups of listeners participated. One group consisted of 30 undergraduate students who received course credit for their participation. The
second group consisted of 14 Indiana State Police officers who participated
in the study as volunteers. All were native speakers of English with no
reported history of speech or hearing disorders. Each listening session lasted
approximately 1 hr. Listeners were presented with eight talkers saying 24
sentences each (192 trials total) from audiotape over headphones in a quiet
room. Listeners were asked to decide whether each sentence heard had been
produced while the speaker was sober or while the speaker was intoxicated;
responses were recorded by circling either S[ober] or I[ntoxicated] on a
response sheet. Additionally, listeners rated their degree of confidence in
their response on a scale from 1 (just guessing) to 5 (very sure).

As might be expected, scores on this single-interval identification task
were lower than those for the A–B paired-discrimination experiment described earlier. Nevertheless, mean percent correct responses were 61.5 for
the students and 64.7 for the police officers; tests of proportions showed
that both groups of listeners performed significantly better than chance.
Mean accuracy for sober sentences was 60.5% and for intoxicated sentences
64.5%. Mean accuracy for the eight talkers ranged from 55% to 71.9%;
tests of proportions showed accuracy for all eight talkers to be significantly
better than chance. A series of t-tests also showed that for six of the eight
talkers, the police officers performed more accurately than the college students, although this difference was not large.

Additional signal-detection analyses assessed discrimination performance while also controlling for response bias (see Green & Swets, 1966). Mean beta (a measure of response bias) and d' (a measure of discrimination performance independent of response biases) were calculated from the proportion of hits (correct identification of an intoxicated sentence) and false alarms (misidentification of a sober sentence as intoxicated). Both beta and d' were higher for the police officers than for the students, but whereas the difference for beta was not significant, d' was significantly higher (as determined by t-test) for the police officers (0.786) than for the students (0.603). This indicated that the police officers were significantly better than the students at discriminating sentences from the two conditions.

The receiver-operating characteristic (ROC) graph in Figure 7.6.1 plots proportions of hits and false alarms for the individual talkers and the police officers and students as listeners (see Swets, 1986a, 1986b). Results for individual talkers were similar across the two groups, but the police officers appeared to apply a stricter judgment criterion for seven of the eight talkers. Finally, percent accuracy across the confidence rating categories is shown in Table 7.6.2. For both listener groups, as confidence increased, accuracy did as well.

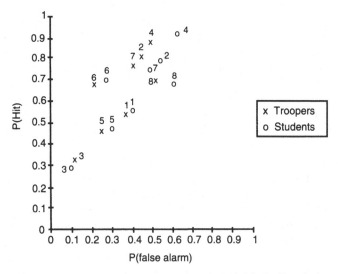

FIGURE 7.6.1 Receiver operator characteristic space for individual talkers by listener group (second perceptual experiment). (From Pisoni and Martin, 1989. Copyright © 1989 by Williams & Wilkins. Used by permission.)

TABLE 7.6.2   Percentage Accuracy across
the Five Confidence Rating Categories
for Trooper and Student Listeners:
Second Perceptual Experiment[a]

	Listener group	
Confidence ratings[b]	Troopers (%)	Students (%)
1	56.9	50.0
2	56.0	53.6
3	61.6	58.7
4	69.5	64.8
5	75.3	72.5

[a] From Pisoni and Martin (1989). Copyright © 1989
by Williams & Wilkins. Used by permission.
[b] 1 = least confident; 5 = most confident.

7.7 JOHNSON, PISONI, AND BERNACKI, 1989

This is a preliminary version of part of an appendix to National Transportation Safety Board (1990) and of K. Johnson et al. (1990). Further discussion
of alcohol and speech in the *Exxon Valdez* grounding can be found in
Chapter 8.

7.8 BEHNE AND RIVERA, 1990

This study continued the series of reports from the Indiana University/
General Motors studies (see section 7.1), reporting acoustic analyses of
segmental and prosodic aspects of isolated spondees (two-syllable words).
Results revealed that under intoxication, second and third formants were
lower, and that mean amplitude and mean frequency were both higher and
more variable. When this report appeared, Dawn Behne and Susan Rivera
were affiliated with the Speech Research Laboratory at Indiana University.

7.8.1 Subjects and Methods

Subjects were six male students from Indiana University, at least 21 years
of age and native speakers of English with no history of speech, hearing,
or language disorders. Subjects were screened using assessment procedures
described in section 7.1.1.2. Table 7.8.1 gives talker characteristics for the
six subjects for this study, including age; BAC at the beginning of recording
(Initial BAC); BAC at the end of the recording session (Final BAC); scores on
the MAST, socialization subscale, and MacAndrew Scale; and self-reported

TABLE 7.8.1   Subjects' Ages, and Blood-Alcohol Levels (BAL) at the Beginning and End of the Recording Sessions.[a, b]

Subjects	Age	Initial BAL (%)	Final BAL (%)	MAST	SOC	MAC	Alcohol intake
1	21	.17	.10	5	30	27	16.80
2	21	.13	.075	4	29	20	5.15
3	22	.15	.085	5	31	27	23.20
4	25	.13	.15	7	33	18	26.99
5	26	.10	.10	2	35	22	6.15
6	22	.16	.10	3	39	23	3.53

[a] From Behne and Rivera (1990). Used by permission.
[a] Also shown are scores on the Michigan Alcoholism Screening Test (MAST), the socialization scale (SOC), and scores on the MacAndrew scale (MAC). Self-reported total alcohol intake during the 30 days prior to recording (converted to ounces of 200-proof alcohol) are shown in the final column.

alcohol consumption during the 30 days prior to the recording session (converted to ounces of 200-proof alcohol). Stimulus material preparation and alcoholization and recording procedures were identical to those described more fully in sections 7.1.1.1 and 7.1.1.2 (some subjects were identical).

For this study, spondees were presented visually on a CRT monitor fed from a PDP 11/34 computer (Digital Equipment Corp.). Presentation rate was determined by the talker, who pressed a button to present the next item and who spoke the word appearing on the screen as quickly as possible. Recordings of spondee productions were made both before and after consumption of alcohol. The specific spondee items used in this study are listed in Appendix 1.

Audio recordings of the spondees were low-pass filtered and digitized at a rate of 20,000 samples/second. SRD (Speech Read) was employed to mark acoustic segments and extract measurements of those marked segments to a parameter file. Information in the parameter file included the duration of the marked segment; and within the marked segment: mean F1, F2, and F3 frequencies; mean FØ and its variability; and mean amplitude and its variability. The following measures were extracted for each of the spondees produced in each of the conditions:

1. Vowel duration: The duration from the beginning to the end of the periodic portion of the vowel in each syllable.
2. Intervowel duration: The duration between the end of the first vowel and the beginning of the second vowel of the spondee.
3. Vowel-to-word duration ratio: The vowel duration divided by the duration of the entire spondee for each syllable.

4. Intervowel-to-word duration ratio: The intervowel duration divided by the duration of the entire spondee.
5. First, second, and third formant frequencies: The mean frequency of the first (F1), second (F2), and third (F3) formants within the vowel of each syllable.
6. Mean amplitude: The mean amplitude within the vowel of each syllable.
7. Amplitude variability: The standard deviation of the amplitude within the vowel of each syllable.
8. Mean fundamental frequency: The mean fundamental frequency within the vowel of each syllable.
9. Fundamental frequency variability: The standard deviation of the fundamental frequency within the vowel of each syllable.

7.8.2 Results

Segmental results included effects for formant frequencies and segment-to-word duration ratios; prosodic results included effects for amplitudes, fundamental frequencies, and durations. ANOVAs were used to compare means for the measurements in the sober and intoxicated conditions.

7.8.2.1 Segmental Effects

Formant frequencies were compared to test the hypothesis that alcohol affects motor coordination and therefore relative placement of articulators. Differences in articulator placement would be manifested acoustically as changes in the formant frequencies of vowels. Measurements were made for the mean frequencies of the first three formants for the first vowel of the spondee (V1) and the second vowel (V2) in both pre- and postalcohol conditions. Table 7.8.2 displays these mean measurements, along with F values.

TABLE 7.8.2   Condition Means, F Values, and Probabilities for Formant Frequencies[a]

Measure	Sober (mean)	Intoxicated (mean)	F Value	p[b]
V1: F1	566 Hz	576 Hz	0.31	n.s.
V2: F1	605 Hz	595 Hz	0.32	n.s.
V1: F2	1992 Hz	1913 Hz	4.27	0.039
V2: F2	1956 Hz	1885 Hz	2.50	n.s.
V1: F3	3377 Hz	3247 Hz	6.52	0.011
V2: F3	3368 Hz	3223 Hz	5.69	0.017

[a] From Behne and Rivera (1990). Used by permission.
[b] n.s., not significant.

ANOVAs revealed alcohol effects for F2 and F3, but not for F1. As Table 7.8.2 indicates, the F2 values for both the first and second vowel were lower in the intoxicated condition, but this difference was significant only for the vowel in the first syllable. There was a consistently lower F2 for both vowels in the intoxicated condition, but this held only for subjects 1, 2, and 3. subjects 4 and 6 showed formant frequency lowering inconsistently, and Subject 5 showed the opposite change, a raising of F2 under intoxication. Lowering of F3 under alcohol occurred consistently for subjects 1, 2, 3, and 4, so that the first three subjects exhibited consistent lowering for both F2 and F3 under intoxication. Subjects 5 and 6 did not conform to this pattern, both showing raising of F3 for at least one of the vowels.

Table 7.8.3 shows duration ratios for (a) first vowel to word, (b) second vowel to word, and (c) intervowel to word. Although there appeared to be a slight increase in mean segment-to-word duration ratios for both V1 and V2, this difference was not significant . On the other hand, the decrease in mean intervowel-to-word duration ratios was significant and suggests that for duration effects under alcohol, there was a difference between consonants and vowels.

7.8.2.2 Prosodic Effects

Behne and Rivera (1990) investigated the effects of alcohol on three prosodic characteristics: amplitude, fundamental frequency (FØ), and duration. Table 7.8.4 shows mean amplitude, amplitude variability, and F values for each of the vowels in the spondee under both conditions. Both mean amplitude and mean amplitude variability of both vowels increased significantly in the intoxicated condition, as shown in Table 7.8.4. As with other measures, however, there was individual variation in both amplitude and amplitude variability. Subjects 1, 2, 3, and 4 exhibited the general pattern of increase in mean amplitude from the sober condition to the intoxicated condition, but subject 5 exhibited inconsistency, that is, an increase in mean amplitude for the first vowel, but a decrease for the second. Finally, subject 6 showed a decrease in mean amplitude for both vowels. There was a consistent increase in mean amplitude variability in both vowels under intox-

TABLE 7.8.3   Condition Means, F Values, and Probabilities for Segment-to-Word Ratios[a]

Measure	Sober (mean)	Intoxicated (mean)	F Value	p[b]
V1/word duration	0.18 ms	0.19 ms	0.85	n.s.
V2/word duration	0.27 ms	0.28 ms	3.08	n.s.
Intervowel/word duration	0.28 ms	0.26 ms	7.76	0.006

[a] From Behne and Rivera (1990). Used by permission.
[b] n.s., not significant.

TABLE 7.8.4   Condition Means, F Values, and Probabilities for Amplitude Measures[a]

Measure	Sober (mean)	Intoxicated (mean)	F Value	p
V1: mean amplitude	79.5 dB	80.9 dB	67.49	0.0001
V2: mean amplitude	75.9 dB	78.2 dB	173.16	0.0001
V1: amplitude var.	74.6 dB	76.4 dB	69.38	0.0001
V2: amplitude var.	71.6 dB	74.0 dB	122.67	0.0001

[a] From Behne and Rivera (1990). Used by permission.

ication for subjects 1 through 5, but an opposite effect, that is, a decrease in variability for both vowels, for subject 6.

Measures of mean FØ and mean FØ variability showed a pattern roughly similar to those for amplitude. As Table 7.8.5 shows, both mean FØ and mean FØ variability increased for both vowels under intoxication. Furthermore, the trend for increase in FØ under intoxication held generally for subjects 1 through 4, held only inconsistently for subject 5, and was reversed for subject 6, who exhibited a decrease in FØ for both vowels under intoxication. Finally, individual means for FØ variability showed that the general increase in FØ variability held across both vowels for subjects 1 through 5 but was inconsistent for subject 6, who increased variability for the first vowel but decreased it for the second vowel.

The final prosodic measurements were of segment durations, three for each spondee: first vowel, second vowel, and intervowel. As mentioned above, vowel durations were measured from the onset to the offset of periodicity, while the intervowel duration was measured from the offset of periodicity for the first vowel to the onset of periodicity for the second vowel. Table 7.8.6 gives means and F values for these three duration measurements under both conditions. As Table 7.8.6 shows, there was no significant change in mean duration for either of the vowels, but mean intervowel duration decreased significantly from the sober to the intoxicated condition.

7.8.3 Discussion

This study examined the effects of alcohol on speech for words produced in isolation, differing from a number of other acoustic analysis studies

TABLE 7.8.5   Condition Means, F Values, and Probabilities for FØ Measures[a]

Measure	Sober (mean)	Intoxicated (mean)	F value	p
V1: Mean FØ	130.6 Hz	139.4 Hz	109.94	0.0001
V2: Mean FØ	113.9 Hz	124.3 Hz	229.57	0.0001
V1: FØ Variability	3.4 Hz	5.0 Hz	14.49	0.0001
V2: FØ Variability	4.1 Hz	5.8 Hz	13.88	0.0001

[a] From Behne and Rivera (1990). Used by permission.

TABLE 7.8.6   Condition Means, F Values, and Probabilities for Duration Measures[a]

Measure	Sober (mean)	Intoxicated (mean)	F value	p[b]
V1 duration	0.09 ms	0.09 ms	0.08	n.s.
V2 duration	0.14 ms	0.14 ms	0.26	n.s.
Intervowel duration	0.15 ms	0.13 ms	9.74	0.002

[a] From Behne and River (1990). Used by permission.
[b] n.s., not significant.

discussed in this chapter (e.g., K. Johnson et al., 1989; Klingholz et al., 1988; Pisoni et al., 1985; Swartz, 1988), because in those studies, words were produced in connected speech. Other studies examined isolated words (e.g., Künzel et al., 1992; Niedzielska et al., 1994), but this study, along with Behne et al. (1991), are the only acoustic investigations specifically of isolated words.

Results showed a number of consistent effects of alcohol on the acoustic speech signal. First, the average frequencies of F2 and F3 were lowered from the pre- to the postalcohol condition, affecting vowel quality. Among durational measurements, both intervowel durations and intervowel-to-word duration ratios were reduced from the pre- to the postalcohol condition; however, vowel durations and vowel-to-word duration ratios did not show significant changes. These results indicate different effects of alcohol on consonants and vowels.

Additional effects of alcohol were found in amplitude and fundamental frequency. Increases from the pre- to the postalcohol condition were found for mean amplitude, amplitude variability, mean FØ, and FØ variability. Previous research showed a decrease, rather than an increase, in overall amplitude under alcohol, but Behne and Rivera attributed the present results to individual differences under extraordinary conditions. The variability, however, was consistent with previous research (e.g., Pisoni et al., 1985), in that variability of both amplitude and FØ increased in all of these studies, despite differences in the stimulus materials.

7.9 JOHNSON, PISONI, AND BERNACKI, 1990

This is the published version of the analysis that also appears as a working paper (see section 7.7) and as an appendix to a report by the NTSB regarding the grounding of the tankship *Exxon Valdez* in 1989. Further discussion of the role of alcohol and speech in the *Exxon Valdez* grounding can be found in Chapter 8.

7.9.1 Methods

The analysis reported here was based on six taped samples of speech produced by Captain Joseph Hazelwood, master of the U.S. tankship *Exxon Valdez* at the time of its grounding near Valdez, Alaska, USA. Five of the speech samples were provided by the United States NTSB, and the sixth sample was recorded from a broadcast television interview (CBS News: *Saturday Night with Connie Chung*) in March of 1990. All six samples were from different times relative to the actual time of grounding of the tankship. Five tapes (designated [−33], [−1], [0], [+1], and [+9]) were excerpted from radio transmissions from the bridge of the *Exxon Valdez* to the United States Coast Guard Vessel Traffic Center facility at Valdez, Alaska. The tape designated [−33] was recorded 33 hr before the grounding, at about 1500 on 22 March 1989, while the *Exxon Valdez* was inbound to Valdez. The [−1] tape was recorded approximately 45 min prior to the grounding, from 2324.50 to 2330.54 on 23 March 1989, during the outbound passage. The tape designated [0] was recorded immediately after the grounding, from 0026.41 to 0038.47 on 24 March 1989, and contains initial reports of the grounding. The tape designated [+1] contains statements made from 0107.29 to 0131.36 on 24 March 1989. Finally, the tape designated [+9] was recorded 9 hr after the grounding, from 0912.00 to 0938.10 on 24 March 1989, and contains statements regarding salvage of the cargo. The final (sixth) recording was taken from a televised interview as noted above.

Two phrases, "*Exxon Valdez*" and "thirteen and sixteen," were used to analyze fundamental frequency and speaking rate. Both phrases were repeated several times in the audiotaped radio transmissions and occupied similar discourse and sentence positions, affording a measure of control over potential variability.

7.9.2 Results

Results were reported as differences between speech signals in recordings made close to the time of the grounding and those made further removed from the time of the grounding. These differences were categorized as gross effects, segmental effects, and suprasegmental effects, as summarized in Table 7.9.1.

7.9.2.1 Gross Effects

Errors in phonetic properties (mispronunciations) or in lexical characteristics were considered gross effects. K. Johnson et al. (1990) cautioned that errors of the type listed in Table 7.9.1 also occur in spontaneous speech whether or not talkers have consumed alcohol. Additionally, because the speech samples were spontaneous, the intent of the talker was a matter of

TABLE 7.9.1   Summary of Phenomena Found in the Analysis
of the National Transportation Safety Board Tapes[a, b]

Gross effects	Revisions
	(−1) *Exxon Ba,* uh *Exxon Valdez*
	(−1) departed disembarked
	(−1) I, we'll
	(−1) Columbia Gla, Columbia Bay
Segmental effects	Misarticulation of [r] and [l]
	(0) northerly, little, drizzle, visibility
	[s] becomes [ʃ]
	Final devoicing (e.g., [z] → [s])
	(−1, 0, +1) Valdez → Valdes
Suprasegmental effects	Reduced speaking rate
	Mean change in pitch range
	(talker-dependent)
	Increased FØ jitter

[a] Numbers in parentheses indicate the time of recording.
[b] From K. Johnson, Pisoni, and Bernacki (1990). Copyright ©
1990 by S. Karger AG, Basel. Used by permission.

conjecture; equally ambiguous was whether or not some utterance or part
of an utterance was in error. Thus, Johnson et al. reported only those
instances in which the speaker corrected himself. On this basis, all gross
effects across the six tapes were found in the tape made at 1 hr prior to the
grounding. The [−1] tape thus contained the entire corpus of effects noticeable by an untrained listener without benefit of measurement instruments.

7.9.2.2 Segmental Effects

Johnson et al. pointed out that the audiotapes used for analysis contained
a large amount of noise and that repeated listenings and transcription were
necessary. This was true for the misarticulations of liquids and for final
devoicing noted in Table 7.9.1 but not for the fricative substitution, several
instances of which were then also subjected to acoustic analysis.

Misarticulation of the liquid consonants [l] or [r] occurred at time [0],
immediately after the grounding. Examples are pronunciations of the words
northerly, little, drizzle, and *visibility.* There was also evidence of final
devoicing in, for example, the word *Valdez,* in which the final *z* had an [s]
substitution. These were noted at times [-1], [0], [+1].

A substitution of the alveolar fricative [s] by the alveopalatal fricative [ʃ]
was revealed by acoustic analysis. Figure 7.9.1 shows power spectra for
typical productions of these two sounds, produced by the first author (K.
Johnson) under controlled conditions with a high SNR ratio and instrument
response up to 5,000 Hz. On these displays, frequency in Hz is displayed

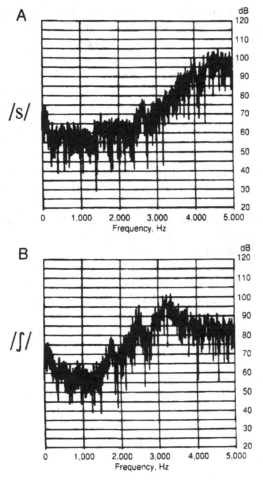

FIGURE 7.9.1   Power spectra of [s] (a) and [ʃ] (b) produced by K. J. in a quiet recording booth with recording equipment responsive up to 5000 Hz. (From K. Johnson, Pisoni, and Bernacki, 1990. Copyright © S. Karger AG, Basel, Switzerland. Used by permission.)

along the ordinate and energy (power) in dB along the abscissa. Differences between the two segments are apparent: whereas [s] shows an energy peak between 4000 and 5000 Hz, the energy peak for [ʃ] is lower, between 3000 and 4000 Hz. Additionally, [ʃ] has a second peak, lower in amplitude, and located between 2000 to 3000 Hz.

Figure 7.9.2 displays power spectra for transmitted productions of [ʃ] in the words *she's* and *shouts* and for background noise from the radio transmissions from the *Exxon Valdez* at time [-33]. As Figure 7.9.2 shows, the lower amplitude energy peak in the 2000–3000 Hz range was present; however, the energy peak in the 3000–4000 Hz range was absent, due to a 3000-Hz band-limit imposed by the radio equipment (energy above 3000 Hz was attenuated at approximately 50 dB per octave with a noise floor 50 dB below maximum signal level). Because the NTSB recordings were gathered under less than ideal conditions,[1] K. Johnson et al. (1990) were concerned about background spectral noise. To assess these differences, they paired each production of [ʃ] in Figure 7.9.2 with spectra of noise recorded during open-microphone pauses to serve as a comparison baseline for the fricative spectra.

Similarly, power spectra of [s] in *sea* or *see* and background noise were compared; average temporal distance of noise from [s] was 1.3 sec. For the [-33] and [-1] productions, the spectral shape of the [s] appeared to mimic that of the noise, leading K. Johnson et al. (1990) to conclude that the spectral energy of the fricative was not within the frequency range of the transmission system. However, the [0] and [+1] spectra showed energy peaks between 2000 and 3000 Hz. This was considered evidence of a change from [s] to [ʃ], as this spectrum more nearly resembled that of the alveopalatal fricative rather than of the alveolar. K. Johnson et al. also noted that evidence for this substitution was lacking from the [-33] to the [-1] recordings. Finally, the [+9] spectrum more closely resembled the [-33] and [-1] spectra in lacking the energy peak between 2000 and 3000 Hz.

7.9.2.3 Suprasegmental Effects

Suprasegmental effects included reduced speaking rate, mean change in pitch range, and increased jitter. Neither amplitude nor long-term average spectra was measured, because the transmission equipment had an automatic gain control, and the microphone-to-mouth distance was presumed to be variable. In making measurements of speaking rate and fundamental fre-

---

[1] All NTSB-provided tapes were originally recorded on the same United States Coast Guard recording equipment. However, the tape designated as [-33] was rerecorded onto a handheld cassette tape recorder prior to being accidentally erased. This second tape was analyzed by K. Johnson et al. (1990) using the same handheld tape recorder that had been used to record it. To investigate the possibility of corruption of the [-33] tape, K. Johnson et al. (1990) analyzed an unidentified background sound that appeared on both the [-33] and the [-1] tape. The [-33] tape had an average FØ of 480 Hz ($n = 4$) and an FØ range of 438–588 Hz, whereas the [-1] tape had an average FØ of 472 Hz ($n = 10$) and an FØ range of 456–481 Hz. Average FØ was thus higher and FØ range greater for the [-33] recording than for the [-1] recording. K. Johnson et al. (1990) determined that the variability in the [-1] recording was too great for that recording to be used as a comparison standard for the [-33] recording. However, they also concluded that the magnitude of potential corruptions of the [-33] tape indicated (corresponding to from -9 to 22% of the measurements) would not have been sufficient to account for speech changes subsequently reported.

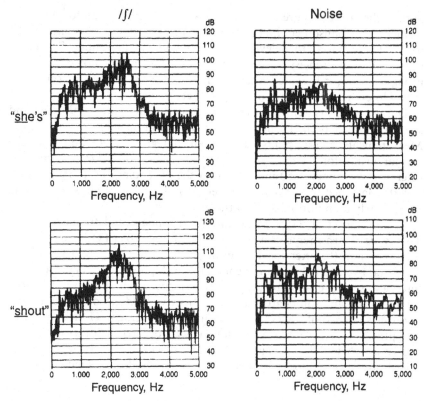

FIGURE 7.9.2 Power spectra of [ʃ] produced by Captain Hazelwood in the words *she's* and *shout* recorded 33 hr before the accident. Each spectrum is paired with a spectrum of the background noise from a nearby open-mike pause. (From K. Johnson, Pisoni, and Bernacki, 1990. Copyright © S. Karger AG, Basel, Switzerland. Used by permission.)

quency, K. Johnson et al. (1990) paid close attention to possible differences in discourse and sentence position and chose the phrases "*Exxon Valdez*" and "thirteen and sixteen" for analysis, because these were repeated a number of times in different transmissions and occurred in comparable discourse and sentence positions.

Separate measurements were made for each of the segments in "*Exxon Valdez*." Means of two occurrences of the utterance from each transmission interval were compared, and it was found that the total duration increased from the [-33] transmission to the [0] transmission and then decreased from there. That is, phrase duration was longer the closer a transmission was to the time of the grounding. Further examination revealed that the effect of increased duration was not equally distributed among the segments in the phrase: the effect was greater for the vowels and the [v] than for the other segments. K. Johnson et al. (1990) further measured one occurrence of the word "*Valdez*" from the televised interview with Connie Chung. The duration for this occurrence is compared with those for transmission occurrences in Figure 7.9.3; it is evident that the duration of the interview occurrence most closely resembled that of the [-33] recording.

Durational measurements were also made for the phrase "thirteen and sixteen," which occurred in discourse-final position in three recordings. Measurements of this phrase are shown in Figure 7.9.4. Similar to the measurements for "*Valdez*" in Figure 7.9.3, the total duration for this utterance was longer at times closer to the grounding. K. Johnson et al. (1990) concluded from these measurements that the captain was speaking more slowly than normal around the grounding.

K. Johnson et al. (1990) also measured fundamental frequency (FØ). Two types of measurements were made: (a) average voice FØ across samples of speech and (b) jitter (peak-to-peak perturbations in FØ). Figure 7.9.5 shows (a) average FØ measurements for two shipboard utterances and one interview sentence and (b) jitter measurements from those same speech samples. The first shipboard utterance, "*Exxon Valdez,*" occurred at least two times in each of the NTSB recordings, and average FØ measurements and jitter measurements over the four vowels occurring in this phrase are shown as filled circles in Figure 7.9.5. Measurements for the second shipboard utterance, "thirteen and sixteen," were based on a smaller number

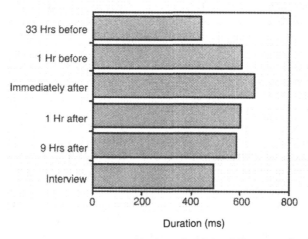

Duration (ms)

FIGURE 7.9.3 Duration of the word *Valdez* from the National Transportation Safety Board tapes compared with the same word produced in a similar discourse position in the televised interview. (From Johnson, Pisoni, and Bernacki, 1990. Copyright © S. Karger AG, Basel, Switzerland. Used by permission.)

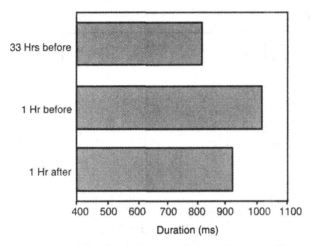

FIGURE 7.9.4 Duration of the phrase *thirteen and sixteen* from recordings made at three times around the time of the accident. (From K. Johnson, Pisoni, and Bernacki, 1990. Copyright © S. Karger AG, Basel, Switzerland. Used by permission.)

of speech samples (mainly because of low amplitudes in a number of renditions), but each measurement in Figure 7.9.5 for this utterance (shown as open triangles) was based on at least two vowels. Average FØ and jitter measurements for a sentence from the March 1990 televised interview are indicated by filled squares in both panels of Figure 7.9.5.

Because of the background noise on the NTSB recordings, K. Johnson et al. (1990) could not employ standard pitch-detection algorithms used for speech recorded in the quiet. Modification of an existing pitch algorithm was therefore used, whereby the signal was rectified and low-pass filtered before any attempt to locate successive pitch periods. Visual confirmation of the algorithm was made prior to calculation of FØ and jitter. Jitter was calculated according to Davis's (1976) *pitch perturbation quotient.* As indicated in Figure 7.9.5(a), average FØs were lower in recordings close to the time of the grounding than in those further removed. Panel (a) also shows the average FØ range for each phrase in each recording. With the exception of the [+9] recording, these FØ ranges are not readily distinguishable from each other, but Figure 7.9.5(b) shows a trend toward more jitter in the recordings around the time of the grounding than in those further removed.

To summarize, K. Johnson et al. (1990) found the following acoustic-phonetic changes in audio recordings made around the time of the grounding as compared to those recordings made further removed from the time of the

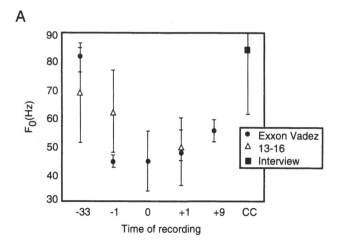

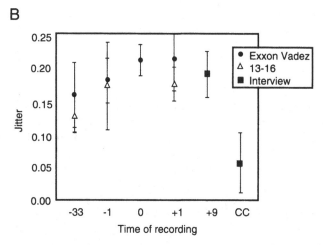

FIGURE 7.9.5 (a) Average FØ in *Exxon Valdez, thirteen and sixteen,* and from one sentence in the televised interview as a function of time of recording. (b) FØ jitter measurements from the same speech samples. (From K. Johnson, Pisoni, and Bernacki, 1990. Copyright © S. Karger AG, Basel, Switzerland. Used by permission.)

grounding: (a) gross effects: revisions; (b) segmental effects: misarticulations, including changes in [r] and [l], changes in [s], and final devoicing; and (c) suprasegmental effects, including reduced speaking rate, lower FØ, and increased FØ jitter.

7.9.3 Discussion

This report represents an application of laboratory research to a real-life situation. The question was whether there was sufficient evidence in voice recordings to indicate intoxication. In that sense, a general question was whether the acoustic signal could in principle contain sufficient evidence, but a specific question was whether a particular person at a particular time under particular circumstances revealed intoxication in those voice recordings.

Although K. Johnson et al. (1990) proposed that alcohol intoxication was the simplest explanation for the speech changes observed in the tape recordings, they also noted three factors limiting their ability to make a conclusive determination. First, gaps in the research literature regarding alcohol and other effects on speech production included a lack of studies of vocal jitter under alcohol, as well as insufficient research regarding other environmental and emotional effects on the speech signal. Second, the available research literature on alcohol and speech reported results from relatively small numbers of subjects. Third, the type and quality of the available tape recordings for speech analysis were limited. This included a lack of information regarding speaking intensity and the presence and variability of background noise. Addtionally, the history of the [−33] tape was a complicated one and could introduce error into the analysis.

7.10 NATIONAL TRANSPORTATION SAFETY BOARD, 1990

This is the report of the NTSB regarding the grounding of the tankship *Exxon Valdez* near Valdez, Alaska, in 1989. Among other safety factors discussed are those regarding the role of alcohol in the grounding. As part of its investigation, the NTSB made available audio recordings of radio transmissions from the *Exxon Valdez* to two sets of researchers in Canada and the United States. Transcripts of these transmissions and reports from both research teams were included in an appendix to the report.

The authors of the first report included in the appendix were Mark B. Sobell and Linda C. Sobell of the Addiction Research Foundation in Toronto, Ontario, and both professors at the University of Toronto. Their primary results were based on an auditory analysis of vocal quality changes present on the transmission tapes occurring between a time roughly 24 hr prior to the grounding to a time roughly 1 hr before the grounding. The results of their analysis are discussed more fully in Chapter 8.

The authors of the second report included in the appendix were Keith Johnson, David B. Pisoni, and Robert H. Bernacki, affiliated with the Speech Research Laboratory at Indiana University in Bloomington, Indiana. Their report has appeared in three versions: (a) the version appearing in Appendix J of the NTSB report, (b) as a working paper in the progress report of the Speech Research Laboratory at Indiana University (K. Johnson et al., 1989), and (c) a published version in the journal *Phonetica* (K. Johnson et al.,

1990). The analysis by these researchers is discussed in section 7.9 (K. Johnson et al., 1990), with further discussion in Chapter 8, where possible forensic application of speech analysis techniques are considered.

7.11 KÜNZEL, 1990

This conference presentation is a short report of the work done in the Federal Republic of Germany reported fully in Künzel et al. (1992). The forensic aspects and applications of the research are apparent both from the author's affiliation with the German *Bundeskriminalamt* (Federal Criminal Police Office) and the forensics conference at which this presentation was made. In this paper, Kuenzel reported on acoustic and phonetic analyses of speech pauses and speaking rate. A full report of this research project was published as Künzel et al. (1992), discussed in section 7.18.

7.12 BEHNE, RIVERA, AND PISONI, 1991

This study continues the research program undertaken at Indiana University under contract with General Motors Research Laboratories. Other studies from that program include Pisoni et al. (1985; see section 7.1), Pisoni et al. (1986; see section 7.2), Pisoni and Martin (1989; see section 7.6), and Behne and Rivera (1990; see section 7.8). In Behne, Rivera, and Pisoni (1991), the authors investigated the effects of alcohol on durational aspects of speech. Results showed sentence durations to be consistently longer under alcohol, but word durations only inconsistently different. All authors were affiliated with the Speech Research Laboratory at Indiana University.

7.12.1 Subjects and Methods

Subjects for this study were nine male volunteers from Indiana University. All were at least 21 years of age and native speakers of English with no history of speech, language, or hearing disorders. Questionnaires were used to assess alcohol consumption and risk for alcoholism, as described in section 7.1.1.2. Scores for subjects used in this study appear in Table 7.12.1. Stimulus material preparation, alcoholization procedures, and recording procedures were identical to those described more fully in sections 7.1.1.1 and 7.1.1.2.

Recordings were low-pass filtered and digitized at a sampling rate of 20 kHz. Durational measurements were made using a waveform editor; word durations were based on monosyllabic words and spondees, whereas sen-

TABLE 7.12.1 Subjects' Ages, and Blood-Alcohol Levels at the Beginning and End of the Recording Sessions[a, b]

Subjects	Age	Initial BAL (%)	Final BAL (%)	MAST	SOC	MAC	Alcohol intake
1	26	.10	.10	2	35	22	6.15
2	22	.16	.10	3	39	23	3.53
3	21	.17	.10	5	30	27	16.80
4	21	.13	.075	4	29	20	5.15
5	22	.15	.085	5	31	27	23.20
6	25	.135	.15	7	33	18	26.99
7	21	.15	.10	6	36	24	8.94
8	21	.15	.095	0	42	22	13.13
9	21	.19	.12	6	34	27	5.54

[a] Also shown are scores on the Michigan Alcohol Screening Test (MAST), the socialization scale (SOC), and scores on the MacAndrew scale (MAC). Self-reported total alcohol intake during the 30 days prior to recording (converted to ounces of 200-proof alcohol) are shown in the final column.
[b] From Behne, Rivera, and Pisoni (1991). Used by permission.

tence durations were measured for isolated sentences, tongue twisters, and sentences within passages.

7.12.2 Results

For each type of utterance, durations were collapsed across subjects, and an ANOVA was used to compare means in the two conditions. Table 7.12.2 gives mean durations for each utterance type in the two conditions, along with F values. Figure 7.12.1 shows mean durations for sentences, measured from tongue twisters, isolated sentences, and sentences within the three connected passages. The effect of alcohol was significant for tongue twisters and isolated sentences. Additionally, there was a reliable effect of alcohol

TABLE 7.12.2 Mean Durations and F Values for Each Utterance Type[a]

	Sober	Intoxicated	F value
Monosyllabic words	521 ms	540 ms	31.80 ($p < .001$)
Spondees	519 ms	529 ms	1.29 (n.s.[b])
Tongue twisters	1920 ms	2130 ms	10.50 ($p < .001$)
Simple sentences	1510 ms	1640 ms	182.67 ($p < .001$)
Grandfather passage	4030 ms	4440 ms	12.65 ($p < .001$)
Victory garden passage	4470 ms	4930 ms	14.62 ($p < .001$)
Rainbow passage	4590 ms	5050 ms	22.68 ($p < .001$)

[a] From Behne, Rivera, and Pisoni (1991). Used by permission.
[b] n.s., not significant.

on sentence durations in the three connected passages. In general, and as illustrated in Figure 7.12.1, sentence durations were longer in the intoxicated condition than in the sober one.

Durations for words were measured for monosyllables and spondees, all produced in isolation. Figure 7.12.2 gives mean durations for the two types of words in the two conditions. Although durations tended to be longer in the intoxicated condition, this difference was statistically reliable only for the monosyllabic words and not for the spondees.

7.12.3 Discussion

The conclusion from this study was that alcohol increases the duration of words and sentences; that is, subjects spoke more slowly after alcohol. Both monosyllabic words and spondees were examined; the lengthening effect of alcohol was reliable for the monosyllabic words but not for the spondees (although these also reflected the trend). For sentences, however, alcohol exerted the effect on all elicited types: tongue twisters, isolated sentences, and sentences in passages. These results were consistent with previous findings for longer durations and slower speaking rates (e.g., Lester & Skousen, 1974; Pisoni et al., 1985, 1986; Pisoni & Martin, 1989; Sobell et al., 1982).

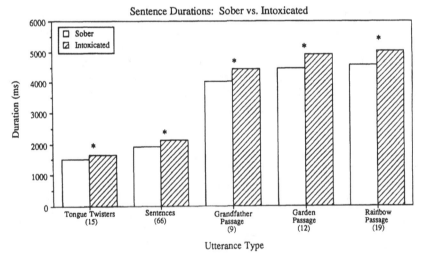

FIGURE 7.12.1 Sentence durations from the sober and intoxicated conditions for the tongue twisters and simple sentences, and for sentences from within the passages. Values in parentheses on the y-axis are the number of sentences contributing to the mean for each utterance type. An asterisk marks means that are reliably different. (From Behne, Rivera, and Pisoni, 1991. Used by permission.)

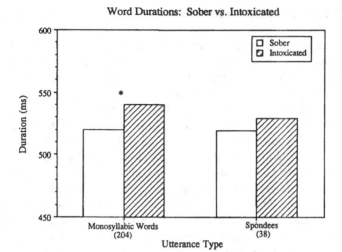

FIGURE 7.12.2 Word durations from the sober and intoxicated conditions for the monosyllabic words and spondees. Values in parentheses on the *x*-axis are the number of words
contributing to the means for each utterance type. An asterisk marks means that are reliably
different. (From Behne, Rivera, and Pisoni, 1991). Used by permission.)

7.13 BRAUN, 1991

This report from the Künzel-Braun-Eysholdt group was presented at the
XIIth International Congress of Phonetic Sciences, in Aix-en-Provence,
France. Angelika Braun was affiliated with the Landeskriminalamt
Nordrhein-Westfalen in Düsseldorf, Germany. Other reports from this same
research project are Künzel (1990, 1992), Eysholdt (1992), and Künzel et
al. (1992). Results were reported for segmental analyses (velar action, slurred
articulations, and segment lengthening) and for "production errors." A full
report of this research project was published as Künzel et al. (1992), discussed in section 7.18.

In discussing velar action, Braun reported that "the denasalization of
vowels implies the nasalization of vowels, i.e. that there is no case of consonant denasalization without vowel nasalization" (p. 147). What was probably meant was that denasalization of *consonants* implies nasalization of
vowels, but even then, the evidence indicated the implication to be the
other way around. That is, at BrACs of 0.12% and above, both consonant
denasalization and vowel nasalization occurred, but below that level, only
consonant denasalization occurred. Also, Braun reported cases of "cluster"
reduction, although some of these may actually have involved a related but
somewhat different process of deaffrication.

7.14 BRENNER AND CASH, 1991

This article reviews the speech analyses informing the finding by the NTSB
that the master of the U.S. tankship *Exxon Valdez* was impaired by alcohol
when the ship grounded on Bligh Reef, near Valdez, Alaska, in March 1989.
Voice recordings were analyzed by three groups: (a) the NTSB's audio
laboratory (NTSB group); (b) Mark B. Sobell and Linda C. Sobell, of the
Addiction Research Foundation in Toronto, Ontario, Canada, as expert
consultants (Toronto group); and (c) Keith Johnson, David B. Pisoni, and
Robert H. Bernacki, of the Speech Research Laboratory at Indiana University, in Bloomington, Indiana, as expert consultants (Bloomington group).
The findings of the last-named group appear elsewhere, including K. Johnson
et al. (1990) and Pisoni et al. (1991). A full discussion of the issues of
alcohol and speech surrounding the *Exxon Valdez* grounding can be found
in Chapter 8. At the time this article appeared, Malcolm Brenner was a
human performance investigator with the NTSB in Washington, DC, and
James R. Cash was a National Resource Specialist, Cockpit Voice Recorder,
with the same agency.

7.14.1 Voice Recordings

The speech materials used for analysis by all three groups were tape recordings of excerpted radio transmissions from the bridge of the *Exxon Valdez*.
The on-board radio transmitter was enclosed in a telephone-style handset
and used FM radio transmission. Transmissions were relayed by microwave
link towers to the U.S. Coast Guard Vessel Traffic Center (VTC) facility at
Valdez, Alaska; there, the transmissions were recorded on a continuously
running multichannel tape recorder (Magnasync Model 2-R/P-30).

A total of 42 transmissions from the master of the Exxon Valdez were
identified from five different periods relative to the time of the grounding:

1. Thirty-three hours prior to the grounding [–33]: recorded at
   approximately 1500 on 22 March 1989 while the *Exxon Valdez*
   was inbound to Valdez.
2. One hour (approximately 45 min) prior to the grounding [–1]:
   recorded from 2324.50 to 2330.54 on 23 March 1989 outbound
   from Valdez.
3. Immediately subsequent to the grounding [0]: recording from
   0026.41 to 0038.47 on 24 March 1989.
4. One hour subsequent to the grounding [+1]: recorded from
   0107.29 to 0131.36 on 24 March 1989.
5. Nine hours subsequent to the grounding [+9]: recorded from
   0912.00 to 0938.19 on 24 March 1989.

Speech analyses by the three research groups were based on composite recordings assembled by NTSB staff.

7.14.2 Results

Results were reported from four areas in which alcohol had previously been found to affect speech: (a) changes in speaking rate, (b) speech errors, (c) misarticulations, and (d) changes in vocal quality.

The investigation of speaking rate was based on the results of previous research demonstrating reduced speech rates under alcohol (Lester & Skousen, 1974; Pisoni & Martin, 1989; Pisoni et al., 1986; Sobell & Sobell, 1972; Sobell et al., 1982). Brenner and Cash reported findings on speaking rate from both the NTSB group and the Bloomington group. The NTSB analyzed 36 of the 42 tape-recorded statements made by the master. The composite tape was digitized at 16 kHz, and the statements were played back and examined both visually using a graphic display of the waveform and auditorily using headphones and speakers. Start and stop times of the statements were recorded to provide duration measurements; these durations and a computation of the number of syllables yielded speaking rate in syllables per second (S/s). Table 7.14.1 summarizes these measures.

Mean speaking rates in syllables per second at the five intervals were: [−33]: 5.1; [−1]: 3.2; [0]: 2.9; [+1 hour]: 3.5; [+9]: 4.4. Speaking rates were thus slower at the intervals closest to the time of the grounding and faster at [−33] and [+9]. An ANOVA showed significant differences between the five intervals, and contrast tests showed that speech 1 hr prior to the grounding was significantly slower than 9 hr subsequent and 33 hr prior.

Duration measurements by the Bloomington group were made on the phrase "*Exxon Valdez*," spoken at least once during each interval. The times required to say the phrase were, at the [−33] interval, 706 ms; at [−1], 934 ms; at [0], 1087 ms; at [+1], 980 ms; at [+9], 883 ms. Similar to the findings of the NTSB group, this measurement showed shorter durations at intervals further removed from the grounding time.

The NTSB group also measured the speech of other persons on the original tape recordings for comparison with the master's speech. Mean speaking rates for these persons were: chief mate, 4.4 S/s; second mate, 5.8 S/s; pilot, 5.7 S/s; VTC watchstander (1 hr prior to the grounding), 6.5. All of these talkers showed speaking rates higher than that of the master, both prior to and subsequent to the grounding.

Speech errors were also present in the tape recordings, but because the intention of the talker was not known for sure in spontaneous speech, they were clearly errors only when the captain corrected himself. At 1 hr prior to the grounding, this occurred in four instances: Statement 3: "*Exxon Ba,*

TABLE 7.14.1   Summary of Speaking Rate Measures for 36 Statements That Provided
Sufficient Data for Analysis (7 or More Spoken Syllables)[a]

Statement number	Number of syllables analyzed	Measured durations	Speaking rate (syllables/s)	Hours with respect to accident
1.	12	2.18	5.5	−33
2.	88	19.28	4.6	−33
3.	11	3.79	2.9	−1
4.	42	16.20	2.6	−1
5.	50	16.16	3.1	−1
6.	48	15.24	3.1	−1
7.	16	4.18	3.8	−1
8.	17	4.35	3.9	−1
9.	78	24.20	3.2	−1
10.	11	3.50	3.1	−1
11.	66	35.43	1.9	0
13.	16	3.83	4.2	0
14.	7	1.67	4.2	0
15.	25	10.36	2.4	0
16.	7	2.56	2.7	0
17.	18	9.54	1.9	0
18.	7	1.94	3.6	+1
19.	58	19.54	3.0	+1
20.	68	17.49	3.9	+1
21.	65	20.34	3.2	+1
23.	15	5.83	2.6	+1
24.	16	4.11	3.9	+1
25.	33	9.06	3.6	+1
26.	15	3.37	4.5	+1
27.	94	22.10	4.3	+9
28.	50	14.05	3.6	+9
29.	39	7.61	5.1	+9
30.	28	6.08	4.6	+9
33.	9	1.86	4.8	+9
34.	21	4.97	4.2	+9
35.	38	10.91	3.5	+9
36.	52	11.73	4.4	+9
37.	48	12.56	3.8	+9
40.	13	2.88	4.5	+9
41.	13	2.81	4.6	+9
42.	7	1.33	5.3	+9

[a] From Brenner and Cash (1991). Copyright © 1991 by Aerospace Medical Association. Used
by permission.

ah, *Valdez*"; Statement 4: "We've, ah, departed the pilot or disembarked
the pilot. Excuse me"; Statement 5: " . . . judging by our radar, I
we'll probably . . ."; Statement 9: '. . . ice out of Columbia Gla . . .
Bay . . . ."

The investigation of misarticulations was based on observations in the literature that misarticulations of certain sounds occur more frequently under alcohol. For instance, Pisoni and Martin (1989) and Pisoni et al. (1986) had observed that certain "difficult" sounds requiring fine sensorimotor control and timing were especially susceptible to misarticulation under alcohol. In the case of the *Exxon Valdez* tapes, the Bloomington group used phonetic transcription and power spectrum displays to identify misarticulated segments in the master's speech. Misarticulations included: (a) misarticulation of the liquids [l] and [r] in such words as *northerly, little, drizzle,* and *visibility*; (2) devoicing of the final consonant in the word "*Valdez,*" and (3) realization of alveolar [s] as the alveopalatal [ʃ] in the word *Exxon* at intervals around the time of the grounding.

Vocal quality was assessed by the Toronto group, who observed changes in the master's speech across the five intervals. Statements from 33 hr prior to the grounding, were "rapid, fluent, without hesitation, and with few word interjections (i.e., ah) in relation to the length of the sample" (National Transportation Safety Board 1990, p. 224). However, around the time of the grounding, changes in the master's speech included considerable word interjections, broken words, incomplete phrases, corrected errors, and increased speaking time and hesitations (National Transportation Safety Board 1990, p. 225). Then, beginning with statements at 9 hr subsequent to the grounding, the researchers observed that "the speaker sounds more fluent (more rapid speech, more responsive) and makes few word interjections (ah)" (National Transportation Safety Board 1990, p. 225).

7.14.3 Other Causes of Speech Changes

Brenner and Cash also considered a number of other factors that might have contributed to the changes in speech observed in the tapes. Among these alternative factors were fatigue, psychological stress, drug effects, and medical problems.

The question of fatigue rested on knowing the master's sleep schedule, specifically during the period preceding the grounding. This was not determined in the investigation, because the master did not have watchstanding duties the night prior to the grounding. It was suggested that the master was continuously active from approximately 1030 on 23 March 1989 until the grounding at approximately 0009 on 24 March 1989; a possible exception was a 1.5-hr period during the outbound passage when the master went to his quarters. Among other evidence, testimony from Coast Guard personnel indicated that the master remained awake from the time of the grounding (approximately 0009 on 24 March 1989) until 1050 on 24 March 1989. Given this, Brenner and Cash took the recording from 9 hr subsequent to the grounding as an example of speech produced under fatigue but found less evidence of speech impairment in that tape than in ones recorded closer to the time of the grounding.

Brenner and Cash also considered the possibility that psychological stress might have been revealed in the tape recordings. Assuming that stress would be a natural result of the grounding itself, the speech samples from 33 hr and 1 hr prior to the grounding were analyzed. Again, the recording from 1 hr prior to the grounding already showed evidence of speech impairment. The researchers also considered drug effects as a cause of speech changes; here, toxicology results showed evidence of only alcohol in the blood and urine samples. Finally, medical causes of speech changes, such as stroke, were considered. Here, health insurance records showed no claims filed in the year preceding the grounding. The only evidence of a medical problem was treatment for alcohol problems in 1985 and arrests for motor vehicle offenses in 1985 and 1988.

7.14.4 Discussion

Both the Toronto group and the Bloomington group independently reported to the NTSB that the speech changes exhibited by the master of the *Exxon Valdez* were consistent with changes observed when a talker is impaired by alcohol, and the NTSB concluded that Joseph Hazelwood was impaired by alcohol at the time of the grounding. A fuller discussion of this incident can be found in Chapter 8.

7.15 PISONI, JOHNSON, AND BERNACKI, 1991

This article reviewed research on alcohol and speech, as well as the specific case of the Exxon Valdez. The general literature summarized included Dunker and Schlosshauer (1964), Klingholz et al. (1988), Lester and Skousen (1974), Pisoni et al. (1986); Pisoni and Martin (1989), Sobell and Sobell (1972), Sobell et al. (1982), and Trojan and Kryspin-Exner (1968). The report on the acoustic analysis of recordings from the *Exxon Valdez* reiterated K. Johnson et al. (1990), discussed in section 7.9. A short discussion of the legal aspects of speech and voice analysis as an indicator of intoxication was based on Tanford, Pisoni, and Johnson (1991), which is more fully discussed here in Chapter 8.

7.16 EYSHOLDT, 1992

This paper continued the series of reports described fully in Künzel et al. (1992). Eysholdt was affiliated with the Department of Phoniatrics and

Pediatric Audiology at the Ear, Nose, and Throat Clinic at the University of Erlangen, Germany. In this report, Eysholdt presented the results of subjective perceptual judgments of clinical voice parameters and of strobo-scopic and endoscopic examination. Eysholdt suggested that acute alcohol intoxication was a model of central dysphonia with increased vocal-fold tonus and disturbance of kinesthetic voice control, further suggesting that various vocal parameters examined could be classified into four groups: (a) unaffected by alcohol: vital capacity; (b) affected by alcohol for short periods of time: glottic closure; (c) affected proportionally to the alcohol level: maximum phonation time, frequency range, fundamental frequency, overall voice quality; (d) affected inversely proportional to the alcohol level: vocal fold amplitude, mucosal waves.

7.17 KÜNZEL, 1992

This report was Hermann Künzel's *Habilitationsvortrag* (roughly, a lecture delivered by a tenure candidate) at the Philipps-Universität in Marburg, Germany. Künzel concentrated on phonetic production characteristics of alcohol-affected speech and perception of alcoholized speech by listeners. Results from these investigations were reported fully in Künzel et al. (1992), discussed in section 7.18.

In a short discussion at the end of this work, Künzel suggested that the effects of alcohol on speech might be understood within the context of gestural or articulatory phonology, as proposed, for example, by Browman and Goldstein (1986, 1989, 1992). This theory suggests that

> gestures are characterizations of discrete, physically real events that unfold during the speech production process. Articulatory phonology attempts to describe lexi-cal units in terms of these events and their interrelations, which means that gestures are basic units of contrast among lexical items as well as units of articula-tory action. (Browman & Goldstein, 1992, p. 156)

Within this theory, articulatory gestures can overlap in time and can more-over have durations longer than the traditional segment. Cases of reductions and substitutions in alcohol-affected speech can thus be accounted for as perturbations in the relative timing of various gestures.

7.18 KÜNZEL, BRAUN, AND EYSHOLDT, 1992

This book is a detailed and exhaustive report of a research project on the effects of alcohol on speech. The three authors were affiliated with forensic and academic institutions in (West) Germany. Hermann J. Künzel was affiliated with the Speaker Identification and Tape Authentication Laboratory (*Fachbereich Sprechererkennung und Tonbandauswertung*) at the German *Bundeskriminalamt* (the federal law enforcement agency comparable to the United States Federal Bureau of Investigation), as well as with the phonetics department at the University of Marburg. Angelika Braun was affiliated with the Speaker Identification Division (*Sachgebiet Sprechererkennung*) of the *Landeskriminalamt* for North-Rhine/Westphalia (comparable to a state criminal investigation department in the United States). Finally, Ulrich Eysholdt was affiliated with the Department of Phoniatrics and Pediatric Audiology at the University Ear-Nose-Throat Clinic (*Abteilung für Phoniatrie und Pädaudiologie der Universitätsklinik für Hals-Nasen-Ohrenkranke*) in Erlangen.

The approach in this study and in this report was interdisciplinary, bringing together practitioners and analyses from phonetics and linguistics, from phoniatrics and logopedics, and from neurology. Other reports from this research project include Künzel (1990, 1992), Braun (1991), and Eysholdt (1992). Note that all reported BrACs are expressed as permillages (‰), as was done by Künzel et al. A review of this book appears as Grassegger (1994).

7.18.1 Subjects and Methods

Subjects were 33 male police officers in training at the Hessian Police School in Wiesbaden, Germany, with a mean age of 23 years (*SD* = 15 months). A questionnaire was used to determine smoking and drinking practices and to identify medical risks. Twenty of the subjects used alcohol regularly, between one and five glasses of beer daily, whereas thirteen claimed to be irregular consumers of alcohol. Twenty of the subjects were nonsmokers, while thirteen smoked between 10 and 20 cigarettes or several pipes per day. No positive results were reported from an ear, nose, and throat (ENT) examination administered immediately prior to the experimental session.

Speech materials for the study consisted of a combination of read text and quasi-spontaneous speech. The text for reading was Aesop's fable "The Northwind and the Sun" (in German; see Appendix for text), which required between 40 and 45 sec to read at a normal rate, while quasi-spontaneous samples were elicited with a picture. Additionally, subjects spoke aloud the sentence *Wir gehen zu Omi nach Hause* and the numbers 21 through 30.

Subjects were first examined before consumption of alcohol. Four research groups worked simultaneously, to assure uniformity in reporting of results. The examinations included linguistic/phonetic analysis of the speech materials, as well as logopedic, phoniatric, and gross neurological examinations. At the end of the assessments in the sober condition, a 90-min drinking period began. The beverage consisted of 40% vodka, which was consumed after fasting, either straight or diluted. Exact dosages were not prescribed, but subjects were informed approximately how many 100-ml containers, based on their weight, were required to achieve the target alcohol concentration of between 1 and 2‰. Thirty minutes after completion of alcohol consumption, and then at 60-min intervals thereafter, breath-alcohol concentration (BrAC) was measured, and linguistic data were gathered. The original research protocol called for five speech samples under alcohol; in practice, this was not possible, as a number of subjects who achieved high alcohol concentrations were either unwilling or unable to continue for the close to 6 hr required to complete the protocol. On the other hand, a number of subjects who had achieved low alcohol concentrations were released when BrACs fell below 0.3‰. On average, then, three samples were elicited, rather than five; in all, the 33 subjects contributed 102 speech samples. Figure 7.18.1 shows the distribution of the 33 subjects in six alcohol concentration categories according to maximum achieved BrACs. Many results were reported for these categories of BrACs rather than for individual subjects; additionally, many results divide the subjects into two major groups: those with maximum BrACs $< 0.8‰$ ($N = 11$) and those with maximum BrACs $\geq 0.8‰$ ($N = 22$).

BrAC was used as the indicator of level of intoxication and was measured using a Siemens-Alcomat, an infrared breath-alcohol analysis device. Phonetic and acoustic measurements were made using a computerized, interactive speech analysis system (Spektro 3000), developed specifically for forensic applications (see Künzel, 1985, 1987, 1988). Particularly useful were color displays of short-term spectrography, long-term average spectrography, and high-resolution waveforms. Analysis could be done in close to real time, and because all three types of displays could appear on the screen simultane-

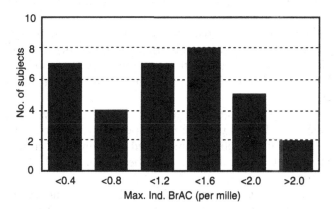

FIGURE 7.18.1 Distribution of the 33 subjects in maximum individual breath-alcohol concentration (BrAC) classes. (From Künzel, Braun, and Eysholdt, 1992. Copyright © 1992 by C. F. Müller Verlag, Hüthig GmbH. Used by permission.)

ously, it was possible to perform a number of durational analyses that depended on segmentation of the speech signal. Fundamental frequency was computed using an inverse filtering algorithm modifed for forensic purposes. Hoarseness was quantified as jitter, using Relative Average Perturbation (RAP; see Baken, 1987, p. 178; Koike, 1973). Using their own transcriptions, two phoneticians with forensic experience performed auditory analyses of such parameters as nasality, lengthening, pause ratios, and vocal quality changes. Error analysis was used to determine linguistic changes. For all measurements, changes due to alcohol were determined by comparing the measurements for the various parameters in the nonalcohol condition to those obtained at the point of maximum BrAC.

A perceptual experiment formed a second component. Speech materials were the first 10–12 sec of the read text from each of the 33 subjects in both the sober condition and the maximum BrAC condition. These 66 stimuli were randomized on digital audiotape (DAT) with a 4-sec interstimulus interval. Listeners were 30 clerical workers, ranging in age from the low 20s to the middle 50s. Instructions were to determine if the speaker of each of the 66 sentences was intoxicated or not (an absolute identification task) and additionally to rate confidence in responses on a scale from 0 (completely unsure) to 4 (completely sure).

The assessment of voice characteristics consisted of a number of clinical measurements; endo- and stroboscopic examination; and gross neurological measures of motor control, coordination, and balance. The clinical measurements included the following:

1. Vital capacity: Measured with a handheld spirometer. Subjects were instructed after two normal breathing cycles to inhale as deeply as possible and then to exhale into the spirometer. The volume of expired air was recorded as the vital capacity.

2. Speaking fundamental frequency (*individuelle Indifferenzlage/mittlere Sprechstimmlage*): Assessed by auditorily comparing the apparent fundamental pitch during recitation of the numbers 21 through 30 with an electronically generated tone. This was not necessarily the same as the measured FØ.

3. Maximum phonation time: Measured with a stopwatch while the subject sang [a] as long as possible in the speaking fundamental frequency.

4. Frequency range of phonation: Elicited by having subjects match tones generated by an electronic device, first to their upper boundary, then to the lower boundary.

5. Vocal attack (*Stimmeinsatz*) and (overall) voice quality (*Stimmklang*): Assessed subjectively by assigning a number ranging from 1 to 5. For vocal attack, 1 = breathy, 2 = soft, 3 = normal, 4 = strong, 5 = hard (*verhaucht, weich, normal, fest, hart*, respectively). For voice quality, the scale ranged from 1 (*aphon* 'aphonic') to 5 (*tönend* 'sonorous').

Laryngoscopic examination at each interval enabled the researchers to examine directly whether observed changes in speech and voice were attributable to local changes in the larynx. These probes were conducted without topical anesthesia to avoid (a) possible interactions between anesthetic and alcohol, (b) aspiration by subjects who continued to consume alcohol, and (c) possible effects on kinesthetic control of the voice mechanism. Alcohol appeared to increase pharyngeal sensitivity in the subjects, so that after the first examination interval, video recordings were discontinued.

Instrumentation for the endoscopic and stroboscopic examination included a Wolf rigid 90° magnifying laryngoscope with two magnification fields, integrated airway, and attached lighting cable. The light source (Timcke Model KQ42) could produce either a sustained or a strobed light. For the stroboscopic examination, the strobe light was synchronized with the vibration rate of the vocal folds as conveyed by a microphone while the subject sang a sustained note. Synchronization of the light with the actual vibration rate produced the illusion of a still image of the vocal folds, but if light and vibration were slightly offset, there was an illusion of slow-motion movement.

The interpretation of laryngoscopy, and especially of stroboscopy, is highly observer-dependent. In this study, two experienced investigators made independent observations, on-line, because of the lack of videotapes. The phoniatric investigators examined spatial and temporal symmetry of vibration, glottic closure, vibration amplitude, and mucosal waves. Each parameter was rated on a scale of either 3 or 5 steps. Vibration amplitude and mucosal waves were assessed on a 5-point scale, vibration symmetry and glottic closure on 3-point scales. Also conducted during endoscopy was an examination of the larynx in terms of laryngeal morphology and placement, symmetry, coloration, and condition of the mucus, and gross motility of the vocal folds; this was conducted to ensure that no patients suffered from injury or acute illness that might prevent further participation. All subjects passed this examination and continued.

A neurological examination of gross and fine motor control, coordination, and balance was conducted. Nine of the subjects were examined at all intervals, and 24 subjects were examined in the sober condition and at the first, third, and fifth interval. The examination consisted of the following tests:

1. Walk-and-turn: Subjects walked a 10-m line with closed eyes and outstretched arms. After walking in one direction, subjects stopped, turned 180°, and walked the other way.
2. Finger-to-finger: While seated with closed eyes and outstretched index fingers, subjects brought the tips of the fingers together.

Performance on each of the three tasks, walking, turning, and finger-to-finger, was assessed on a 3-point scale. The following two neurological tests were measured for duration.

3. Path tracing: Subjects used a pen to trace seven printed paths of increasing difficulty without touching the printed boundaries. The time required to complete the task was recorded with a stopwatch; each instance of touching the line was counted and classified according to the level of difficulty.
4. Provocation (postrotational) nystagmus: Subjects stood in place and spun themselves three times. Nystagmus was then observed and its duration measured with a stopwatch.

Results of the phoniatric/logopedic examinations were reported in a number of ways. A value for each parameter for each subject was determined using the sober value as a reference point and assigning a value of 100% to that condition for each subject. The problem of wide dispersion of the data was thus mitigated and general tendencies could be noted. One series of measurements was based on the time course of the changes. Intervals in this series were offset by approximately 30 min from those used for the phonetic results and are thus expressed as whole hours. A second series of mesurements was based on BrAC in intervals of 0.2‰. This was measured independent of the maximum BrAC. In these results, two measurements within the same BrAC class could come from two subjects at widely disparate time intervals, and more than one measurement could be reported for each subject. A third series of results was based on the changes observed at the point of maximum BrAC, which occurred approximately 30 min after cessation of alcohol consumption.

7.18.2 Results

Results for this study can be divided into four broad categories: speech, perception, voice, and neurological results.

7.18.2.1 Speech Results

7.18.2.1.1 **Error Analysis**   Two types of speech analyses were performed: a linguistic error analysis and an acoustic-phonetic analysis. The error analysis was considered an indicator of both the planning stages of language and their motor implementation. The present study differed from a number of others in using read text rather than spontaneous speech, so that an error could be defined operationally as a deviation from the prepared text.

Künzel et al. used the following typology for error types and error levels: error types were insertions, omissions, substitutions, and repetitions; error levels were segment/syllable, (single) word, word order, and line. Segments and syllables were grouped together, because errors committed at these levels were not unambiguous; the omission of a segment, for instance, could also constitute omission of a syllable. The category "line" was included because of the nature of the task (reading text), and errors included both skipping and repeating a line (or a portion of a line).

Figure 7.18.2 shows the mean number of errors committed in the sober condition and at each of the maximum alcohol levels. Künzel et al. noted that the mean number of errors in the sober condition (2.9) might appear somewhat high, especially compared to the next two levels, but they pointed out that the count included intonation errors as well as segmental and lexical errors, and that the reading in the sober condition was the subjects' first contact with the text. The fact that changes in number of errors at the two maximum BrACs below 1.2‰ were small and statistically nonsignificant was attributed to a small practice effect. Above maximum BrACs of 0.8‰, however, there was an increase in the number of errors, and another, very large, increase beyond 1.6‰. Insertions were relatively rare in comparison to sober measurements at BrACs below 1.2‰; above that point, there was a relatively large increase. Omissions increased after BrACs of 0.8‰. Up to BrACs of 1.2‰, substitutions occurred even less often than in the sober condition, but at higher BrACs rose dramatically. The number of repetitions increased only for the BrAC classes of <2.0‰ and >2.0‰. Table 7.18.1 shows the relative proportion of each of the four error types as a function of maximum individual BrAC. As Table 7.18.1 shows, in the sober condition, substitutions accounted for over half the errors, whereas insertions accounted for just over 8%. But at 0.4‰ BrAC, substitutions and insertions were about equal, each accounting for a third of the errors. At the next higher level (0.8‰), omissions accounted for half the errors, while insertions and substitutions each accounted for a quarter. At 1.6‰ and 2.0‰ BrAC,

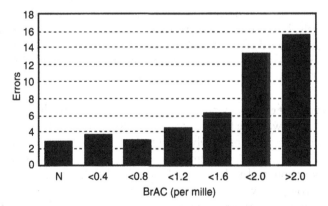

FIGURE 7.18.2   Increase in the number of errors under the influence of alcohol (N = sober value). (From Künzel, Braun, and Eysholdt, 1992. Copyright © 1992 by C. F. Müller Verlag, Hüthig GmbH. Used by permission.)

TABLE 7.18.1   Relative Proportions of 4 Error Types as a Function of
Alcoholization Level[a]

	Maximum individual breath-alcohol concentration (‰)						
	Sober	<0.4	<0.8	<1.2	<1.6	<1.8	>2.0
Insertions	8.3	33.3	25.0	19.0	21.2	20.7	26.3
Omissions	22.2	16.7	50.0	42.9	18.2	13.1	36.8
Substitutions	55.6	33.3	25.0	23.8	60.6	50.0	31.6
Repetitions	13.9	16.7	0.0	14.3	0.0	15.2	5.3

[a] From Künzel, Braun, and Eysholdt (1992). Copyright © 1992 by C. F. Müller Verlag, Hüthig
GmbH. Used by permission.

substitutions again accounted for at least half of the errors. At the highest
BrAC (two subjects) substitutions and omissions each accounted for about
a third of the errors, with insertions accounting for about a quarter.

At lower BrACs (0.4, 0.8, 1.2‰), the only linguistic level noticeably
affected was segments/syllables. Errors affecting single words, in fact, were
below the sober level at 0.8‰. A noticeable increase in single-word errors
first occurred above 1.2‰, whereas word order and line errors increased
above 1.6‰. In the 1.6, 2.0, and >2.0‰ BrAC classes, the level showing
the greatest increase in errors was the single word, with segment–syllable
errors second. Neither word order nor line errors were as frequent as seg-
ment/syllable and single-word errors.

The greatest proportion of errors at lower BrACs was at the segment–
segment syllable level, accounting for at least half of the errors in BrAC
classes 0 (sober), 0.4, 0.8, and 1.2‰. At 0.8‰, in fact, segment–syllable
errors accounted for all of the speech errors. Second in proportion were
single-word errors, with very few if any errors commited at the word-order
or line levels. Beginning with BrAC class 1.6‰ and continuing in the higher
BrACs, single-word errors accounted for the greatest proportion of errors,
with segment–syllable errors second. At the two highest BrACs, 2.0
and >2.0‰, there were some, but few, errors at the word order and line
levels.

Correction of errors tended to decrease from the nonalcohol to the alcohol
condition. This was true for both apparent willingness to correct and success-
ful correction. Even at relatively low BrACs, there was a decrement in both
awareness of error and willingness to correct. At higher BrACs, there was
further reduction, and at the highest BrACs (>2.0‰), these abilities appeared
to be lost completely.

The largest class of errors were intonation errors, and with but a single
exception, these remained uncorrected. Intonation errors were of three types:
(a) incorrect rising intonation at the end of a declarative sentence, (b) incor-

rect falling intonation within a complex sentence, and (c) contour breaks. These could be either syntactically or semantically unnecessary abrupt contour deviations or pausal interruptions. Figure 7.18.3 shows how the number of intonation errors increased as BrAC increased. As Figure 7.18.3 shows, at BrACs above 0.4‰, there was a constant rise in the number of intonation errors, following the increase in BrAC. At BrACs above 2.0‰ (two subjects), the number of intonation errors was over twice the number committed at the next lower BrAC.

7.18.2.1.2 Phonetic/Acoustic Analysis The phonetic analysis undertaken by Künzel et al. revealed a number of systematic changes in nasality, segment lengthening, incomplete articulations, segment substitutions, fundamental frequency (FØ), jitter, speaking rate, and pauses. These were characterized by Künzel et al. as changes in "articulatory setting" (see Laver, 1979, 1980).

Of the 33 subjects in Künzel et al.'s study, 22 showed some change in nasality in the alcohol condition, and this appeared to be related to BrAC. Of 11 subjects with maximum BrACs < 0.8‰, 3 (27%) showed changes, but of the 22 subjects with maximum BrACs > 0.8‰, 19 (86%) showed changes. Additionally, of the 22 subjects displaying nasality effects, all showed denasalization of nasal consonants, but a subset of these, 15 subjects, also showed nasalization of oral vowels. Figure 7.18.4 shows the percent subjects who nasalized vowels or denasalized consonants in each of the BrAC classes. As Figure 7.18.4 shows, at lower BrACs, denasalization of nasal consonants occurred to the exclusion of nasalization of vowels. Above 0.8‰, however, both nasalization and denasalization occurred.

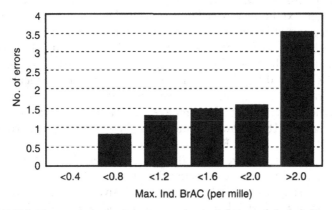

FIGURE 7.18.3   Increase in intonation errors under the influence of alcohol. (From Künzel, Braun, and Eysholdt, 1992. Copyright © 1992 by C. F. Müller Verlag, Hüthig GmbH. Used by permission.)

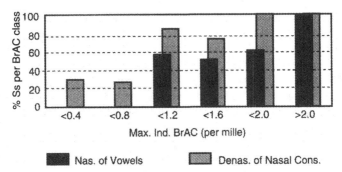

FIGURE 7.18.4   Nasalization of vowels and denasalization of consonants. (From Künzel, Braun, and Eysholdt, 1992. Copyright © 1992 by C. F. Müller Verlag, Hüthig GmbH. Used by permission.)

An analysis of segmental lengthening was conducted on the sentence *Der Nordwind blies mit aller Macht* from the text. For subjects in the <0.4‰ BrAC class, only consonantal lengthening occurred. Beginning with the 0.8‰ BrAC class, however, subjects exhibited both consonantal and vocalic lengthening. Although the peak effect of consonantal lengthening occurred in the 1.2‰ BrAC class, vocalic lengthening affected a greater percentage of subject as BrACs increased, until all subjects were affected at the very highest BrACs. The authors proposed that segmental lengthening was a result of a reduced rate of movement in the articulatory organs (especially the tongue).

Considered 'incomplete articulations' (*unvollständige Artikulationen*) were those that were "reduced," for example, spirantization of stops, as in the case of *bass* for *bat*. Other examples from the literature included those articulations exhibiting reduced precision cited by Pisoni and Martin (1989) and Lester and Skousen (1974), and characterized as slurred articulations, cluster reduction, and deaffrication. In Künzel et al.'s study, these appeared to affect almost all of the subjects, including those at lower maximum BrACs. At BrACs below 0.8‰, the mean number of incomplete articulations per subject was 1.0, but at BrACs above 0.8‰, the mean was 4.5; for both groups, the mean number of incomplete articulations in the sober condition was 0. Figure 7.18.5 shows the mean number of incomplete articulations in each of the maximum BrAC classes. From Figure 7.18.5, it can be seen that there were large increases in the mean number of reductions at BrACs above 0.8‰, with another dramatic rise above 2.0‰.

Reductions appeared to affect almost exclusively alveolar segments with various manners of articulation. Examples included the following: (a) in the sequence [stʃtr] in the phrase *Einst stritten,* there was incomplete closure for one or both of the [t]s or incomplete articulation for the [s], resulting

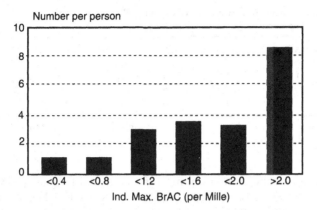

FIGURE 7.18.5 Average number of incomplete articulations. (From Künzel, Braun, and Eysholdt, 1992. Copyright © 1992 by C. F. Müller Verlag, Hüthig GmbH. Used by permission.)

in a lack of frication; (2) in the phrase ". . . *der den Wanderer zwingen* . . . ," there was incomplete articulation of any of the three [d]s; (3) in the phrase *desto fester,* there was incomplete closure for one or both of the [t]s. In some cases, reductions made it difficult or impossible to segment waveforms and spectrograms.

Substitutions were differentiated from incomplete articulations, in that the former, although not in the text, were nevertheless correctly produced sounds of the language. With only one exception, substitutions affected only consonants. In general, it was front (labial and alveolar) consonants that were affected by substitutions, both as substituted and substituting segment. Five pairs of segments were in mutually substituted/substituting relationships: [p] and [t], [d] and [n], [b] and [v], [l] and [n], and [t] and [n]. The segments most often replaced by another were [n] and [s], and the segment most often substituting for another was [s]. Other, unidirectional, substitution patterns were [θ] for [t], [s] for [d], [β] for [v], [ŋ] for [m], [m] for [n], [d] or [s] for [l], [θ] for [s], [s] for [r], and [x] for [ç]. Thus, very often affected were segments requiring full oral cavity closure: stops, nasals, and laterals. Over two-thirds of the substitutions involved a change in place of articulation or manner of articulation, but not both. Voicing differences occurred in fewer than 20% of the cases.

Substitution patterns appeared to include a degree of language specificity. Lester and Skousen (1974) and K. Johnson et al. (1989) had reported a substitution pattern replacing [s] with [ʃ], but Künzel et al. did not find this substitution. Rather than attribute this to a general articulatory constraint, however, Künzel et al. noted similar substitutions in their own data, those of [s] by [θ] and of [z] by [ð]. Although substitutions were relatively rare, Künzel et al. did note a general trend for them to increase with higher BrACs.

TABLE 7.18.2 Fundamental Frequencies of 33 Talkers in Sober and Alcoholized Condition[a]

Maximum BrAC	<0.4	<0.8	<1.2	<1.6	<2.0	>2‰
Number of subjects	7	4	7	8	5	2
FØ sober (Hz)	120.4	128.5	120.0	130.8	116.4	132.0
FØ alcoholized (Hz)	123.3	129.5	127.8	135.9	122.4	135.5
Difference	2.9	1.0	7.8	5.1	6.0	3.5

[a] From Künzel, Braum, and Eysholdt (1992). Copyright © 1992 by C. F. Müller Verlag, Hüthig GmbH. Used by permission.

In the nonalcohol condition, mean fundamental frequency (FØ) for the talkers was 123.9 Hz, with a range from 100 to 149 Hz. At maximum BrAC, mean FØ was 128.5, but the difference of 4.6 Hz was not significant. From the sober condition to the point of maximum alcohol level, mean FØ increased for 25 of the subjects, decreased for 7 of the subjects, and remained unchanged for 1 subject. The magnitude of changes was somewhat less for the increases in FØ than for the decreases, so that no subject decreased more than 9 Hz, but seven subjects increased FØ by between 11 and 19 Hz. The mean increase in FØ was 7.5 Hz, whereas the mean decrease was 4.3 Hz. Table 7.18.2 gives mean FØ for each of the six BrAC classes in both conditions. As shown in Table 7.18.2, all six BrAC classes increased mean FØ under alcohol, with larger increases above 0.8‰.

Pitch variability was assessed by computing standard deviations of the FØ. Standard deviations increased for 24 of the subject talkers, decreased for 5, and remained the same for 4. Mean standard deviation for all subject talkers was 17.6 Hz in the nonalcohol condition and 20.2 Hz at maximum BrAC, a significant difference. Figure 7.18.6 shows changes in the standard

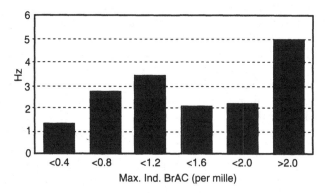

FIGURE 7.18.6 Change in standard deviation of fundamental frequency (0 = sober value). (From Künzel, Braun, and Eysholdt, 1992. Copyright © 1992 by C. F. Müller Verlag, Hüthig GmbH. Used by permission.)

deviation in Hz (where 0 = the sober value) for each each of the six BrAC classes. As Figure 7.18.6 shows, for all BrAC classes, standard deviation of FØ increased; additionally, it also shows that, although the increase in variability was highest for the highest BrAC class, there was no linear relationship between standard deviation change and BrAC class.

One of the quantitative analogs to the subjective determination of "hoarseness" is "jitter," or slight perturbations of frequency (see Baken, 1987, pp. 166ff). The algorithm used to determine jitter was based on Relative Average Perturbation (RAP; see Koike, 1973), which measures the deviation of a period from the average value of that period and its immediate (or very close) neighbors. Adjustments to the basic RAP algorithm accommodated the types of speech samples generally available for forensic analysis; whereas clinical measurements are based on sustained vowels, forensic samples are generally much shorter. Analysis of jitter here involved estimating the long-term fundamental using cepstrum analysis. The deviation of the fundamental or period of each cycle from the long-term fundamental was then measured. The analysis was thus based on an optimized FØ time course and a comparison with the actual time course and calculation of deviations.

Jitter was measured for the long vowel [iː] in the word *blies* 'blew,' appearing twice in the text (see Appendix 2). Regardless of condition, measurements were widely dispersed (by as much as double), probably because samples were taken from running speech, rather than from sustained vowels. Figure 7.18.7 displays the mean (of the two occurrences) jitter indices in the sober and maximum BrAC conditions across BrAC classes. As Figure 7.18.7 shows, jitter values in the sober condition across all BrAC classes ranged from just above 0.6% to just above 0.8%; these values corresponded to findings for nonpathological male voices (e.g., Horii, 1979; Takahashi & Koike, 1975). Additionally, Figure 7.18.7 shows that in all BrAC classes,

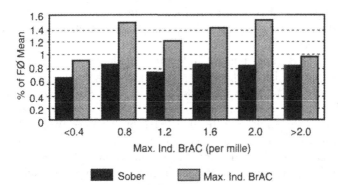

FIGURE 7.18.7   Average jitter indices: sober and at maximum individual BrAC. (From Künzel, Braun, and Eysholdt, 1992. Copyright © 1992 by C. F. Müller Verlag, Hüthig GmbH. Used by permission.)

jitter increased from the sober to the maximum BrAC condition, with increases ranging from 16-84% of the sober measurements. There was no linear relationship between proportion of increase in jitter and alcohol level: in both the lowest and the highest BrAC class, percentage increase was comparatively small compared with the increases in the midrange BrAC classes. Likewise, individual results showed that 26 of the 33 subjects had increased jitter in the alcohol condition as compared with the sober condition, but again, increases in jitter were not proportional to BrAC.

Seven subjects decreased jitter from the sober to the alcohol condition. Two had maximum BrACs below 0.8‰ and showed decreases of 0.19 and 0.10% from the sober value; the remaining five were at higher BrACs and showed decreases ranging from 0.03-0.15%. One characteristic of these seven subjects was that all had very high jitter measurements in the sober condition, only slightly below, or even above, the 1% suggested as the "hoarseness threshold." For the entire subject group, mean jitter in the sober condition was 0.77% and in the alcohol condition 1.27%, a significant difference. For subjects with maximum BrACs below 0.8‰, mean jitter values were 0.73% in the sober condition and 1.12% in the alcohol condition. For those with maximum BrACs above 0.08‰, these were 0.79% in the sober condition and 1.32% in the intoxicated condition. Both differences were significant.

Two measures of speaking rate were made: syllable rate, the number of syllables spoken per unit of time, and articulation rate, the number of syllables spoken per unit of time after subtracting pauses. The latter was suggested by Goldman-Eisler (1968) as a more precise measure of the movement of articulatory organs. In previous work, Künzel (1987) had determined an average articulation rate of between 4.4 and 6 syllables per second (S/s) for adult speakers of German. In determining articulation rate, signal interruptions of more than 100 ms were considered pauses, as long as they were also perceived as such by trained listeners. This avoided the problem of including among pause measurements certain voiceless or devoiced portions of speech.

Figure 7.18.8 shows both syllable and articulation rate changes for each of the maximum BrAC classes. As shown in Figure 7.18.8, for all BrAC classes above 0.4‰, there was a decrease in both syllable and articulation rate. The slight increase in syllable rate for BrACs below 0.4‰ was not significant. Some subjects' rates increased, but none of these subjects had maximum BrACs above 0.8‰. The mean syllable rate for all subjects was 4.9 S/s ($SD = 0.4$ S/s) in the nonalcohol condition and 4.4 S/s ($SD = 0.65$ S/s) in the alcohol condition, a significant difference. For subjects with maximum BrACs below 0.8‰, mean syllable rate was 5.0 S/s in the nonalcohol condition and 5.0 S/s in the alcohol condition (no difference). For subjects with maximum BrACs above 0.8‰, mean syllable rate was 4.9 S/s in the

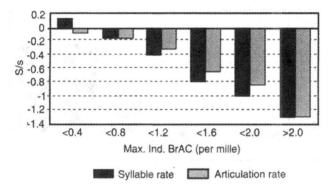

FIGURE 7.18.8   Changes in syllable rate and articulation rate. (From Künzel, Braun, and Eysholdt, 1992. Copyright © 1992 by C. F. Müller Verlag, Hüthig GmbH. Used by permission.)

sober condition and 4.1 S/s in the alcohol condition, a significant difference. Moreover, changes in syllable rate correlated highly with maximum BrAC ($r = 0.80$).

Recall that articulation rate measures syllables produced per unit of time (here, seconds), after subtracting pauses. Mean articulation rates for the entire group were 6.0 S/s ($SD = 0.4$ S/s) in the sober condition and 5.6 S/s ($SD = 0.6$ S/s) in the maximum alcohol condition, a significant difference. As seen in Figure 7.18.8, articulation rate decreased at a maximum BrAC (0.4‰) that was lower than that of the initial decrease in syllable rate (0.8‰). For those subjects with maximum BrACs <0.8‰, mean articulation rate was 6.1 S/s in the sober condition and 6.1 S/s in the alcohol condition. However, for those subjects with maximum BrACs >0.8‰, there was a significant difference between mean articulation rate in the sober condition (6.0 S/s) and in the alcohol condition (5.3 S/s). As with syllable rate, changes in articulation rate also correlated highly with maximum BrAC ($r = 0.75$).

Künzel et al. differentiated three types of speech pauses: structural, planning, and hesitation pauses. Structural pauses occur between clauses, and the text used in this study contained 16 such pauses. Planning pauses are encountered in spontaneous speech, when, for example, a speaker is deciding what to say next. Hesitation pauses occur between or within syntactic units smaller than the clause, that is, not at major syntactic boundaries. Examples of hesitation pauses (indicated by a virgule) were as follows (p. 53): . . . *desto fester / hüllte sich der / Wanderer* . . . and . . . *nun erwärmte / die Sonne / die Luft / mit ihren / freundlichen Strahlen.*

Predictions regarding pauses were first, that planning pauses would not occur, since the spoken text was read (samples of spontaneous speech were recorded but not analyzed). Second, at least in the sober condition, structural pauses would be used to parse the sentence for content or to inhale. Addition-

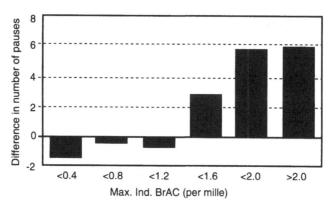

FIGURE 7.18.9   Changes in number of pauses (0 = sober value). (From Künzel, Braun, and Eysholdt, 1992. Copyright © 1992 by C. F. Müller Verlag, Hüthig GmbH. Used by permission.)

ally, it was predicted that one effect of alcohol might be an increase in the number and perhaps the duration of structural pauses. Third, it was predicted that under alcohol, hesitation pauses would increase, indicating reduced ability to process the visual written form into the spoken form.

Contrary to expectations, the mean number of pauses for all 33 talkers was higher in the sober condition (mean = 16.6, SD = 3.3) than in the maximum BrAC condition (mean = 15.9, SD = 5.2), although the difference was not significant, and the authors suggested a possible practice effect. Figure 7.18.9 shows the difference in number of pauses (where 0 is the value in the sober condition) as a function of maximum BrAC class. As can be seen in Figure 7.18.9, pauses in the lowest BrAC classes were lower in the alcohol condition than in the sober condition. At higher BrACs, however, the number of pauses increased from the sober condition to the alcohol condition, and for the highest two BrAC classes, there was a particularly marked increase. Table 7.18.3 lists mean number of pauses according to type and BrAC either above or below 0.8‰. As Table 7.18.3 shows, there

TABLE 7.18.3   Mean Number of Structural and Hesitation Pauses[a]

	Structural pauses		Hesitation pauses	
	Sober	Alcohol	Sober	Alcohol
Talkers with <0.8‰ BrAC (n = 11)	12.1	10.3	2.1	1.8
Talkers with >0.8‰ BrAC (n = 22)	12.5	12.6	2.3	4.7
Weighted mean of all 33 talkers	12.4	11.8	2.2	3.7

[a] From Künzel, Braun, and Eysholdt (1992). Copyright © (1992) by C. F. Müller Verlag, Hüthig GmbH. Used by permission.

was a slight decrease for the entire group in the number of structural pauses from the sober condition to the maximum alcohol condition, but there was also an increase in the number of hesitation pauses. For those subjects with maximum BrACs <0.8‰, there were decreases in both structural and hesitation pauses. For subjects with maximum BrACs >0.8‰, however, there were increases in the mean number of both structural and hesitation pauses (the latter more than doubled).

Mean duration of pauses was 478 ms in the nonalcohol condition and 587 ms in the maximum alcohol condition, an increase of 23%. For those subjects with maximum BrACs below 0.8‰, mean pause durations were 480 ms in the sober condition and 510 ms in the alcohol condition. For those with BrACs above 0.8‰, mean durations were 478 ms in the sober condition and 626 ms in the alcohol condition, a significant difference. All of the maximum BrAC classes in fact showed some increase in mean duration of pauses.

7.18.2.1.3 Elimination Phase Speech Results

Data were available from 12 of the subjects with maximum BrACs of at least 0.8‰ who were available at least 6 hr after completion of alcohol consumption. Seven had maximum BrACs between 1.5 and 1.9‰, and five had BrACs of at least 1.0‰ at the end of the 6 hr.

Table 7.18.4 gives the number of subjects showing alcohol effects for nasality, segmental lengthening, incomplete articulations, and sound substitutions at 0.5 hr subsequent to alcohol consumption and then at 1-hr intervals thereafter. In all cases in Table 7.18.4 except sound substitutions, no values are given for the sober condition, because the type of analysis performed here (characterizing a subject as either showing an effect for the parameter or not) used the sober condition as a reference point. In Table

TABLE 7.18.4 Temporal Course of Alcohol Effect on Various Parameters in Number of Affected Subjects ($n_{max} = 12$)[a]

	Sober	Hours after end of drinking period					
		0.5	1.5	2.5	3.5	4.5	5.5
Denasalization of nasal consonants	b	12	11	11	10	9	7
Nasalization of oral vowels	b	7	4	3	1	1	0
Lengthening of vowels	b	12	8	7	7	6	2
Lengthening of consonants	b	8	7	9	4	2	1
Incomplete articulations	b	12	11	9	5	5	2
Sound substitutions	2	1	7	7	5	4	1

[a] From Künzel, Braun, and Eysholdt (1992). Copyright © 1992 by C. F. Müller Verlag, Hüthig GmbH. Used by permission.

[b] No sober values available; see text.

7.18.4, data are given separately for denasalization of nasal consonants and nasalization of oral vowels. One-half hour after alcohol consumption, all 12 subjects exhibited denasalization, while 7 showed nasalization. The number of subjects exhibiting denasalization remained high for the entire elimination period, and at 5.5 hr after consumption, over half of the original 12 subjects still showed denasalization. This contrasts with the subjects exhibiting nasalization: there was a steady decrease in the number of subjects affected over the postconsumption period, and at the final interval, no subjects showed nasalization of oral vowels.

Lengthening showed similar differential effects for consonants and vowels. As Table 7.18.4 shows, at 0.5 hr after consumption, all 12 subjects exhibited vocalic lengthening, but the number of affected subjects decreased to 8 at the 1.5-hr interval and then decreased steadily throughout the elimination period. On the other hand, although only 8 of the 12 subjects exhibited consonantal lengthening at 0.5 hr, there was little change through the 2.5-hr interval, when the number began to decrease. All 12 subjects exhibited incomplete articulations at the 0.5-hr interval, but from that point there was a steady decrease across the elimination period.

Sound substitutions constituted an exceptional class of speech changes. Among the parameters in Table 7.18.4, data from the nonalcohol condition were available only for substitutions, exhibited by two of the subjects. Furthermore, at the point of maximum BrAC, one-half hour after cessation of alcohol consumption, only one subject displayed substitutions. This was in contrast to all other parameters, which showed alcohol effects for the greatest number of subjects at that interval. Substitutions showed the largest effects only at the next two intervals, with seven subjects affected 1.5 and 2.5 hr after alcohol consumption. From that point, there was a steady decrease across the remaining elimination period.

Table 7.18.5 shows results during the elimination phase for several other speech parameters, expressed as means rather than number of subjects affected. The number of errors remained higher than the sober value for the first three postconsumption intervals but began to decrease after that and returned to the sober value by the final interval. The number of pauses was elevated for the first two postconsumption intervals[2] but resumed its sober level at the 2.5-hr interval; from there, the number of pauses fell below the sober level and continued to decline throughout the postconsumption period. At maximum BrACs (0.5 hr postconsumption), mean pause duration was elevated 38% above the sober level; from that point, there was a steady decline through the rest of the elimination period, although mean pause duration at the final interval still remained 10% above the sober level.

---

[2] A value of 5.8 at the 1.5-hr interval in Künzel et al.'s (1992, p. 62) original table appears to be a typographical error (cf. *Abbildung 25a* in Künzel et al., 1992, p. 63).

TABLE 7.18.5   Mean Parameter Values for Talkers during Observation Period[a]

| | Sober | Hours after end of drinking period | | | | | |
		0.5	1.5	2.5	3.5	4.5	5.5
Number of errors	2.2	6.2	6.8	6.4	4.8	2.9	2.2
Number of pauses	15.1	17.1	5.8	15.1	13.7	12.9	12.3
Duration of pauses in ms	466	643	612	562	587	542	514
Syllable rate	4.9	4.2	4.5	4.6	4.6	5.0	4.8
Articulation rate	6.0	5.5	5.7	5.8	5.9	6.0	5.7
Fundamental frequency (Hz)	122	131	127	129	124	123	124
Standard deviation of fundamental frequency (Hz)	17.5	20.3	20.2	19.1	18.3	18.0	17.9
Jitter (% of fundamental frequency)	0.83	1.67	1.11	1.50	1.48	1.19	1.30

[a] From Künzel, Braun, and Eysholdt (1992). Copyright © 1992 by C. F. Müller Verlag, Hüthig GmbH. Used by permission.

Mean syllable rate was reduced for the first four postconsumption intervals, but this returned to normal levels around the 4.5- and 5.5-hr intervals. Reduction in articulation rate also occurred at maximum BrAC, but appeared to remain depressed throughout the postconsumption period. The difference in changes in syllable rate and articulation rate could be attributed to the elevated pause durations throughout the observation period.

Mean FØ reached its highest value at maximum BrAC (0.5 hr postconsumption) and, although reduced from its maximum level, remained above the sober value throughout the postconsumption period. Standard deviation of FØ was elevated from the sober value at maximum BrAC and then declined steadily until it was close to the sober level at the final interval. Jitter (expressed as a percent of FØ) was 0.83% in the sober condition. At the 0.5-hr interval, the point of maximum BrAC, this was more than doubled at 1.67%. From that point, there was a gradual but inconsistent decrease across the observation period. As indicated in Table 7.18.5, the 1.5-hr interval showed a lower value for jitter than either of the surrounding intervals. The authors cautioned that at this interval, three of the most highly alcoholized subjects were unable to provide measurements, so that the jitter mean at this interval was based on only nine subjects. At the last interval, jitter was still above the sober level, at 1.30%.

7.18.2.2 Perception Results

Methods for the perceptual assessment are described in section 7.18.1. This component consisted of an identification task and a confidence rating. Upon presentation of a recorded sentence, listeners were asked to determine whether the sentence was or was not produced in the intoxicated condition and further to indicate their confidence in that response.

The overall percent correct judgments for sentences produced in both conditions was 66.8%. For sentences produced under alcohol, percent correct scores ranged from 51.1% to 95.8%. Figure 7.18.10 shows the percent correct judgments as a function of maximum BrAC under which sentences were produced. As Figure 7.18.10 shows, percent correct increased as a function of increasing BrACs. Up to a BrAC of 0.8‰, both correct and incorrect responses had equal confidence ratings of 2.5 (on a scale from 0 to 4). For talkers with BrACs above 0.8‰, however, confidence in correct responses increased as BrAC increased, whereas confidence in incorrect responses decreased as BrAC increased. For all of the responses, the mean confidence ratings were 2.7 for correct responses and 2.2 for incorrect responses, a significant difference.

To investigate listeners' decision criteria, the authors used an ROC to measure listener biases toward either sober or intoxicated responses (also see discussion in section 7.6.2). An ROC graph plots the probability of hits against the probability of false alarms. The ROC graph for this study is given as Figure 7.18.11. In this figure, the probability of correct identification of a sentence produced under alcohol (P ["A"/A] or a hit) is plotted along the ordinate, while the probability of incorrectly identifying a sentence actually produced in the sober condition as having been produced under alcohol (P ("A"/N) or a 'false alarm') is plotted along the abscissa. The "guessing line" emanates from the 0-point as a 45° diagonal. Each of the remaining six curves on the graph indicates the ROC for one of the six maximum BrAC classes. The closer the ROC curve is to the diagonal line, the less good the identification is, and the farther the curve is from the diagonal, the better the identification. As shown in Figure 7.18.11, the ROC curve for the lowest BrAC (0.4‰) very nearly approximated the chance line, but with increasing

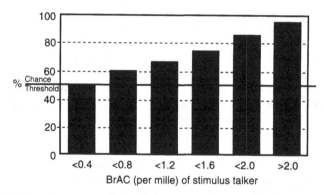

FIGURE 7.18.10   Percent correct listener judgments as a function of breath-alcohol concentrations (BrAC) of stimulus talkers. (From Künzel, Braun, and Eysholdt, 1992). Copyright © 1992 by C. F. Müller Verlag, Hüthig GmbH. Used by permission.)

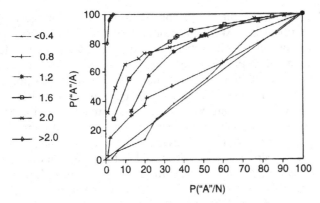

FIGURE 7.18.11 Receiver-operator characteristic curves for listeners as a function of breath-alcohol concentrations of the stimulus talkers. (From Künzel, Braun, and Eysholdt, 1992). Copyright © 1992 by C. F. Müller Verlag, Hüthig GmbH. Used by permission.)

BrACs, the ROC curves moved further toward the upper left corner of the space.

Three similar perceptual experiments had been conducted previously, reported in Klingholz et al. (1988), in Pisoni et al. (1985), and in Pisoni and Martin (1989). The experiment reported by Klingholz et al. used twelve speech therapists as listeners and included two tasks: an identification task like the one used here and a discrimination task in which listeners heard pairs of sentences, that is, the same sentence produced in both the sober and the intoxicated condition (in either order). In the latter task, listeners had to decide which of the two presented sentences was produced under alcohol. In the identification task, 54.0% of the intoxicated sentences were identified correctly, as compared to the present study, in which 66.8% of both alcohol and nonalcohol sentences were correctly identified (range in the present study: 51.1 to 95.8% correct). In the discrimination task of Klingholz et al., 61.1% of the sentences produced under alcohol were correctly identified; responses further showed a relationship to BAC, such that correct responses were 54.2% for BACs <0.1% and 82.0% for BACs >0.1%.

Pisoni et al. (1985) conducted a discrimination experiment using two groups of listeners: six laboratory staff members (experienced listeners) and 21 undergaduate students (naive listeners). Both groups performed the same task, determining which of two presented sentences had been recorded while the talker was intoxicated. For the experienced listeners, percent correct scores ranged from 66.2 to 92.6% (mean = 82.4%, SD = 10.2%). For the naive listeners, scores ranged from 64.0 to 85.3% (mean = 73.8%, SD = 6.5%).

Both Künzel et al. and Pisoni and Martin (1989) pointed out that an absolute identification task might more nearly approximate real-world forensic situations, in which (sober) comparison utterances would not be available. In an identification task, Pisoni and Martin used two sets of listeners: 30 undergraduate students (naive listeners) and 14 police officers (trained listeners). Listeners heard 24 different sentences, half produced by sober talkers and half by intoxicated talkers. Listeners determined whether a sentence was produced in the sober or the intoxicated condition. Mean correct responses across all sentences was 61.5% for the students and 64.7% for the police officers. Sentences produced in the sober condition were correctly identified 60.5% of the time, and those in the intoxicated condition 64.5%. Mean accuracy for different talkers ranged from 55–71.9%. Both listener groups performed significantly better than chance, and accuracy for all talkers was also significantly better than chance.

Table 7.18.6 shows mean percent correct scores from the various perceptual experiments reported in the four studies under discussion. As Table 7.18.6 shows, the highest scores were for trained listeners in a discrimination task, reported in Pisoni et al. (1985). Scores from Künzel et al. for untrained listeners in an identification task were similar to those for both trained and untrained listeners reported by Pisoni and Martin, whereas scores from Klingholz et al. for trained listeners and sentences under intoxication only were somewhat lower. Similarly, scores for trained listeners and sentences under intoxication from Klingholz et al. were lower than for untrained listeners and both types of sentences from Pisoni et al. and Pisoni and Martin.

7.18.2.3 Voice and Neurological Results

This section reports on the phoniatric, logopedic, and neurological examinations conducted as part of this study. General methods are described in section 7.18.1.

7.18.2.3.1 Voice Results   Voice quality was assessed subjectively. Under alcohol, voice was judged to be hoarse and somewhat aperiodic. Voice

TABLE 7.18.6 Comparison of Perception Experiment Results in Percent Correct from Four Studies

	Discrimination		Identification	
	Trained listeners	Naive listeners	Trained listeners	Naive listeners
Klingholz et al. (1988)	61.1[a]	—	54.0[a]	—
Künzel et al. (1992)	—	—	—	66.8
Pisoni et al. (1985)	82.4	73.8	—	—
Pisoni & Martin (1989)	—	—	64.7	61.5

[a] Sentences produced under alcohol only

quality was worst when BrACs were highest, at the first interval after cessation of alcohol consumption. From that point, mean voice quality improved through the remainder of the observation period, just as mean BrAC decreased throughout that same period. No direct relationship was found between voice quality and BrAC alone. One observed phenomenon was that voice quality appeared to more nearly approximate the sober value for those subjects with BrACs over 1.8‰; the authors attributed this to alcohol tolerance. Thus, although alcohol did appear to affect voice to the extent that it was noticeable to trained observers, individual differences were so great, that the specific effects of alcohol on this parameter could not be considered predictable.

Vocal attack was not significantly affected by alcohol. There was no relationship between vocal attack and time of testing or maximum individual or mean BrAC. Examination of frequency range of phonation required subjects to sing sustained notes at the high and low extremes of their frequency range. The lower boundary was little affected by alcohol, but the upper boundary was raised by more than a half octave. The entire range was thus widened but began to decrease after the first interval as a function of time. A relationship between frequency range and BrAC appeared to hold only between 0.8 and 1.8‰, where frequency range, both as a percent of the sober value and its absolute value, tended to increase with increased BrACs. There were also deviations at the highest BrACs, which the authors attributed to the small number of subjects in those ranges and to tolerance.

Speaking fundamental frequency (mean speaking frequency) was measured subjectively during running speech (while the subjects recited the numbers 21 through 30) by auditory comparison with an electronic tone generator. Speaking fundamental frequency was highest at the first interval (1 hr postconsumption), when it was 8% above the sober value; at 2 hr postconsumption, it returned to normal levels. No specific relationship was found between speaking fundamental frequency and either maximum individual BrAC or collective BrACs. Similarly, vital capacity was not significantly different under alcohol.

Maximum phonation time increased by approximately 13% at the first interval and decreased from that point, approximately following the BrAC curve, but returning to the sober level only at the last interval, 5 hr postconsumption. Maximum phonation times increased significantly only in the BrAC range of from 0.7 to 1.6‰. The authors attributed phonation times in the normal range at relatively high BrACs to the small number of subjects at these levels and possible alcohol tolerance. The combined results of increased maximum phonation times and unchanged vital capacity was explained by the authors as a sign of decreased glottic flow; this in turn could be a result of a shortened glottal open-phase, a smaller effective glottal surface, or both, and both could be the result of increased vocal-fold tonus.

7.18.2.3.2 Endoscopic and Stroboscopic Results   Because of elevated oral and pharyngeal sensitivity, it was not possible to make endoscopic and stroboscopic video recordings at any interval after the sober condition. One purpose of the physical examination was to look for changes in laryngeal morphology, specifically edema as the result of hyperemia in the larynx due to asymmetrical muscle tonus. Such morphological changes were not found upon endoscopic examination, and there was thus no evidence for local bases of the observed changes in speech and voice resulting from alcohol consumption or intoxication.

The size of the greatest displacement of the vocal folds during horizontal excursion is the maximum amplitude; maximum amplitudes were determined subjectively and qualitatively by assigning them to categories on a 5-category scale. Amplitudes decreased to a maximum reduction at 2 hr postconsumption and then rose again from that point, approaching close to the sober level at 5 hr postconsumption. The concept of mucosa as a "cover" for the vocal folds is attributable to Hirano (1974). During vibration, waves travel on this mucosa from the inferior to the superior surface of the vocal fold; a pliable mucosa is necessary both for the occurrence of the mucosal wave and for normal phonation. In the present study, mucosal waves were assessed on a 5-point scale. One hour after cessation of consumption, mucosal waves were significantly reduced but returned to normal (sober) levels 3 hr later. There was no significant relationship between measurements for mucosal waves and either maximum individual or collective BrAC. During normal phonation, maximum closing of the glottis during a vibratory cycle should result in complete closure, whereas incomplete glottal closure indicates abnormal phonatory functioning. Glottal closure was assessed on a 3-point scale and was maximally disturbed 1 hr after cessation of consumption but returned to normal levels 2 hr later. The most commonly observed change was insufficient adduction, resulting in a chink in the posterior third of the glottis, while mid and anterior closure insufficiency were observed in only two cases.

7.18.2.3.3 Neurological Results   Neurological data from all intervals were available for only 9 of the 33 subjects. In the walk-and-turn task, five of these nine showed noticeable changes during the walk portion, whereas only three showed changes during the turn portion. The number of affected subjects was thus sufficient to cause a significant rise in the mean across all nine subjects. Under maximum individual BrAC, errors in the walk portion increased only at levels above 2.0‰. For the turn portion, similarly, there were no significant changes at maximum individual BrAC, and only the two subjects with BrACs above 2.0‰ displayed exceptional behavior.

Performance on the finger-to-finger task was not shown to be dependent upon BrAC. There was, in fact, some slight mean improvement at lower

BrACs, which could indicate a practice effect. Performance was significantly impaired only at maximum individual BrACs above 1.5‰. Two measurements were made for the path-tracing task: time required to complete the task and number of errors. Although the time required to complete the task was not altered significantly under alcohol, the error rate showed a significant increase with increases in BrAC. There was a weak correlation ($r = 0.58$) between error rate and maximum individual BrAC. Although error rates were quite high at the first interval, there was a decrease as a function of time; this was attributed to practice and compensatory effects.

Neither a practice effect nor compensation was possible in the test of induced nystagmus. Mean duration of nystagmus in the sober condition was 6 sec. For the nine subjects who were measured at all available intervals, durations more than tripled under intoxication and were approximately proportional to BrAC. Measurements for the whole group at the first interval showed no clear tendencies.

7.18.3 Discussion

In general, observed changes in the various speech parameters were larger for the phonetic and linguistic parameters than for the phoniatric ones. Table 7.18.7 presents a chronology of phonetic and linguistic changes at increasing BrACs. As Table 7.18.7 shows, phonetic changes were evident even at the lowest BrACs (below 0.4‰), although no speech errors were recorded at that point. At the lowest level, denasalization, consonant lengthening, and jitter increase were already evident. At the next level (0.4–0.79‰) BrAC, lengthening was extended to vowels, jitter continued to increase, and speech rate began to decrease. At the third level (0.8–1.19‰ BrAC), incomplete articulations and nasalized vowels appeared, and FØ changed. At the fourth level (1.2–1.59‰ BrAC), pauses increased, and at the fifth level (1.6–1.99‰ BrAC), all subjects denasalized consonants, lengthened vowels, and continued to increase the number of pauses. For speech errors, there was a steady increase in both the number and number of types from the lowest BrAC level to the highest. Additionally, at higher BrACs, correction attempts decreased, and unsuccessful corrections increased.

Phoniatrically, the most noticeable change was the increase in the frequency range of phonation by as much as a half-octave, the result of a raising of the upper boundary. Künzel et al. atttributed a number of observed changes to an increase in laryngeal tonus, among these the increase of frequency range, changes in pitch and fundamental frequency, as well as the endoscopically observed decrease in vibration amplitude. Apparently not a cause was change in the mucous membrane. No morphological changes such as edema were evident.

TABLE 7.18.7   Chronology of Alcohol-Determined Changes in Linguistic and Phonetic Parameters (Künzel, Braun, & Eysholdt, 1992)

Up to 0.39‰ BrAC[b] (7 subjects)
  Error analysis:
  Phonetic analysis:

- Negative
- Appearance of denasalized nasal consonants
- Appearance of segmental lengthening in consonants
- Increase in jitter

0.4–0.79‰ BrAC (4 subjects)
  Error analysis:

  Phonetic analysis:

- Appearance of intonation errors, particularly in the form of incorrect lowering
- Considerable increase in lengthening of vowels (half of all subjects affected)
- Drastic increase in jitter
- Beginning of continual reduction in speech tempo, extending to all BrAC levels

0.8–1.19‰ BrAC (7 subjects)
  Error analysis:
  Phonetic analysis:

- Rise in general error rate, particularly omissions
- Clear increase in incomplete articulations (of consonants)
- Increase in denasalized nasal consonants, as well as frequent appearance of nasalized oral vowels
- Further clear increase in lengthening of vowels and consonants (almost all subjects affected)
- Clear rise in fundamental frequency

1.2–1.59‰ BrAC (8 subjects)
  Error analysis:

  Phonetic analysis:

- Substantial increase in insertions and substitutions
- With intonation errors, large increase in breakings, with concomitant relative decrease in incorrect lowering
- Considerable presence of word errors (from here on more prevalent than segmental errors)
- Considerable increase in number of pauses

1.6–1.99‰ BrAC (5 subjects)
  Error analysis:

  Phonetic analysis:

- Further considerable increase in general error rates, in particular substitutions and repetitions; also higher level word order and line level are affected; correction attempts—also multiple corrections—mostly unsuccessful, so that coherent meaning of the text to a certain extent cannot be conveyed
- All subjects exhibit denasalized nasal consonants
- All subjects exhibit lengthening of vowels
- Disproportionate increase in hesitation pauses in comparison to syntactic constituent pauses
- Clear increase in the proportion of pauses in the speech signal

(continues)

TABLE 7.18.7 *(continued)*

Greater than 2.0‰ BrAC (2 subjects)	
Error analysis:	• Further increase in the number of segmental errors
	• Deviations from norms on all grammatical levels causes coherence of the text to be lost
	• Correction attempts no longer undertaken
Phonetic analysis:	• Further considerable increase in incomplete articulation
	• Further considerable increase in average fundamental frequency, as well as increase in variability

[a] From Künzel, Braun, and Eysholdt (1992). Copyright © 1992 by C. F. Müller Verlag, Hüthig GmbH. Used by permission.
[b] BrAC, breath-alcohol concentration.

Results from the perceptual experiment were consistent with the findings of other studies (e.g., Pisoni & Martin, 1989): listeners could reliably identify speech produced under alcohol. These results are especially striking because the listeners were untrained, and exposure to the speech material from an individual talker was extremely brief.

The most important implication of this research for possible forensic applications is that there did not appear to be a well-defined linear relationship between any specific parameter and level of intoxication (BrAC), but if taken collectively, these parameters did appear able to index some unspecified degree of alcohol intoxication. An extremely important consideration was the high degree of individual variability among both the subjects and the speech parameters. All of this means that it would be difficult to define a single speech measure that could serve as an index of alcohol intoxication.

The authors believed that the types of measures used here could in fact be used to establish alcohol intoxication, with the following caveats: (a) intoxication could be established only for a particular individual in a particular instance, and (b) these measurements could not establish a specific BAC or BrAC. Most useful would be a combination of the types of speech and voice measurements used here and other perceptual-motor tests of nonverbal functions. Further, at least the following conditions would have to obtain: (a) the speech sample must be compared with a sample taken when the subject is sober; (b) the speech samples must be of sufficient quantity, duration, and quality; (c) the time course of alcohol intake during the period in question must be established; (d) the usual drinking behavior of the subject must be established; especially crucial would be determining whether or not alcoholism is present; (e) external factors present during the time the speech sample is recorded must be established; these might include other drugs, illnesses, and emotional and physical state; (f) all possible relevant parameters must be measured.

7.19 SWARTZ, 1992

This article reports the major results from the author's doctoral dissertation, discussed in section 7.5. Sixteen subjects recorded exemplars of the alveolar stops [d] and [t] in both a nonalcohol and an alcohol condition. Measurement of VOTs for both stops indicated that, although there were consistent time-dependent variabilities, VOT variability was resistant to the effects of alcohol. A discussion of this research appears in section 7.5.

7.20 JOHNSON, SOUTHWOOD, SCHMIDT, MOULI, HOLMES, ARMSTRONG, CRITZ-CROSBY, SUTPHIN, CROSBY, MCCUTCHEON, AND WILSON, 1993

This study introduced the use of electropalatography (EPG) and electroglottography (EGG) to research on the effects of alcohol on both speech and voice. Speech was collected from one prealcohol interval and four postalcohol intervals and subjected to acoustic, EPG, and EGG analysis. K. Johnson et al. (1993) concluded that articulatory effects of alcohol are best characterized as sporadic incoordination and that a simple tally of inarticulate episodes more clearly reflects alcohol effects than averages across all utterances. At the time this paper was presented, Keith Johnson and most of the remaining authors were affiliated with the Department of Biocommunication at the University of Alabama at Birmingham (Birmingham, Alabama).

7.20.1 Subjects and Methods

Subjects for this study were two men and two women volunteers reporting normal speech and hearing abilities; no medical conditions or medications contraindicated alcohol consumption.

Equipment included instruments to measure BAC and BrAC, to collect and store speech samples, and to collect and store physiological data. Breath-alcohol concentration was measured with a Lion Laboratories (Cardiff, Wales, UK) Alcolmeter (Model SD-2), an electrochemical oxidation/fuel cell sensor device. The EGG signal was collected by a Kay Elemetrics Laryngograph (Model 6094), with output and an accompanying acoustic signal collected from a head-mounted microphone (Shure SM10A) by a DAT recorder (Panasonic SV-255). EPG data were collected by a Kay Palatometer

(Model 6300), with a simultaneous acoustic signal collected by a Kay Computerized Speech Lab (Model 4300); digitization and storage of both signals was on a Gateway 486/50.

EGG (Fabré, 1957; see Baken, 1987; Colton & Conture, 1990; Titze, 1990, for overviews) is an indirect and noninvasive method of assessing laryngeal function, specifically adduction of the vocal folds. It is based on the principle that human tissue is a moderately good conductor of electricity and is a better conductor of electricity than air is. Thus, for an electrical current flowing between two electrodes placed on opposite sides of the neck (e.g., over the alae of the thyroid cartilage), resistance is increased when the vocal folds are abducted and decreased when they are adducted (i.e., conductance is increased by adduction and decreased by abduction). The output display, a waveform of the glottal cycle, is thus a time-varying record of the conductance of electricity through the larynx (technically not just through the glottis, as the name would imply).

Palatography (see Baken, 1987) is a method for investigating tongue–palate contact. The traditional method, dating back to the nineteenth century, involves placing a colored paste or powder either directly on the palate or on a fitted pseudopalate. Articulation of a single sound segment results in the removal of the substance from wherever the tongue contacts the palate; a record is made by either drawing or photographing either the palate itself or the prosthesis. Obvious disadvantages of this method include the fact that it can record only single articulatory events and that reapplication of the coating is necessary after each trial (a further drawback is that many of the coating mixtures are, so to speak, unpalatable).

EPG (see Baken, 1987), on the other hand, requires no repreparation after each contact, making recording of continuous speech possible. EPG, like EGG, is based on the conductance of tissue. In EPG, a subject is fitted with a pseudopalate holding exposed electrodes; when the tongue contacts an electrode, an electrical circuit is completed, which is detected by the palatometer. Any number of electrodes can be activated, and the resulting display shows the lingual–palatal contact configuration for a particular articulation. The pseudopalate used in this study in conjunction with the Kay Palatometer held 96 electrodes, whose grid-like pattern was divided into three regions: (a) the anterior-most 12 electrodes, corresponding (roughly) to the alveolar ridge; (b) the middle 23 electrodes, corresponding to the anterior section of the palatal dome; and (c) the posterior-most 61 electrodes, corresponding to the posterior region of the palatal dome. As with most EPG pseudopalates, no electrodes corresponded to either the teeth or the velum. The device sampled at 100 samples per second and stored the patterns to disk together with a time-aligned acoustic signal.

The sampling rate of the acoustic signal gathered together with EPG data was only 10 kHz, too low for analysis of fricatives, and thus the speech sample gathered by the DAT recorder was redigitized at a rate of 22 kHz. For the voice analysis of [a], the speech and EGG waveforms were sampled with the Kay Computer Speech Lab package at 51.2 kHz, and the EGG signal was used for identification of pitch periods. Recording levels were set at the first data-collection session and maintained throughout subsequent sessions.

Speech materials for this study were (a) words containing [s] and [ʃ], (b) words containing [l], and (c) a prolonged [a]. The sibilant-containing words were chosen to examine the observation (see Lester & Skousen, 1974; Trojan & Kryspin-Exner, 1968) that [s] is commonly affected by alcohol. Because production of [s] can vary according to phonetic environment, words were chosen with this sound in different word positions, word-prosodic environments, and sentence-prosodic environments. The set of words consisted of three subsets: (1) s-words: *saw, possible, possibility, posterior*; (2) s-ch-words: *postulate, posturing, postulatable*; and (3) sh-words: *shah, posh*. Groups 1 and 2 differ in that all of the [s]s in the latter group are followed by an affricated /t/. Because the change in [s] commonly associated with alcohol is backing, the words in Group 3 were included for comparison purposes. To test for different word-prosody effects on [s], the pairs *possible—possibility* and *postulate—postulatable* were included; within each pair, the stress (primary or secondary) preceding the [s] is different for each word. To examine effects of sentence prosody, pairs of sentences were constructed in which emphatic stress fell either on the test word or on a word preceding the test word, for example, "I didn't say likelihood, I said POSSIBILITY" as opposed to "Instead of time travel, only SPACE travel is a possibility."

All test words were contained in sentences, which were printed on individual sheets of white paper. In addition to the measurements made for the test words, productions of [l], which occurred both in test words and in sentence contexts, were examined. Finally, a 5-sec sustained production of [a] was elicited to examine further possible changes in vocal function.

All four subjects were examined in a single session lasting approximately 4 hr. Total alcohol doses of approximately 1 g alcohol per kg body weight were administered at regular intervals to achieve peak BACs of 0.1%. The preparations were 100-proof straight liquor: vodka for subjects PC and KJ, tequila for subject SS, and whiskey for subject BC. All subjects followed an identical schedule of consumption, absorption and distribution, and data collection in five sessions: one before consumption of alcohol and four after. Each data-collection session lasted approximately 10 min and (except for the last) was immediately followed by a consumption session lasting approximately 20 min. In the first three consumption sessions, subjects consumed one-third of the total dose of alcohol; in the final consumption session, subjects consumed a nonalcoholic beverage and some food. There was a

30-min interval after the completion of each consumption session and before commencement of the data session.

Prior to the first data-collection session, subjects practiced speaking with the pseudopalate in place by reading aloud a short passage. Also at this session, the EGG electrodes were fitted and their positions marked for subsequent replacement in later sessions. At each data-collection session, the EPG system was calibrated, productions of test sentences were digitized to the Gateway, and EGG and acoustic data from sustained [a] were recorded.

7.20.2 Results

7.20.2.1 Blood-Alcohol Concentrations

Alcohol concentrations were measured immediately prior to collection of speech samples at each data session. Session 1 was not preceded by alcohol consumption, and the consumption interval immediately preceding Session 5 was limited to a nonalcoholic beverage and food. Alcohol levels for each of the four subjects, as well as averages, are given in Figure 7.20.1. As Figure 7.20.1 shows, all subjects were at 0.00% BAC at Session 1, and all subjects had lower BACs at Session 5 than at Session 4. In general, there was a session-to-session increase in BAC from Session 1 through Session 4. This general trend was borne out both by the average BAC and by three of the four subjects; Subject BC also showed the general trend, although the reported BACs for this subject for Sessions 3 and 4 were equal. For Session 2, BACs ranged from 0.035– 0.065%; for Session 3, from 0.065–0.115%; for Session 4, from 0.11–0.13%; and for Session 5, from 0.085–0.115%.

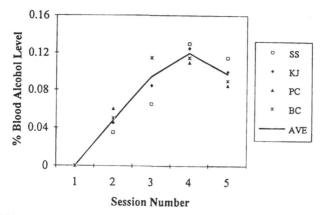

FIGURE 7.20.1 Blood alcohol level measurements for all four speakers at each of the five recording sessions. These measurements were taken immediately before speech data were collected in each of the five sessions. (From K. Johnson et al., 1993. Used by permission.)

The greatest range in BACs was observed for Session 3, with a difference of approximately 0.05% BAC between the lowest and highest BACs. At all other postalcohol sessions, differences were between 0.02 and 0.03%. There was some session-to-session overlap in BACs, such that one subject in Session 3 had a BAC equal to or higher than two subjects (including himself) in Session 4, and two subjects in Session 4 had BACs equal to or lower than one subject in Session 5.

7.20.2.2 Effects of Alcohol on Speech

Figure 7.20.2 shows the first spectral moment results for the three types of sibilants, averaged across talkers and word/sentence stress conditions. Of the three types of sibilants examined, alcohol appeared to affect only those in *s-ch*-words. As shown in Figure 7.20.2, the spectral center of gravity (the first spectral moment) for both the *s* and *sh* words remained unchanged across sessions, but for *s-ch*-words, there was a drop in Session 3, resulting in a more [ʃ]-like sibilant. However, the spectral center of gravity for this sound segment rose again for Sessions 4 and 5. This lowering in Session 3 and return in Sessions 4 and 5 was observed in both the averaged data and individual data and was attributed to a compensatory strategy, especiallly since BACs were higher in Sessions 4 and 5 than in Session 3.

EPG results for the sibilants were as in Figure 7.20.3 as the percent electrodes contacted (averaged across talkers and stress conditions) in the three regions of the pseudopalate. As indicated in Figure 7.20.3, productions of [s] were characterized by more front contact than mid or back, whereas [ʃ] productions showed more mid- and back contact than front. Furthermore,

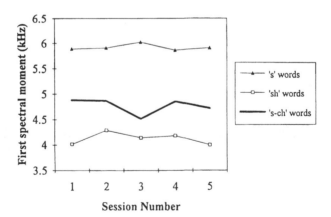

FIGURE 7.20.2   Average spectral center of gravity by recording session and word type. These data are averaged across speakers and stress conditions. (From K. Johnson et al., 1993. Used by permission.)

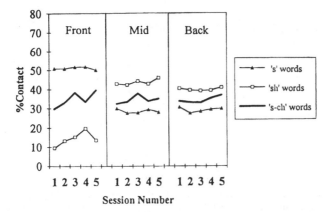

FIGURE 7.20.3 Average percent electrodes contacted in three regions of the palate for the three classes of fricatives across recording sessions. Data as in Figure 7.20.2 are averaged across speakers and stress conditions. (From K. Johnson et al., 1993. Used by permission.)

productions of [s] differed from [ʃ] mainly in having more front contact. In all three regions of the pseudopalate, the sibilant in the *s-ch* showed contact patterns between those of the other two. Across sessions, changes occurred in the front region for sibilants in the *sh-* and *s-ch*-words and in the midregion for the *s-ch*-words. These changes did not correlate simply with the changes in the first spectral moment noted above. Also, the front region of the pseudo-palate held only 12 electrodes. Better correlated with the first spectral moment results was the pattern of change for midelectrode contact for the sibilant in the *s-ch*-words. The EPG results showed specifically a retraction in Session 3; that is, a greater percentage of the electrodes in the midregion were contacted in comparison to other sessions.

For both first spectral moment and EPG results, measurements were averaged across talkers and stress conditions. A second type of analysis involved a simple count of speech errors committed in the different sessions. Two types of errors were examined: (a) misarticulation in the sequence [st] in *postulate* and (2) misarticulation of [l]. Examination of waveforms of words containing [st] revealed an error pattern involving failure to produce stop closure. Figure 7.20.4 shows the percent errors committed on this sequence as a function of time, in both stressed and unstressed position. As Figure 7.20.4 shows, in unstressed cases, the rate of [st] errors correlated with BAC, that is, increases for both through Session 4, and decreases between Sessions 4 and 5. In stressed cases, the relationship was not as clear: first, there was a decrease in [st] errors from Session 1 (prealcohol) to Session 2 (first postalcohol), and second, although BACs increased between Sessions 3 and 4, the percentage of [st] errors decreased.

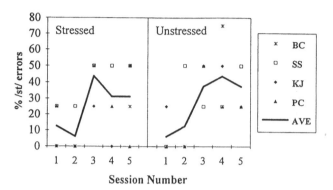

FIGURE 7.20.4   Percent [st] errors produced by the four speakers by session and sentence type. (From K. Johnson et al., 1993. Used by permission.)

Examination of alcohol effects on [l] was based on the words *possible, possibility, postulate, postulatable* and on the word *law,* occurring in two sentence contexts. Two types of errors were noted in the EPG analysis: (a) failure to achieve front contact for [l]; and (b) coalescence of adjacent alveolar articulations ([l] and [t]) in *possibility.* Figure 7.20.5 shows error rates for productions of [l], initial in *law* and noninitial in both stressed and unstressed positions, as a function of session number. As Figure 7.20.5 shows, no subject produced errored initial [l], but noninitially, as with [st], error rates tended to be higher when BACs were higher, especially in unstressed cases.

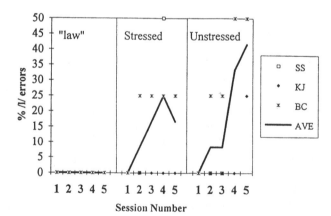

FIGURE 7.20.5   Percent [l] errors produced by the four speakers by session and sentence type. (From K. Johnson et al., 1993. Used by permission.)

K. Johnson et al. (1993) offered two tentative conclusions: (a) misarticulation effects of alcohol on speech are sporadic rather than ubiquitous; and (b) BAC correlates better with the number of inarticulate episodes than with averages across all utterances. K. Johnson et al. (1993) suggested that the sporadic nature of alcohol effects could be accounted for by a random noise model incorporating these characteristics: (a) effects of alcohol on nervous system function could be modeled as an increase in random noise in the system, so that increasing BAC would be modeled as increasing random noise; and (b) greater attention to speaking could compensate for alcohol effects, and this would be modeled as selective reduction in the amount of noise in the system.

7.20.2.1 Effects of Alcohol on Voice

A number of measurements assessed alcohol effects on voice. A specific hypothesis was that whereas articulation effects were due to changes in central nervous system (CNS) functioning, changes in vocal function might be attributable to morphological changes in the vocal folds, specifically edema and swelling. This hypothesis was first examined in Dunker and Schlosshauer (1964), considered in Klingholz et al. (1988), K. Johnson et al. (1990), and Watanabe et al. (1994), and rejected by Künzel et al. (1992).

Using productions of sustained [a], K. Johnson et al. (1993) measured these phonatory parameters: jitter, shimmer, harmonics-to-noise ratio, open quotient, pitch breaks, and root-mean-square (RMS) amplitude. Jitter, shimmer, and harmonics-to-noise ratios were measured using postprocessing analysis capabilities of the Kay Computerized Speech Lab, based on the acoustic signal and the EGG waveform. Jitter and shimmer were measured as Relative Average Perturbation (Davis, 1976; Koike, 1973), and the harmonics-to-noise ratio was calculated according to Yumoto (1987) and Yumoto, Sasaki, and Okamura (1984). Figure 7.20.6 shows jitter as a function of session; jitter tended to increase through sessions, although this tendency was small and inconsistent. Figure 7.20.7 shows shimmer measurements as a function of session. As with jitter, shimmer also tended to increase slightly in Session 5. It was noted that although articulatory effects occurred by Session 3, increases in jitter and shimmer were delayed until Session 5, suggesting that if increases in jitter and shimmer were due to morphological changes in the vocal folds, such changes were delayed relative to neurological effects.

K. Johnson et al. (1993) found that the harmonics-to-noise ratio tended to decrease for some talkers in the alcohol condition, consistent with findings by Klingholz et al. (1988). Mean and individual harmonics-to-noise ratios are shown in Figure 7.20.8; changes in the harmonics-to-noise ratio were similar to those for jitter and shimmer: Different talkers were affected to different degrees. On the whole, the jitter, shimmer, and harmonics-to-noise

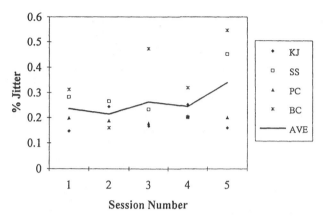

FIGURE 7.20.6 Jitter measurement during sustained [a] by speaker and recording session. (From K. Johnson et al., 1993. Used by permission.)

ratio measurements did not clearly support the hypothesis that phonatory effects were due to morphological changes to the vocal cords. These indirect measures showed changes that were at best small and inconsistent across talkers.

K. Johnson et al. (1993) further tested the morphological-change hypothesis by measuring open quotient (see Baken, 1987, pp. 210ff) in the EGG signal. Each glottal wave cycle (T) consists of an open phase (Op) and a closed phase (Cp). The open quotient (Oq) is equal to Op/T; if there is no glottal closure, then Oq = 1. The prediction tested by K. Johnson et al.

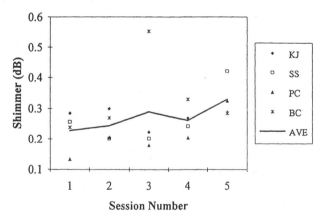

FIGURE 7.20.7 Shimmer measurement during sustained [a] by speaker and recording session. (From K. Johnson et al., 1993. Used by permission.)

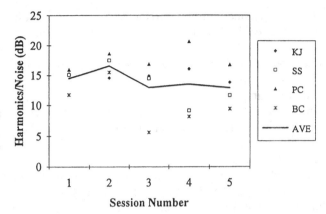

FIGURE 7.20.8 Harmonics-to-noise ratio during sustained [a] by speaker and recording session. (From K. Johnson et al., 1993. Used by permission.)

(1993) was that if the vocal folds suffered edema or swelling, then both Op and Oq would be reduced. Using the differentiated EGG signal for sustained [a], K. Johnson et al. (1993) measured 10 randomly chosen pitch periods at intervals of approximately 400 ms. Figure 7.20.9 shows average Oq as a function of session; Oq tended to increase across the five sessions, but three of the talkers decreased Oq in Session 3. For all talkers, however, Oq increased again from Session 3 to Session 4. K. Johnson et al. (1993) interpreted this effect as compensatory, possibly the result of vocal-fold edema around Session 3. If compensation was a factor here, then the effects could

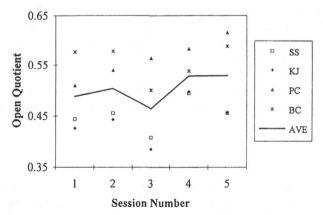

FIGURE 7.20.9 Open quotient measurements taken from EGG plotted by speaker and recording session. (From K. Johnson et al., 1993). Used by permission.)

not have been large, since, in comparison to Session 1 values, Session 3 values were higher for three of the talkers, and Session 5 values were higher for all talkers.

Two other apparent effects of alcohol on voice were examined: the tendency for voices to "break" and the tendency for speech to be louder. An examination of the amplitude envelope and calculated FØ for the sustained [a] from one of the talkers (SS) in Session 4 revealed marked fluctuations (episodic, rather than period-to-period) in both amplitude and frequency. Measures of FØ during sustained [a] revealed no consistent changes as a function of session number.

The general lack of change in FØ was consistent with findings from other studies (e.g., Pisoni et al., 1986), but still other studies found either increases (e.g., Behne & Rivera, 1990) or decreases (e.g., Watanabe et al., 1994). In those studies that have examined variability of FØ, however, results consistently show increased variability (measured as the standard deviation of FØ) as a function of alcohol (see, e.g., Behne & Rivera, 1990; Klingholz et al., 1988; Künzel et al., 1992; Pisoni et al., 1986). K. Johnson et al.'s (1993) measurement of the standard deviation of FØ conformed to this general pattern.

To examine the perception of loudness in alcohol-affected speech, K. Johnson et al. (1993) measured the RMS amplitude of a 200-ms span of sustained [a] approximately 200 ms into the vowel. RMS amplitude increased as BAC increased, with a return to prealcohol levels for some talkers in Session 5. K. Johnson et al. (1993) proposed two possible explanations. First, talkers might increase amplitude in later sessions to compensate for reduced motor control. Second, the amplitude increase in the measured portions of the vowel might reflect directly a loss of motor control, especially of respiration, resulting in overly high subglottal pressure and increased amplitude at the onset of the vowel. To test the latter possibility, K. Johnson et al. (1993) compared the RMS amplitude of the onset of the vowel with that of the entire vowel. Through successive sessions, the difference between the RMS amplitude of the onset and that of the entire vowel became greater. This tended to confirm the hypothesis that respiratory control was diminished at high BACs, such that talkers initiated the vowel with a higher amplitude than was sustainable throughout the duration of the vowel.

7.20.3 Discussion

The EPG and EGG methods employed in this physiological study of alcohol effects on speech and voice are unique in the literature and provided both independent confirmation of previous results and a different way of studying alcohol effects. Decrements in motor control of both articulatory and phonatory aspects of speech were found, which were more readily apparent when tallies of errors were considered rather than averages across all utterances. K. Johnson et al. (1993) proposed a qualitative model of these effects involving addition of random noise to normal speech processes as well as the compensatory effect of selective attention to reduce that noise. Decrements in motor control were best considered as sporadic rather than as all-encompassing. This view of alcohol effects on speech and voice was supported by the lack of clear evidence that alcohol-induced morphological changes of the phonatory apparatus, especially the vocal folds, lay at base of the changes. Further evidence against morphological changes was talkers' apparent ability to compensate for alcohol effects within approximately 40 min. Given these results, specifically the sporadic nature of inarticulate effects, K. Johnson et al. (1993) held out little hope that a detection system for alcohol intoxication based on speech and voice would be feasible.

7.21 NIEDZIELSKA, PRUSZEWICZ, AND SWIDZINSKI, 1994

This study was conducted by a team of scientists from the University of Medical Science in Lublin, Poland (Niedzielska), and the University of Medical Science in Poznan, Poland (Pruszewicz and Swidzinski). It investigated the hypothesis that alcohol induces changes in laryngeal function, including phonatory disorders. This was tested using acoustic analysis of the speech of alcohol-addicted subjects.

7.21.1 Methods

The subjects for this study included 10 control and 30 experimental subjects. Control subjects exhibited no alcohol addiction, whereas the experimental subjects were divided into two groups: Group 1 ($N = 19$) exhibited alcohol addiction from 1 to 10 years; Group 2 ($N = 11$) had been addicted to alcohol between 11 and 20 years. Daily alcohol consumption for most subjects in Groups 1 and 2 ranged from 500 to 1000 ml of 45% vodka. Linguistic material for recording and analysis consisted of sentences, words, vowels, and a read text.

Recorded speech material was analyzed for acoustic markers indicating laryngeal function changes using digital analysis of spectral and temporal characteristics on an IBM/AT microcomputer and TRA-14A software. Values for the following parameters were calculated (p. 116): (a) "medium and maximum jitter values, i.e. the variability in length of vibration periods of vocal folds from one cycle to another" (calculated according to Hollien, Michel, and Doherty's (1973) "jitter factor"); (b) "harmonic structure of speech signal"; (c) "variable distribution of periodicity of vowel courses";

(d) "noise content in the individual threads of analysis"; (e) "intonation course variability character."

7.21.2 Results

Results for the three groups for the speech parameters are summarized in Table 7.21.1. In the table, harmonic structure is characterized as rich (harmonic structure above 2500 Hz), medium rich (harmonic structure up to 2500 Hz), or poor (harmonic structure up to 1500 Hz). Periodicity and noise interference of periodicity are inverses of each other, and intonation variability is characterized as well-differentiated, medium differentiated, barely differentiated, and (with) little differentiation.

As indicated in Table 7.21.1, both mean and maximum jitter factor values were higher for Group 1 than the control group and higher for Group 2 than for either of the other two groups. The harmonic structures of all subjects in the control group were characterized as either rich or medium rich. For Group 1, rich/medium rich harmonic structures were attributed to 58% of the subjects and poor harmonic structure to 42%. For Group 2,

TABLE 7.21.1 Summary of Results[a]

	Control group	Group 1 (1–10 yr)	Group 2 (11–20 yr)
Number of subjects	10	19	11
Mean jitter	119 ± 0.35%	199 ± 0.27%	4.20 ± 1.98%
Maximum jitter	11.31 ± 3.0%	19.6 ± 8.1%	32.5 ± 7.6%
Harmonic structure	Rich or medium rich	3 Ss: rich 8 Ss: medium-rich 8 Ss: poor (ranging below 1500 Hz)	No Ss: structure > 2500 Hz 5 Ss: medium rich (up to 2500 Hz) 6 Ss: poor (up to 1500 Hz)
Periodicity course of vowels	70–90%	13 Ss: 30–50% 6 Ss: 60–80%	3 Ss: 20–40% 8 Ss: 50–70%
Periodicity course interfered by wideband noise	10–30% of vowel duration	13 Ss: 50–70% 6 Ss: 20–40%	8 Ss: 30–50% 3 Ss: 60–80%
Intonation course variability	Medium and well differentiated	3 Ss: well differentiated 4 Ss: medium differentiation 12 Ss: barely differentiated	No well-differentiated melodic courses 7 Ss: medium differentiation 4 Ss: little differentiation

[a] From Niedzielska, Pruszewicz, and Swidzinski (1994).

less than half (45%) of the harmonic structures were characterized as medium rich, and 55% were characterized as poor. On the measure of the
proportion of periodicity during vowel production, a maximum of 90%
was reported for the control group, with maxima of 80 and 70% respectively
for Groups 1 and 2.

Intonation variability for the control group was characterized as either
well-differentiated or medium-differentiated for 100% of the subjects. For
Group 1, intonation variability was characterized as well-differentiated for
16% of the subjects, medium-differentiated for 21%, and barely differentiated for 63%. For Group 2, intonation variability was characterized as
medium-differentiated for 64% of the subjects; 36% showed little differentiation and no subjects showed well differentiated intonation variability.

The authors maintained that the results, particularly for jitter, indicated
incipient functional laryngeal changes for Group 1. For Group 2, results
indicated functional changes for all subjects and for four subjects with mean
jitter values above 5%, early organic changes as well.

7.21.3 Discussion

This work applied methodology suggested in Pruszewicz et al. (1991) for
the differential diagnosis of organic and functional dysphonia using acoustic
analysis. In that pilot study, differential diagnoses of organic and functional
laryngeal disturbances were established by phoniatric examination, and
these results were compared to a number of acoustic measures. Results
indicated that it was possible to use acoustic analyses to differentiate between
functional and organic disorders of the larynx.

Niedzielska et al. maintained that differences in the acoustic signal between the control group and both alcohol groups indicated at least some
functional changes in the larynx, and in some cases in Group 2, organic
changes as well. It is true that there were differences among the groups in
terms of jitter, harmonic structure, vowel periodicity, and intonation, but
whether these changes could be considered significant or reliable enough to
clearly differentiate the three groups is not clear. There were, in fact, some
methodological and analytical difficulties or at least reporting oversights
that need to be taken into account when interpreting the results of this study
and possibly those of Pruszewicz et al. (1991).

Subjects were divided into three groups: a control group with no alcohol
addiction, subjects with 1–10 years of alcohol addiction, and subjects with
11–20 years of alcohol addiction. Other subject information that would
help in interpreting the results would be age and sex of the subjects. Additionally, the derived datum of average FØ would be useful; this would be
especially helpful in interpreting the harmonic structure/noise results. The
authors used the landmark frequencies of 1500 and 2500 Hz to differentiate

rich, medium-rich, and poor harmonic structure, but there is a difference between males and females, given different mean FØs. Other necessary but missing methodological information included exact recording techniques, especially microphone placement. For instance, one figure, a spectrogram of a sentence produced by a Group 2 subject, appears to show almost no energy above about 1000 Hz and is intended to exemplify lack of differentiation in intonation variability. However, it is almost impossible for there to be absolutely no energy above 1000 Hz, even in severely disordered voices. It is not impossible that something was wrong with placement or use of the microphone during recording or with the analysis equipment used to generate the spectrograms.

One would also like further information regarding measurement and analysis techniques. A basic question concerns the use of the speech materials; it was not always clear which of the various speech materials were used for the different analyses. The difference, for instance, between connected speech and isolated vowels might influence the measurements for periodicity during vowel production; aperiodicity in vowels embedded in connected speech might arise from contextual sources such as surrounding fricative segments. Furthermore, in this regard, there was no report of the criteria used for determining onset and offsets of vowels or for determining whether a given portion of the speech waveform was considered periodic or not. Finally, the proportion of periodicity to nonperiodicity is very dependent on the particular vowel.

Methods for determining intonation differentiation are also not explicitly given. Intonation is a fairly complex phenomenon whose linguistic implications and acoustic correlates are far from clear. Intonation appears to be a combination of at least the acoustic parameters of FØ, intensity, and duration (see Kent & Read, 1992, p. 149), and these are measurable instrumentally. However, which, if any, of these, were actually measured is unclear, and it is also unclear how precisely the reported degrees of intonation differentation were determined.

7.22 WATANABE, SHIN, MATSUO, OKUNO, TSUJI, MATSUOKA, FUKAURA, AND MATSUNAGA, 1994

This study examined the relationship between changes in phonetic function and physiological changes in hypopharyngeal and laryngeal mucosa after ingestion of alcohol. Hiroshi Watanabe, Takemoto Shin, Hiromichi Matuso, and Junichi Fukaura were affiliated with the Department of Otolaryngology–Head and Neck Surgery at Saga Medical School, Saga, Japan. Fumio Okuno was in the Department of Internal Medicine at the University of

Occupational and Environmental Health, in Fukuoka, Japan; Tsutomu Tsuji was affiliated with the Department of Forensic Science at Wakayama Medical College, in Wakayama, Japan. Midori Matsuoka and Hisashi Matsunaga were affiliated with Saga Medical School, in Saga, Japan: Matsuoka with the School of Nursing, and Matsunaga with the Hospital Pharmacy.

7.22.1 Methods

Subjects were 48 medical student volunteers (37 males and 11 females), ranging from 25– 37 years of age. A preparation consisting of 40% vodka mixed with an equal volume of orange juice was administered over a 30-min period to achieve a concentration of 1 g alcohol/kg body weight. BAC was measured before consumption of the beverage and every 30 min after consumption for 2.5 hr. In addition to this measure, the following measures were also made: (a) acetaldehyde in blood using high-pressure liquid chromatography; (b) percutaneous changes in the face, abdomen, and legs, using reflectance spectrophotometry (Sumitomo Denkoh Co.); (c) FØ, intensity, and mean flow rate using a phonation analyzer (Nagashima PS-77) with attached camera (Asahi Pentax PE-2); (d) classification of subjects as "flushing" or "nonflushing," based on an aldehyde dehydrogenase (ALDH2) phenotype screening questionnaire; (e) spectral measurements of five Japanese vowels [a e i o u] from spectrograms (Kay Elemetrics).

7.22.2 Results

Initial determination of alcohol levels was made using observation of spontaneous nystagmus, an optokinetic nystagmus test, and an eye-tracking test.

Mean fundamental frequency (FØ) for males was 115 ± 28 Hz before consumption of alcohol and 108 ± 25 Hz 1 hr later. For females, mean FØ was 262 ± 31 Hz before alcohol and 246 ± 36 Hz 1 hr later. Thus, for both males and females, mean FØ decreased after alcohol consumption. Subjects tended to be able to phonate at both higher and lower frequencies after alcohol intake than before, but neither of these differences was significant. However, as a whole, the increase in frequency range of phonation was significant, and the tendency to expand the pitch range appeared to be more prominent in the female subjects.

Table 7.22.1 displays results of the phonetic function tests before and after alcohol for two "typical" subjects, one male and one female. Both subjects listed in Table 7.22.1 illustrate the tendency toward lowered FØ after alcohol. Mean intensity results were reported for only these two subjects, but it could be inferred that any differences between conditions were not large. Finally, for flow rate, it was noted that "during phonation after alcohol ingestion, the mean airflow was varied and became rough" (p. 344).

TABLE 7.22.1   Results of Phonetic Function Test from a Male Subject (28 years old) and
Female Subject (25 years old), Pre- and Postalcohol[a]

	Male		Female	
	Prealcohol	Postalcohol	Prealcohol	Postalcohol
Fundamental frequency in Hz	111	104	264	239
Intensity in dB SPL	73	71	64	63
Mean flow rate in mL/sec	194	185	282	234

[a] From Watanabe et al. (1994).

Fiberscopic examination revealed some changes in the larynx concomitant
with the observed voice changes. In one male, there were injections occurring
in the anterior commissure, arytenoid regions, ventricles, and free margin
of the vocal folds 1 hr after alcohol consumption, as well as redness in the
vocal folds. Other observations included a shortening of the anteroposterior
diameter of the larynx. In one female, 1 hr after alcohol, there were injections
in the anterior commissure, arytenoid regions, and ventricles, but not in the
vocal folds. Subglottic injection and edema appeared to be similar in the
male and female subject.

This article contained a rather lengthy discussion of the "flushing syndrome" to which some Asians are prone (see also Mizoi, Rukunaga, &
Adachi, 1989). "Flushing" covers a number of signs and symptoms, including facial flushing, flushing elsewhere on the body, dizziness, headaches,
perspiring, palpitations, and nausea. The relevance of flushing to vocal-cord
injections and pitch changes can only be inferred, as no direct comparison
was made between the "flushing" results and the voice and vocal organ
results. One assumes that most if not all of the subjects investigated in this
study were Asian, and that some would "flush" after consuming alcohol.
The vocal organ redness noted for some subjects might be related to this.
However, Watanabe et al. appeared to have evaluated flushing and voice
changes separately, although neither data nor results from any of the flushing
measures were reported. Similarly, the abstract mentions that rhinography
was performed on subjects who complained of nasal congestion after ingesting alcohol, but no results for this measure were reported. Relevant results
from this study are thus the changes in fundamental frequency, in frequency
range of phonation, and in appearance of the hypopharyngeal and laryngeal mucosa.

7.23   DUNLAP, PISONI, BERNACKI, AND ROSE, 1995

This study was part of a research project conducted at the Alcohol Research
Center (Indiana University School of Medicine and Indiana University—

Bloomington) investigating the transmission of genetic risk for alcoholism and the identification of biobehavioral markers for assessing individual susceptibility to accute alcohol effects. This particular study investigated the possibility that changes in speech could act as such markers, permitting reliable assessment of individual risk. All four authors were affiliated with the Department of Psychology at Indiana University, in Bloomington, Indiana, as well as with the Alcohol Research Center at the Indiana University School of Medicine (Indianapolis, Indiana) and Indiana University—Bloomington.

7.23.1 Subjects and Methods

Subjects were 24 male social drinkers, ranging in age from 21–23 years. Sessions were held on two different days, 12 to 16 days apart. Two speech samples were elicited in the first session and three in the second. In each session, subjects shadowed sentences when BrAC was .000% and then again after alcohol had been consumed and a predetermined BrAC (0.5% ± .005%) had been reached. At the end of the second session, subjects shadowed a fifth time, with instructions to speak "as if they had not consumed alcohol." Stimulus materials were presented over headphones, and responses were spoken into an attached boom microphone. Utterances were digitized, and waveforms were measured to determine durations for nine sentences.

7.23.2 Results

Mean sentence durations across the nine sentences and all subjects for the five conditions are given in Table 7.23.1. Multiple ANOVA was used to test effects of alcohol (prealcohol vs. postalcohol) and session (first vs. second). There was a main effect for alcohol but no main effect for session or an interaction. A paired t-test of the second session postalcohol and "fake–good" durations showed no significant difference between the two. The correlation of duration from the first session to the second session was $r = -.134$; p not significant.

TABLE 7.23.1   Mean Sentence Durations[a]

Condition	Mean sentence duration in ms
Session 1: Prealcohol	1599
Session 1: Postalcohol	1625
Session 2: Prealcohol	1589
Session 2: Postalcohol	1632
Session 2: "Fake–Good"	1652

[a] From Dunlap, Pisoni, Bernacki, and Rose (1995).

These results indicated a reliable increase in sentence durations when subjects were administered alcohol to .05% BrAC. The test–retest results, and instructions to subjects to speak as though they had not consumed alcohol, indicated that subjects were unable to control the durational aspects of speech that changed under alcohol. Although the authors concluded that acoustical measurements of speech might hold promise as a biobehavioral marker for alcoholism, wide variation between subjects in sentence duration changes was observed, and there was a lack of consistency in changes in duration within subjects across sessions. These results might have been due to the relatvely low alcohol concentrations used or to the small number of sentences analyzed. Finally, there appeared to be no consistent correlations of changes in sentence duration with personality dispositions or alcohol expectations.

7.24 HOLLIEN AND MARTIN, 1996

This work reports from a project supported by the National Institute on Alcohol Abuse and Alcoholism and conducted in Gainesville, Florida, by Harry Hollien, Camilo A. Martin, and their associates. H. Hollien (personal communication, October 1995) has provided the following summary of this research:

> Research on the effects of intoxication on speech and voice suffers from two problems: the lack of financial support for basic research and the limited interest in the area by qualified scientists. Little wonder, then, that less than 20 publications can be found on this issue and, indeed, fewer than 10 actual investigations have been reported. Supported by the National Institute of Alcohol Abuse and Alcoholism (grant AA-09377), Hollien, Martin and their associates are attempting to obtain systematic and controlled data on the subject. The project is organized into four core phases. The first of these is focused on research design: 1) precise control of subjects (drinking history, condition at time of experiment, etc.), 2) the control of intoxication levels (trials for all subjects are at the same level) and 3) materials (specified speech/voice tests). This phase of the grant was completed in 1994. The second phase involves the confirmation of the physiological measures with behavioral (primarily aural-perceptual judgments); 14 experiments have been completed (as of 1995). The third and fourth lines of inquiry involve traditional analyses of the segmentals of speech and the suprasegmentals of voice.

Some of the results reported in this work were also reported at meetings of the International Association of Forensic Phonetics and the Acoustical Society of America (Alderman et al., 1995; DeJong et al. , 1995; Hollien & Martin, 1995). Harry Hollien has been affiliated with the University of Florida and Camilo A. Martin with the Veterans Administration Medical Center, both in Gainesville, Florida.

7.24.1 Subjects and Methods

Subjects were 16 young adults (11 males, 5 females) between the ages of 21 and 32 years. None exhibited speech or hearing disorders, and all had to speak a general American dialect. None of the females was pregnant. Thirteen subjects were experimental and three control subjects. Alcohol consumption patterns served as both dependent and independent variables, and special procedures were employed to screen subjects. These included adaptations of the Michigan Alcoholism Screening Test (Pokorny et al., 1972), Cahalan et al. (1969), and a psychiatric interview. Subjects were classified as light, medium, and heavy drinkers, and persons who were nondrinkers, alcoholic or problem drinkers, or drug users were not used in the study.

Important to this research was determining methods for controlling and systematizing levels of intoxication. In other studies, alcohol administration has been based on estimates of the dose required to achieve a target concentration; after a standard time interval, alcohol concentration is measured and tasks are carried out. One problem with this method has been wide variation in achieved concentrations at the time of testing. In this study, target BrAC windows were predetermined, and testing occurred only when subjects were within these windows: 0.00, 0.04–0.05, 0.08–0.09, 0.12–0.13, and, during elimination, 0.09–0.08. Constant monitoring after alcohol consumption used one or two AlcoSensor IV (Alcopro, Inc.) breath-alcohol analysis devices, electrochemical oxidation/fuel cell sensors. The methodology employed required relatively fast recovery times for the devices, which was approximately 2 min.

Alcohol was originally prescribed as 0.45 g of 78% alcohol per kg body weight mixed with four parts tonic water administered in three doses over 15 min. This mode of administration, however, often resulted in discomfort, nausea, and erratic increases in BrAC. A modified procedure called for a dose containing one-third 40% rum or vodka, one-third Gatorade (a potassium-containing sports beverage), and one-third orange juice or cola, which resulted in more even absorption without discomfort or nausea.

Speech materials included (a) extemporaneous responses to simple questions, (b) the Rainbow Passage (Fairbanks, 1960), (c) sentences from Fisher and Logemann (1971), and (d) diadochokinetic syllables (modified from Fletcher, 1978, plus the forms *shapoopie* and *buttercup*). Subjects recorded these materials twice when sober and four times after ingesting alcohol. Two simultaneous recordings were made of each trial, with one microphone placed in a positioner at a constant distance of 6 in. from the subject's mouth, and the other positioned in a headband. Each microphone was connected to a separate TEAC-300R tape recorder.

Two types of studies were conducted: (a) correlations between physiological and behavioral measures and (b) analysis of suprasegmental properties of the recorded speech. For assessing physiological-behavioral correlations, one scaling study and three sorting studies were conducted. In the scaling study, the first three passage sentences from eight talkers in both sober and intoxicated conditions were randomized and presented to 50 listeners, who assessed sentences on a 5-point scale ranging from 1 (sober) to 5 (highly intoxicated). In the three sorting tasks, diadochokinetic speech samples from the 0.00 and 0.12 BrAC conditions were presented. In the first procedure, 27 listeners sorted samples into two categories, unspecified except insofar as members of one set should be the same as each other but different from the other set. In the second task, 12 listeners were told that half the samples were produced while talkers were intoxicated and the other half when the same talkers were sober. In the third task, 18 listeners sorted samples into three categories: intoxicated, sober, and no decision.

Both speaking fundamental frequency (SFF) and passage duration were assessed from the passage using the IASCP Fundamental Frequency Indicator (FFI-12; Hollien, 1990), and the number of diadochokinetic gestures produced in 10 sec was measured.

7.24.2 Results

Results of the scaling study were reported for eight talkers (mostly light and moderate drinkers) from the 0.00 and 0.12–0.13 BrAC conditions. All talkers showed a positive shift in ratings from the 0.00 to the 0.12–0.13 condition; additionally, the mean shifted from 1.81 to 3.11, although there was no significant correlation ($r = 0.34$) between BrAC and this measure. In fact, most of the change was accounted for by half of the talkers (means = 1.62 and 3.84). Finally, nonalcohol sentences from at least one subject were consistently perceived as being produced under intoxication, exhibiting a number of dysfluencies.

In the first sorting task, listeners placed 66% of the sober stimuli into one category and 45% of the intoxicated ones into the other category; overall percent correct was somewhat over 60%. In the second sorting task, in which listeners knew the differences between stimuli, overall correct scores were slightly higher, but chi-square tests showed the relationships not to be significant. The best scores were obtained in the third sorting task, which allowed no decision responses (used about 6% of the time). Overall correct scores in this task were the highest of the three, about 64%. In general, results from these sorting tasks were consistent with other studies (e.g., Pisoni & Martin, 1989).

Suprasegmental analyses were conducted on the speech of six of the subjects. On the basis of the scaling experiment, at 0.12–0.13 BrAC, three of these subjects were considered to sound intoxicated and three not to. In the first group (A), there was a mean increase in SFF of 0.2 semitones and for the second group (B) a mean increase of 0.1 semitones. Group A subjects showed mean passage reading times of 22.8 sec in the sober and 26.4 sec in the intoxicated condition, a difference of +3.6 sec (an increase of approximately 16%). Group B subjects had mean reading times of 27.2 sec in the sober and 27.6 sec in the intoxicated condition, a difference of +0.4 sec (an increase of between 1 and 2%). In addition to this difference, a count of articulatory errors showed that Group A committed over eight times more of these than Group B. A measure of diadochokinetic units produced showed mean decreases from sober to intoxicated for both groups, with the effect larger for Group A than for Group B; there was, however, a good degree of individual variation, including opposite effects for some subjects.

7.24.3 Discussion

In addition to fairly straightforward measuring of various speech parameters, this initial report from an ongoing project at the University of Florida addressed a number of methodological questions surrounding the study of alcohol effects on speech. These include subject characteristics, control of intoxication levels, and choice of speech materials. Especially important are the attempts to control fluctuations (Dubowski's "steepling" effect) on the uptake limb of the alcohol curve and to ensure concentration uniformity at time of testing by defining precise requisite BrAC windows. In perceptual and suprasegmental measures, trends were in expected directions, although correlations were often not statistically significant and effects not robust. It is to be hoped that future research from this project will continue to address the important methodological and theoretical issues surrounding research on alcohol and speech.

7.25 CUMMINGS, CHIN, AND PISONI 1996

This paper reported from a research project investigating effects of alcohol on glottal excitation and other acoustic characteristics of speech. The project involved a reanalysis, using novel digital signal processing techniques, of the database collected for the research project described in section 7.1. The first type of analysis considered parameters determined directly from the acoustic speech waveform, whereas a second type of analysis used parameters determined from extracted glottal waveforms (only source characteristics). Cummings et al. reported preliminary results for the first type of analysis from four subjects and results for the second type (from extracted glottal waveforms) for two subjects. Kathleen Cummings was affiliated with the School of Electrical and Computer Engineering at the Georgia Institute of Technology in Atlanta, Georgia, USA, while Steven Chin and David Pisoni were affiliated with the Speech Research Laboratory at Indiana University in Bloomington, Indiana.

7.25.1 Subjects and Methods

Speech materials for this investigation consisted of the digitized speech database constructed for the research on alcohol and speech conducted at Indiana University in the 1980s under contract with General Motors Research Laboratory. Descriptions of the subjects involved and of the elicitation and digital storage techniques can be found in sections 7.1.1. and 7.12.1. Cummings et al. reported results from up to four subjects.

Acoustic speech waveform parameters were determined on vowels from eight isolated words in a nonalcohol condition and an alcohol condition. Each utterance was pitch-marked using a semiautomatic cepstrum-based pitch detector. Boundaries of voiced sections were marked and a pitch contour determined. Extraction of parameters used the original utterance, the voicing boundaries, and the pitch contours. Sample distributions were determined for each parameter, for each subject, and in both conditions; statistical information was calculated for each sample distribution and used for comparison of speech produced in the two conditions.

The parameters used in this analysis were a combination of those used to distinguish among different speaking styles (see Cummings, 1992) and several new distinguishing parameters. These parameters typically involved measures of energy in a given segment of speech and of the pitch period. The measurement of energy involved deriving RMS intensity, a common specification for AC signals. This involved taking the square of the wave amplitude at each point in time, determining the mean of the squared values, and then taking the square root of the mean. Five measurements of each pitch period were made, and from these, fifteen parameters based on either RMS intensity or pitch were determined.

The first measurement was for RMS intensity per pitch period during the vowel segment of each of the isolated words, providing a measure of the total energy generated in each pitch period. Four of the analysis parameters were based on this measurement: (a) [mean (RMS)], the average of the RMS intensity per pitch period for the entire utterance; (b) [max (RMS)], the maximum RMS intensity per pitch period generated at some point in the utterance; (c) [mean (RMS)/(average pitch)], the RMS intensity per pitch period divided by the average length of the pitch period (a normalized RMS intensity); and (d) [max (RMS)/(pitch duration at max location)], the maximum RMS intensity per pitch period divided by the length of the pitch period for which the maximum RMS intensity occurs (another normalized RMS intensity measure).

The second value determined from the acoustic speech signal was the difference in RMS intensity per pitch period in adjacent pitch periods. This measured the variability of energy generated and was a rough estimate of shimmer, or amplitude perturbation (see also Baken, 1987, pp. 113ff). A difference value was calculated for each pair of adjacent pitch periods in the vowel segment. Three parameters based on this change measure were then calculated: (e) [mean (abs(RMSchange))], the mean of the absolute value of the difference in RMS intensity per pitch period in adjacent pitch periods; (f) [mean (RMSchange)], the mean of the total difference in RMS intensity per pitch period in adjacent pitch periods; and (g) [number of sign changes, RMSchange], the number of times RMSchange goes from a positive value to a negative value or vice versa.

The third measurement, pitch contour, was the duration of each pitch period (in samples) over the vowel segment of each isolated word. Two parameters were determined from this measurement: (h) [mean (pitch contour)], the average pitch for the vowel segment; and (i) [(duration of last pitch period—duration of first pitch period)/(average pitch)], a measure of the shape of the pitch contour.

The fourth value measured change in pitch duration from pitch period to pitch period and therefore provided an estimate of jitter (frequency perturbation). This was determined by measuring the difference in pitch duration between adjacent pitch periods. From this value, three paramaters were determined: (j) [mean (Pchange)], the average value of the difference in pitch duration in adjacent pitch periods; (k) [mean (abs (Pchange))], the average value of the absolute value of the difference in pitch duration in adjacent pitch periods; and (l) [number of sign changes, Pchange], the number of times Pchange goes from a positive value to a negative value or vice versa (cf. Hecker & Kreul's (1971) directional perturbation factor). The fifth value was another rough estimate of shimmer, as was the second value, but for this measurement, the RMS intensity over a pitch period was divided by (normalized by) the duration of that pitch period in samples. The value was calculated for each pitch period by calculating the total RMS intensity over each pitch period, dividing by the duration of that pitch period in samples, then calculating the difference in this number for adjacent pitch periods. Three parameters were derived from this measurement: (m) [mean (abs (NormRMSchange))], the mean of the absolute value of the difference in normalized RMS intensity per pitch period in adjacent pitch periods; (n) [mean (NormRMSchange)], the mean of the total difference in normalized RMS intensity per pitch period in adjacent pitch periods; and (o) [number of sign changes, NormRMSchange], the number of times that NormRM-Schange goes from a positive value to a negative value or vice versa.

Glottal waveform extraction was performed on the speech of two of the subjects in both conditions using an adaptation of Wong's closed-phase glottal inverse-filtering method (see Cummings & Clements, 1990, 1992, 1993, 1995; Wong, Markel, & Gray, 1979). Extracted glottal waveforms were marked into four segments: closed, opening, top, and closing. Statistical analysis was then performed for six parameters: closed duration, opening duration, top duration, closing duration, opening slope, and closing slope, and statistical comparisons were made between conditions.

7.25.2 Results

Preliminary results for two subjects were based on a comparison of means and standard deviations of the fifteen parameters for speech produced with and without alcohol for each talker. Identification of a parameter as a possible marker of intoxicated speech required observation of a trend for each speaker, as well as a significant difference in the mean and standard deviation. The following parameters revealed significant differences between the two conditions:

1. (a) *mean (RMS)*: the sober condition for both talkers was slightly lower on average and more clustered than in the intoxicated condidtion.
2. (i) *(duration of last pitch period—duration of first pitch period)/ (average pitch)*: the pitch contour in the sober condition was more flat on average than in the intoxicated condition.
3. (j) *mean (Pchange)*: the average value of the change in adjacent pitch period duration was lower on average and more clustered in the sober condition than in the intoxicated condition.
4. (k) *mean (abs (Pchange))*: the average value of the absolute value of the change in adjacent pitch period duration was lower on average and more clustered in the sober condition than in the intoxicated condition.
5. (l) *number of sign changes, P change*: there were more sign changes in the sober condition than in the intoxicated condition.
6. (n) *mean (NormRMSchange)*: change in normalized RMS intensity was slightly lower on average in the sober condition than in the intoxicated condition.
7. (o) *number of sign changes, NormRMSchange*: there were slightly fewer sign changes in the sober condition than in the intoxicated condition.

As these results indicate, the main differences between speech produced with and without alcohol were to be found in measurements of pitch-period-to-pitch-to-pitch-period variability, that is, jitter (parameters j–l) and shimmer, using normalized RMS intensity.

Preliminary results for the glottal waveform analysis showed similar global patterns for the waveforms from both conditions (i.e., both started as "fatter" pulses and both ended sinusoidally); such characteristics generally hold, however, for any utterance. On the other hand, local characteristics (on a per-waveform basis) did show a number of differences. First, glottal waveforms from speech in the nonalcohol condition showed more distinct beginnings and endings of glottal closure than those from speech produced with alcohol. Second, waveforms from speech produced with alcohol showed more ripple concentrated just during closure, whereas waveforms for speech produced without alcohol showed ripple affecting the entire glottal wave-shape. The ripple found in the alcohol waveforms is considered by some researchers to be a direct result of source-tract interaction. Finally, the entire system was less stationary for the waveforms produced under alcohol, showing more change from pitch period to pitch period than the waveforms from speech produced without alcohol. Similarly, it was possible to extract more of the waveforms from speech in the nonalcohol condition using a single inverse filter, indicating that both the vocal tract and the relationship between the vocal tract and glottal excitation were more stationary.

7.25.3 Discussion

The research conducted by Cummings et al. represents the use of digital speech files for analysis long after they were constructed and points out the usefulness of computer storage and analysis. As indicated in earlier studies (e.g., K. Johnson, et al., 1993; Künzel et al., 1992), perceptible changes occurring after consumption of alcohol are in part due to pitch-period-to-pitch-period variability, as shown by both the acoustic and the glottal waveform analyses.

7.26 SUMMARY

The research discussed in this chapter demonstrates a clear trend toward instrumental analysis of various types in studying the effects of alcohol on speech. For the most part, researchers have examined various "traditional" acoustic parameters to determine what may lie at the base of perceptible changes in speech and voice after consumption of alcohol. Other parameters appear to be amenable to laboratory-based, instrumental analysis, however, as exemplified by the studies by Eysholdt (stroboscopy) and by K. Johnson and his colleagues (EPG and EEG). The development of new techniques in the study of speech and voice will most assuredly reveal further ways in which the relationship between alcohol and speech can be investigated.

CHAPTER **8**

Case Study: The U.S. Tankship *Exxon Valdez* and Novel Scientific Evidence

8.0 INTRODUCTION

In this chapter, we discuss an application of speech analysis as a determinant of alcohol intoxication to a specific real-world situation, the grounding of the oil tanker *Exxon Valdez* in March 1989.

8.1 THE GROUNDING AND THE QUESTION OF ALCOHOL

Unless otherwise indicated, the summary in this section is based on the Marine Accident Report issued by the National Transportation Safety Board (NTSB) (National Transportation Safety Board, 1990). Discussion is confined to that of alcohol use by the captain of the Exxon Valdez.

At approximately 12:09 A.M. (all times given as Alaska Standard Time) on 24 March 1989, the U.S. tankship *Exxon Valdez*, a 987-foot (just over 300 m) oil tanker loaded with approximately 1,263,000 barrels (53,046,000 U.S. gallons or just over 200 million L) of North Slope crude oil, grounded on submerged rocks of Bligh Reef in Prince William Sound, near Valdez, Alaska (USA). The grounding caused the rupture of eight cargo tanks, resulting in the discharge of 258,000 barrels (10,836,000 U.S. gallons or just over 41 million L), the largest oil spill in U.S. history.

The master of the tanker at the time was Captain Joseph Hazelwood, who had been employed by Exxon Shipping Company or its predecessor company since 1968. At approximately 11:53 P.M. on 23 March 1989, Captain Hazelwood left the bridge of the *Exxon Valdez* and turned control of the vessel over to the third mate. Thus, when the ship actually ran aground, the third mate, rather than Captain Hazelwood, had actual bridge control.

At approximately 3:35 A.M. on 24 March, the *Exxon Valdez* was boarded by two investigators from the Coast Guard's Valdez Marine Safety Office. The investigators reported smelling alcohol on Hazelwood's breath when they met with him on the bridge, and when asked about this, Hazelwood told them that he had drunk two Moussy beers (0.05% alcohol) after returning to the ship from Valdez the evening before (at 8:24 P.M., according to the security log at the terminal gate). One investigator reported the smell of alcohol on Hazelwood's breath to the Commanding Officer of the Marine Safety Office, who telephoned an Alaska State police officer, requesting that he conduct alcohol testing at the vessel. The police officer arrived at the *Exxon Valdez* about 6:30 A.M., but did not have the necessary equipment to conduct testing or to collect samples for later testing. At about 10:00 A.M., it was ascertained by the Coast Guard officers that equipment for obtaining toxicological samples was on board, and urine samples were obtained from the third mate and the two able seamen (ABs) on watch at the time of the grounding. Although Captain Hazelwood was also asked to provide a urine sample, he said that he was unable to urinate at that time.

In the meantime, a Coast Guard health services technician was instructed at about 8:30 A.M. to go to the *Exxon Valdez* to take blood and urine samples. He boarded the vessel at about 10:30 A.M. and obtained both a blood sample and a urine sample from Captain Hazelwood. The third mate and two ABs also provided blood samples about this time, and because the urine sample provided earlier by the lookout AB was not sealed properly, a second sample was taken. Toxicological testing of the samples showed no ethanol in either the blood or the urine samples from the third mate and the two ABs. Hazelwood's blood sample (recorded as taken at 10:50 A.M., 24 March 1989) showed an ethanol concentration of 0.061%, while the urine sample showed an ethanol concentration of 0.094%. An independent analysis was performed on a portion of Hazelwood's sample and showed a blood-alcohol concentration (BAC) of 0.06% and a urine alcohol concentration of 0.1%.

The NTSB report contains testimony from witnesses who were in contact with Hazelwood and focuses on the question of whether or not Captain Hazelwood consumed alcohol during the hours preceding the grounding and whether or not he appeared intoxicated to the witnesses around the time of the grounding. The security logbook showed that Hazelwood, the chief engineer, and the radio electronics officer departed the terminal gate at 10:59 A.M. on 23 March to meet with the ship's agent in Valdez. After meeting for approximately 45 min the three crew members were picked up by the inbound pilot, who drove them to a restaurant where the four had lunch. According to the chief engineer, the lunch lasted about 1.5 hr. The chief engineer and the radio electronics officer testified that the pilot and Captain Hazelwood drank nonalcoholic beverages with their lunch, but Hazelwood told the Coast Guard investigating officer that he had had a beer.

After lunch, the pilot drove the three crew members to a shopping center, where the three separated. The owner of a gift store where Captain Hazelwood ordered flowers testified that Hazelwood did not appear to have been drinking. The three were to meet later at a bar, and the engineer testified that he arrived alone at about 4:00 P.M. and that Captain Hazelwood arrived about one-half hour later. However, Captain Hazelwood told the Coast Guard investigator that he arrived at about 3:00 P.M. The radio electronics officer testified that when he arrived at about 4:30, both Hazelwood and the chief engineer were already there. The radio electronics officer testified that each of the three purchased one or more rounds of drinks and said that he drank beer, the chief engineer gin and tonic, and Hazelwood a "clear" (National Transportation Safety Board, 1990, p. 29) beverage. The chief engineer testified to drinking three gin and tonics but did not recall how much Captain Hazelwood drank.

The chief engineer testified that the three left the bar about 7:00 P.M., going to a restaurant to order food to take back to the ship. While they waited for the food to be prepared, they went to an adjacent bar. The chief engineer and the radio electronics officer testified separately that each of the three had one drink during this time, and the radio electronics officer testified further that Captain Hazelwood had drunk vodka. The food was ready at approximately 7:30 P.M., and the three men took a cab back to the ship. The cab driver testified that none of the passengers appeared to be "under the influence of alcohol" (National Transportation Safety Board, 1990, p. 30). The security log at the terminal gate recorded the arrival of the cab at 8:24 P.M. Terminal security officers testified that all persons arriving in cabs were required to walk through a metal detector and that they did not believe any of the people arriving at that time were intoxicated.

The three crew members boarded the ship together, and the ship's agent met with Captain Hazelwood after his arrival. She testified that the captain did not appear intoxicated, although his eyes were watery. The outbound pilot testified that he smelled alcohol on Hazelwood's breath upon the latter's return to the ship, but that his impression was that "the master's behavior and speech were unimpaired" (National Transportation Safety Board, 1990, p. 30). According to the pilot, the captain left the bridge after the ship had gotten underway and did not return until called about 1.5 hr later, just before the pilot disembarked. The pilot testified that the captain returned to the bridge soon after the call and also that he again smelled alcohol on the captain's breath, but again that "the master's speech and behavior gave no indication of impairment" (National Transportation Safety Board, 1990, p. 30).

Two further considerations regarding Captain Hazelwood's use of alcohol are described in the NTSB report, although these considerations do not refer specifically to events transpiring on 23–24 March 1989. First, the president of Exxon Shipping Company testified that while on leave, Hazelwood had entered a hospital for treatment of an alcohol problem in April of 1985. Second, the NTSB investigated the captain's automobile driving record, which showed two convictions for driving while intoxicated, the first in 1985 (from an incident occurring in September 1984) and the second in 1988.

The possible involvement of alcohol in the grounding of the *Exxon Valdez* gained public attention as early as 26 March 1989, two days after the grounding, when the president of Exxon Shipping Company revealed Captain Hazelwood's alcohol treatment program in 1985 (C. Smith, 1992). Two days later, on 28 March 1989, the *Anchorage* (Alaska) *Daily News* and the *New York Times* both reported that Hazelwood's driver's license had been suspended three times for driving while intoxicated and was in fact currently under suspension (C. Smith, 1992). Characterizations of the incident in the press at the time notwithstanding, it needs to be emphasized that the grounding was never really a question of someone getting drunk and steering a ship onto a reef, like a drunk driver steering an automobile into a tree. It was acknowledged from the earliest that the third mate and helmsman were actually controlling the ship's movements, according, in part, to information provided by the lookout. Rather, the question regarding alcohol and the captain was one of impairment of judgment in leaving the bridge at the time he did and leaving navigational control to the third mate, as well as other decision-making issues after the ship ran aground.

8.2 SPEECH SAMPLES FROM THE CAPTAIN OF THE *EXXON VALDEZ*

In late 1989, the NTSB undertook analysis of audiotape recordings of radio transmissions from the bridge of the *Exxon Valdez* around the time of the grounding. As reported in Brenner and Cash (1991) and reviewed in section 7.14, a radio microphone on the bridge of the *Exxon Valdez* was contained in a handheld telephone-style transmitter using FM transmission. These transmissions were relayed by means of microwave towers in the vicinity to the United States Coast Guard Vessel Traffic Center (VTC) at Valdez,

Alaska, and recorded on a multichannel tape recorder (Magnasync Model 2-R/P-30). Forty-two statements by the captain of the *Exxon Valdez* were identified. In addition to performing its own analysis of the speech recorded on the tapes (see Brenner & Cash, 1991; National Transportation Safety Board, 1990), the NTSB elicited the assistance of two groups of researchers who had contributed to the scientific research literature on alcohol and speech. The first group was Dr. Mark B. Sobell and Dr. Linda C. Sobell, located at the Addiction Research Foundation (ARF) in Toronto, Ontario, Canada (see sections 6.5, 6.13). The second group of researchers consisted of Dr. Keith Johnson (a linguist and phonetician), Prof. David B. Pisoni (a psychologist and speech scientist), and Mr. Robert H. Bernacki (an audio electronics and biomedical systems engineer), located at the Speech Research Laboratory at Indiana University in Bloomington, Indiana, USA (see sections 7.1, 7.2, 7.6).

Along with cassette tapes of the radio transmissions, the NTSB also provided the consultants with typewritten transcripts of the 42 statements from the captain of the *Exxon Valdez*. The statements, as transcribed by the NTSB, formed part of the official report. The statements were grouped into five sets of transmissions, each identified by the approximate time relative to the grounding that they were recorded. The first set of statements (Statements 1–2) was recorded approximately 33 hr before the grounding (designated [–33] by Johnson et al., 1990, and Pisoni et al., 1991), or at about 3:00 P.M. on 22 March 1989, as the *Exxon Valdez* was inbound to Valdez, Alaska. The second set of statements (Statements 3–9) was recorded approximately 1 hr before the grounding (designated [–1] by K. Johnson et al., 1990, and Pisoni et al., 1991), or from approximately 11:25 to 11:31 P.M. on 23 March 1989, as the *Exxon Valdez* was outbound. In this set, the captain reported the disembarking of the State pilot and informed the Coast Guard Vessel Traffic Center (VTC) that the *Exxon Valdez* might cross over into the inbound lane because of ice in the outbound lane. The third set of statements (Statements 10–17) was recorded immediately after the grounding (designated [0] by K. Johnson et al., 1990, and Pisoni et al., 1991), or from approximately 12:27 to 12:38 A.M. on 24 March 1989. This set contained the initial report of the grounding by the captain to the VTC. The fourth set of statements (Statements 18–26) was recorded approximately 1 hr after the grounding (designated [+1] by K. Johnson et al., 1990, and Pisoni et al., 1991), or from approximately 1:07 to 1:31 A.M. on 24 March 1989. In this set, the captain informed the VTC that he was attempting to work the tanker off the reef. Finally, the fifth set of statements (Statements 27–42) was recorded approximately 9 hr after the grounding (designated [+9] by K. Johnson et al., 1990, and Pisoni et al., 1991), or from approximately 9:12 to 9:38 A.M. on 24 March 1989. In this set, the captain discussed salvage of the cargo, including directions to other tankers on their approach to the *Exxon Valdez.*

The text of the NTSB report proper described the analysis by the NTSB acoustics laboratory, as well as summaries of the analyses performed by the Addiction Research Foundation (ARF) and Indiana University (IU) groups. Appendix J to the NTSB report contained the NTSB- produced transcription of the radio transmissions and the full reports from the outside consultants at the ARF and at IU. The full report from the researchers at IU was published in the journal *Phonetica* as K. Johnson et al. (1990).

The primary motivation for conducting the analyses of the captain's speech was to fulfill the NTSB's responsibility, as mandated by the Transportation Safety Act of 1974, "to assess and reassess techniques and methods of accident investigation" (88 Stat. 2168, 49 U.S.C. 1903). The evidence regarding the possibility of intoxication was of three types: (a) testimony of eyewitnesses, (b) toxicology results, and (c) speech analyses. Of these three, the discussion of the speech analyses is the longest and most detailed. One reason for this may have been the relative novelty of this type of analysis.

The NTSB report discussed four main effects of alcohol on speech: (a) slowed speech, (b) speech errors, (c) misarticulation of difficult sounds, and (d) changes in vocal quality. The NTSB's own analysis investigated speaking rate for 36 of the 42 statements by the captain. Excluded from analysis were relatively short statements such as "Very well" (Statement 39). Details of this analysis can be found in Brenner and Cash (1991), which is discussed in section 7.14. There were statistically significant differences among the five different intervals, and contrast tests showed that the captain's speech approximately 45 min before the grounding was significantly slower (as measured in syllables per second) than both 33 hr before and 9 hr after the grounding. This change in speaking rate was confirmed by the IU group's duration measurements of the phrase "*Exxon Valdez*" at each of the five intervals. Durations for this phrase were 706 ms at the [−33] interval, 934 ms at [−1], 1087 ms at [0], 980 ms at [+1], and 883 ms at [+9].

Speech errors, the second type of effect, were noted only during the [−1] interval. Because the true linguistic intent of the talker (the captain) was unknown, this category was limited to those errors that were immediately corrected by the talker himself. Four obvious errors were noted in the NTSB report (cf. the "gross effects" noted by K. Johnson et al., 1990, discussed in section 7.9.2.1):

Statement 3:   "*Exxon Ba* ah *Valdez*"

Statement 4:   "We've ah departed the pilot or disembarked the pilot. Excuse me."

Statement 5:   "by our radar, I we'll probably"

Statement 9:   "ice out of Columbia Gla . . . Bay"

The third category, misarticulation of difficult sounds, was based on findings from the researchers at IU, who referred to them as segmental effects (K. Johnson et al., 1990). Their analysis was based on a combination of phonetic transcription (auditory analysis) and acoustic measurements. Examples of misarticulations included (a) errors in the production of [l] and [r], (b) devoicing of the final segment in the word *Valdez*, (3) misarticulation of [s] as [ʃ] in the word *Exxon*.

The fourth category of speech effects examined by the NTSB was called "vocal quality changes," although this use of "vocal quality" differed somewhat from that in the voice literature. In the clinical-scientific literature, this term refers to, for example, "the perception of the physical complexity of the laryngeal tone modified by cavity resonation" (Aronson, 1990, p. 5); Colton and Casper (1990) enumerate a number of attributes of pathological voice quality: hoarseness and roughness, breathiness, tension, tremor, strain/struggle behavior, sudden interruption of voicing, and diplophonia (pp. 17–18).

The use of the term *vocal quality* in the NTSB report appears to be based on its use by the researchers at the ARF, whose assessment of the tapes appears as part of Appendix J to the NTSB report. Important changes in vocal quality noted by these researchers included word interjections, broken words (e.g., the speech errors in Statements 3 and 9 noted above), incomplete phrases, corrected errors (e.g., the speech errors in Statements 4 and 5 noted above), and increases in speaking time (cf. the first category, or speaking rate, discussed above) and hesitations.

The ARF researchers noted "dramatic vocal quality changes" over the course of the tapes. Statements made at the [−33] interval appeared "rapid, fluent, without hesitation, and with few word interjections (i.e. ah) in relation to the length of the sample" (National Transportation Safety Board, 1990, p. 224). In the transmissions made at the [−1] interval, however, they noted "a marked difference in the vocal sample which we evaluate as having characteristics of a speech sample recorded under the influence of ethanol" (National Transportation Safety Board, 1990, p. 224). They suggested that the apparent degree of impairment was so great that crew members in contact with the captain should have been able to notice the changes. A second change took place commencing at the [+9] interval, when the captain sounded "more fluent (more rapid speech, more responsive) and makes fewer word interjections (ahs)" (National Transportation Safety Board, 1990, p. 225).

The report from the ARF researchers served as an outline of the types of analyses that needed to be conducted in order to address the question of the captain's intoxication, although the researchers themselves did not attempt all of them. They pointed out that the published research generally evaluated alcohol effects on speech in two ways, either by human perceptual judgments or by acoustic analysis. They noted that some phrases (e.g., "thirteen and sixteen") were repeated in the relevant audiotapes and that these would be appropriate for acoustic analysis (which, in fact, was subsequently undertaken by the IU researchers). The ARF researchers considered an alternative explanation for these speech changes under which these could be attributed to either fatigue or stress and anticipated the observation later stated explicitly by K. Johnson et al. (1990) that speech changes occurring at the [-1] interval could certainly not be attributed to grounding-induced stress, because these changes occurred in Captain Hazelwood's speech before the grounding. They suggested that other contextual errors, aside from the corrected ones, might be present in the transmissions. The NTSB report subsequently noted that the captain's description of the grounding site ("north of Goose Island off Bligh Reef") was inaccurate. Finally, they observed that there probably existed no "perfect measures," but rather that conclusions could be based on a "convergence of indicators," including human perceptual judgments, acoustic analyses, and the presence of errors in behavior and judgment (National Transportation Safety Board, 1990, pp. 225–226).

8.3 SPEECH ANALYSIS IN THE LEGAL SETTING

8.3.1 *Alaska v. Hazelwood* and the U.S. Coast Guard Hearing

The Executive Summary of the NTSB report stated the probable cause of the grounding as follows (National Transportation Safety Board, 1990, p. v):

> The National Transportation Safety Board determines that the probable cause of the grounding of the EXXON VALDEZ was the failure of the third mate to properly maneuver the vessel because of fatigue and excessive workload; the failure of the master to provide a proper navigation watch because of impairment from alcohol; the failure of Exxon Shipping Company to provide a fit master and a rested and sufficient crew for the EXXON VALDEZ; the lack of an effective Vessel Traffic Service because of inadequate equipment and manning levels, inadequate personnel training, and deficient management oversight; and the lack of effective pilotage services.

In a broad sense, then, the NTSB found that alcohol had contributed to the grounding, but this factor was only one of many. The determination that the captain was impaired by alcohol was based on both toxicological and speech evidence, the testimony of eyewitnesses notwithstanding. Furthermore, although blood and urine samples were collected, this was done only after approximately 10 hr subsequent to the grounding; determination of the captain's BAC at the actual time of the grounding could be made only by retrograde extrapolation, at best a controversial procedure (see Dubowski, 1985, and section 2.2.5). The audio recordings of the radio transmissions from the bridge thus constituted the sole physical evidence available from near the time of the grounding.

Captain Hazelwood faced a number of administrative, civil, and criminal challenges subsequent to the grounding. First, when the results of the toxicological analysis were released by the NTSB on 30 March 1989, Hazelwood was dismissed by Exxon Shipping. Second, Hazelwood was charged by the State of Alaska with three misdemeanors (reckless endangerment, operating a vessel while intoxicated, negligent discharge of oil) and one felony (criminal mischief); this criminal trial ran from 5 February through 23 March of 1990. Third, the U.S. Coast Guard held hearings in late July 1990 to determine whether Hazelwood's captain's license should be revoked. Fourth, a large number of fishermen, property owners, and Alaska natives filed a civil lawsuit against Hazelwood and the Exxon Corporation, maintaining that they were liable for the grounding, for the resulting spill, and for subsequent losses suffered. This case was heard during the summer of 1994 in U.S. District Court in Anchorage, Alaska.

Although the NTSB determined that the captain was impaired from alcohol at the time of the grounding, and although this finding was based to a large extent on analysis of the speech record, nevertheless, the findings of the NTSB did not carry the force of law and in fact could not be used in court cases. This statutorily imposed limitation on the use of the NTSB findings would have been irrelevant to the criminal case against Captain Hazelwood, as the NTSB report did not appear until July 1990 (although the report from the ARF researchers was dated 13 November 1989 and that of the IU researchers, 10 May 1990), while the Alaska criminal case ran from 5 February to 23 March 1990.

At some point, however, both prosecutors and defense counsel in the Alaska case were aware of the IU analyses. The *New York Times* reported on 25 February 1990 ("A Question Recurs," 1990) that Brent Cole, an assistant district attorney, had proposed bringing in the researchers from the ARF and IU. Bishop (1990) reported that Mary Anne Henry, an assistant district attorney in Anchorage, stated that the prosecution had become aware of this research only after the trial was underway and had decided against introducing the findings as evidence because of the strategic factors involved in interrupting the trial with an evidentiary hearing. She was quoted as saying, however, "But if we had known it sooner, we would have" (Bishop, 1990, p. B6). Defense counsel was also aware of the acoustical analysis being conducted at IU; Michael G. Chalos, an attorney representing Captain Hazelwood, was quoted as referring to the speech-analysis techniques as "voodoo stuff" and was further quoted as saying "It's never been introduced as evidence. It's not even in the experimental stage; it's in the exploratory stage, which is even less. It's not accepted" (Bishop, 1990, p. B6). In reply, Prof. David B. Pisoni, one of the IU researchers, said "We have models of how speech functions, and this is the leading edge. The legal community is reluctant to embrace scientific data" (Bishop, 1990, p. B6).

The question of alcohol intoxication hinged on two types of evidence: the toxicological results and the testimony of witnesses. As mentioned above, the toxicological analysis of the body fluid samples showed ethanol concentrations of .061% in the blood and .094% in the urine. Establishing alcohol levels at the time of the grounding had to be done by retrograde extrapolation, which one prosecution expert witness did, testifying that the captain's BAC would have been about .14% at the time of the grounding ("Valdez Jurors Face Basic Questions," 1990). Understandably, the defense questioned the use of retrograde extrapolation. In all, 21 witnesses testified that Hazelwood had shown no visible signs of alcohol impairment the night preceding the grounding. In March, then, Hazelwood was convicted of one of the misdemeanor charges, negligent discharge of oil; he was acquitted on the one felony charge and on the remaining two misdemeanor charges.

The U.S. Coast Guard scheduled master's license revocation hearings for late July of 1990. Hazelwood faced four specific charges: consuming alcohol within 4 hr of taking command of the *Exxon Valdez,* operating the vessel with a BAC exceeding 0.04%, turning control of the vessel over to an unqualified crew member, and negligence in leaving the bridge of the vessel. At the hearing before an Administrative Law judge on 25 July 1990, Hazelwood pleaded no contest to the misconduct charge of consuming alcohol within 4 hr of taking command and the negligence charge for departing the bridge. The Coast Guard, in turn, dismissed the charges of operating the vessel with a BAC exceeding 0.04% and of negligence in relinquishing control of the tanker to the improperly licensed third mate. Hazelwood's license was revoked for 12 months, with 3 months' credit.

8.3.2 Tanford, Pisoni, and Johnson (1991)

Between the end of the U.S. Coast Guard hearings in July of 1990 and the start of the civil lawsuit in May 1994, the NTSB issued its ruling and recommendations. Additionally, two articles appeared in the literature regarding the speech analyses done at the ARF and IU. The first article, Tanford et al. (1991), was written by a law professor at Indiana University (Tanford) and two of the researchers who had performed the speech analyses for the NTSB (Pisoni and Johnson). The second article, Hollien (1993), was written by Prof. Harry Hollien of the Institute for Advanced Study of the Communication Processes at the University of Florida, in Gainesville, Florida.

Tanford et al. (1991) appeared in the *Journal of Criminal Law and Criminology,* a legal journal edited at the Northwestern University School of Law (Evanston, Illinois). The article addressed both the general question of the admissibility of novel scientific evidence in courts of law and the specific question of the admissibility in court of the speech analyses conducted in the *Exxon Valdez* matter. The first part of the article was a summary of the results of the analyses conducted by the IU researchers for the NTSB. These results are reported in K. Johnson et al. (1990), National Transportation Safety Board (1990), and Pisoni et al. (1991) and are discussed in section 7.7.

The second section of the article discussed the legal standard for admitting novel scientific evidence. At issue here was the procedural rule, announced in *Frye v. United States*, 293 F. 1013 (D.C. Cir. 1923), which established the "general acceptance" test as the standard for admissibility of scientific evidence. Under the *Frye* test, scientific evidence is presumed to be excluded from the courtroom, until it has gained general acceptance in relevant fields. Two general criticisms of the *Frye* standard have been that: (a) it excludes scientific theories that, although not yet meeting the general acceptance principle, are nonetheless credible, and (b) that it allows courts unnecessarily wide latitude in rendering decisions simply according to how they determine what the relevant scientific fields are. Tanford et al. discussed the *Frye* standard in terms of three basic criticisms: that is, that the *Frye* test is (a) bad science, (b) bad law, and (c) premised on bad psychology.

Tanford et al. noted that the *Frye* test was designed to help courts separate scientifically reliable evidence from "quackery" but also called "dubious" the assumption that general acceptance of a procedure is synonymous with scientific accuracy. They noted that widespread use of a procedure conveys an appearance of general acceptance without addressing the basic question of whether the procedure is scientifically reliable. Conversely, reliable scientific procedures might not yet have found general acceptance, so that *Frye* induces a "cultural lag" problem.

Second, Tanford et al. argued that *Frye* is bad law, because "its terms are vague and ambiguous, and judges have difficulty applying it to novel scientific evidence" (p. 593). The major difficulty lies in defining the relevant scientific field; a court might define it either too broadly or two narrowly. In the former case, Tanford et al. cited *People v. King*, 266 Cal. App. 2d 437; 72 Cal. Rptr. 478 (1968), which involved the admissibility of spectrographic evidence in voice identification. The relevant field was defined by the judge as encompassing anatomy, physiology, physics, psychology, and linguistics. The analysis results were excluded because general acceptance within all of these disciplines could not be proven. On the other hand, in *People v. Williams*, 164 Cal. App. 2d Supp. 858; 331 P.2d 251 (Cal. App. Dep't Super. Ct. 1958), which involved a controversial test for detecting narcotics use, the relevant field was defined as "those who would be expected to be familiar with its use." Test results were therefore admitted, although the evidence indicated that the general population of medical professionals was completely unfamiliar with the procedure.

Tanford et al. further argued that *Frye* is bad law because it does not set forth specific foundation requirements. Specific points include a lack of restrictions on who may be called as a witness; lack of specificity regarding whether a single witness can establish general acceptance; lack of specificity regarding whether general acceptance can be a matter merely of expert opinion or whether a minimal level of conditional fact is required. Further, they argued, *Frye* requires that some "thing" have gained general acceptance but does not further define that thing, leaving open the question of whether general acceptance applies to a theory, a technology, a procedure or technique, an instrument, or some combination of these. In general, Tanford et al. argued, the *Frye* test places a burden of decision regarding the admissibility of scientific evidence on judges who are ill equipped to make that decision because of their lack of scientific training.

Third, Tanford et al. argued that the premise in *Frye* that jurors would be overawed by expert testimony is dubious. They cited studies in social psychology finding that "people generally *undervalue* scientific data, misunderstand and under-utilize statistics, rely on anecdotes and emotion rather than empirical scientific evidence when making important decisions, and persistently hold beliefs contrary to scientific logic and mathematics" (Tanford et al. 1991, p. 596).

In a third section, Tanford et al. considered alternative legal standards to the *Frye* test; these would either modify *Frye* or replace it with a relevancy test. Suggested modifications have included (a) substituting substantial acceptance or reasonable acceptance for general acceptance, although Tanford et al. argued that these would still be ambiguous and would still fail to distinguish reliable from unreliable new techniques; (b) modifying the definition of *field* to include acceptance within a narrow specialty, although again Tanford et al. argued that this would still fail to address the question of reliability; and (c) modifying the requirement of general acceptance of a technique to general acceptance of the underlying scientific principles.

Tanford et al. noted, however, that the trend has been toward replacing *Frye* rather than modifying it. Specifically, legal scholars have advocated replacing the general acceptance principle with one of basic relevancy. Advocates of this type of test have suggested five criteria for the admission of scientific evidence: First, the evidence should be introduced by a qualified expert. Qualification could be by "knowledge, skill, experience, training, or education" (Federal Rules of Evidence 702), but Tanford et al. noted that in some instances (e.g., the Hazelwood case), a fully educated scientist might be required. Second, the expert testimony must assist the jury. This might seem obvious, but it goes to the question of whether or not the jury is presumed competent to draw its own conclusions. In some jurisdictions, scientific evidence has been presumed to be inadmissible and would be permitted only if the material was "completely beyond the understanding and common experience of the average juror" (Tanford et al. 1991, p. 599). The more contemporary view is that of "presumptive admissibility," which allows such evidence if the jury can be assisted in comprehending the evidence or drawing conclusions.

The third criterion is that any equipment used be in good working order. This includes both instrumentation and human operators (e.g., laboratory personnel). The fourth criterion is that the scientific evidence must be relevant under basic relevancy rules (e.g., it will assist the jury in its determination of facts, as under Federal Rules of Evidence 401–402) and must be reliable. Tanford et al. cited Gianelli (1980), who argued for a three-part test of reliability: (a) the scientific community must consider the underlying principles to be valid; (b) the application of the principle must be scientifically reliable; and (c) the technique must have been properly applied in the particular case. The standard created by a relevancy test is one of presumptive admissibility, and such evidence would be excluded only if it was not supported and if it would not actually assist the jury. Finally, the fifth criterion is that the probative value of the scientific evidence must outweigh its potential prejudicial effect; juries must not be misled by an exaggerated sense of scientific infallibility.

Tanford et al. next considered the admissibility of acoustic-phonetic evidence in the *Exxon Valdez* case. They conceded that the analyses conducted at IU would probably not be admissible under the *Frye* test, because the particular application had not gained general acceptance in the scientific community. It would also probably be inadmissible under two *Frye* test modifications: those (1) establishing a criterion of substantial acceptance and (2) specifying a narrow field test. However, under a relevancy test such as the five-part one discussed above, the acoustic-phonetic evidence might be admissible.

First, Tanford et al. suggested that the type of scientific evidence under discussion here would have to be introduced by an expert witness, specifically a researcher in the field of speech science. Qualifications within this field would include a graduate degree in an underlying discipline (e.g., linguistics, psychology, speech and hearing science, electrical engineering), training or experience in speech science, affiliation with a speech science laboratory in either an academic or an industrial setting, membership in the Acoustical Society of America, and familiarity with the alcohol and speech literature. Second, the introduction of this type of expert testimony would assist the jury in providing nonredundant information. That is, in addition to the auditory observations regarding speech produced under alcohol that would be shared by both expert and jury, the expert could provide further information regarding instrumental measures of such parameters as pitch, duration, and amplitude. Third, and this addressed the *Exxon Valdez* case directly, Tanford et al. were satisfied that the relevant equipment was in good working order. Tanford et al. noted that the acoustic-phonetic analysis depended not on absolute measurements, but rather relative ones, that is, comparisons of measurements across speech samples obtained at different times. Thus, if the same recording and playback equipment was used for both comparison samples, equipment irregularities should appear equally on both control and test recordings. Possible instrument-specific fluctuations were dealt with by comparing tape-to-tape samples of the speech of the Coast Guard radio operator and of background noise. In the laboratory, independent multiple measurements were made, and no errors were found.

Fourth, Tanford et al. argued that the acoustic-phonetic evidence could withstand the tests of scientific reliability and relevance. They noted that both the underlying principles of speech science (particularly acoustic-phonetic analysis) and the effects of alcohol on motor function (specifically speech motor control) were scientifically valid and uncontroversial (citing, e.g., Borden & Harris, 1984, for speech science, and Berry & Pentreath, 1980, for alcohol effects). The publication of some of the research on alcohol and speech in peer-reviewed scientific journals was also cited as evidence of the validity of this approach, as was also the lack of any published literature inconsistent with the published findings. Tanford et al. further noted that the general acoustic-phonetic techniques employed in this analysis enjoyed widespread use throughout the various disciplines comprising speech science, and that previous research had proven to be reliable and valid measures. Additionally, they noted that a number of controlled laboratory studies had established acoustic changes as reliable measurements of changes in speech induced by alcohol.

Finally, Tanford et al. argued that because the scientific evidence was reliable, there should be little danger that its prejudicial effect would outweigh its probative value. Important was the uniqueness of the acoustic-phonetic evidence to the central question of intoxication; the results of the acoustic-phonetic analyses constituted the only unbiased physical evidence available. Furthermore, there was little danger of misleading the jury by an aura of infallibility, since this type of analysis would be unfamiliar to most of the public.

Tanford et al. thus concluded that the scientific evidence of intoxication in the *Exxon Valdez* case was sound and reliable, and that furthermore, such evidence should be admissible under new relevancy tests for scientific evidence.

8.3.3 Hollien, 1993

A decidedly different point of view from that taken by Tanford et al. appeared in Harry Hollien's "An oilspill, alcohol and the captain: A possible misapplication of forensic science," published in 1993 in *Forensic Science*

International. In this article, Hollien considered the possibility that the research conducted by the NTSB and its ARF and IU consultants (see section 8.2) was a misapplication of scientific procedures to the forensic question of intoxication.

Hollien cited the following studies as constituting essentially the whole body of research on the relationship between intoxication and speech: Andrews et al. (1977), Beam et al. (1978), Dunker and Schlosshauer (1964), Hollien (1985), Klingholz et al. (1988), Künzel (1990), Lester and Skousen (1974), Natale et al. (1980), Pisoni et al. (1986), Pisoni and Martin (1989), Sobell and Sobell (1972), Sobell et al. (1982), and Trojan and Kryspin-Exner (1968). Hollien's general characterization of these articles was that "most are sharply limited in scope" (1993, p. 98). More specifically, though, he also mentioned a high degree of variability in the studies, much of it in experimental designs. He indicated that "few, if any investigators have controlled for drinking habits, or studied increasing vs. decreasing BAL, or investigated the effects of effort, or employed blind controls or contrasted intoxication with other physiological/psychological states" (Hollien, 1993, p. 99). Additionally, he suggested that changes in speech due to other factors (e.g., stress and fatigue) were another confounding dimension. Finally, he cited the additonal complicating factor of apparent improvement in speech measures at low alcohol levels. He cited findings from Hollien (1985) and Künzel (1990) indicating increased "speaking precision" at "low levels of intoxication." Hollien (1985) showed an increase in "speech precision" at about the 0.02% level, which was based on "informal speech measures" (Hollien, 1993, p. 100). Künzel (1990; discussed in section 7.11) included measurements of pauses and speaking rate. At 0.04 and 0.08% maximum breath-alcohol concentrations (BrACs), subjects showed a decrease in the number of speech pauses from the nonalcohol measurement, and at 0.04% increased the number of syllables produced per second.

Hollien reported that the NTSB researchers performed two studies of Hazelwood's speech, limiting their measurements to syllable rate. In the first study, the researchers compared syllable rate measurements across the five time intervals and found a decrease of approximately 40% from the first recording to the one made immediately after the grounding. Hollien argued that slow speaking rates could also be observed during the television interviews in March and August 1990; however, this observation was, according to Hollien, "subjective" (1993, p. 101). The second set of measurements by the NTSB researchers compared Hazelwood's speaking rate to that of four other personnel recording around the same time; speaking rates for all five were about the same in the first and last recordings, but Hazelwood's speech was slower in the middle, around the time of the grounding. Hollien cited as major problems the limited scope of analysis, the lack of control samples, and the lack of comparison with other emotional and physical states. According to Hollien, the approach used by the ARF researchers "while subjective, can be fairly robust if applied properly" (1993, p. 101). Hollien further observed that "their efforts suffered scientifically and the conclusions they drew appear deficient" (1993, p. 101), although he provided no specific objective criticisms.

Hollien described the techniques used by the IU researchers as "fairly sophisticated" (1993, p. 101), but he did have reservations about the conclusions. First, Hollien noted that the IU researchers reviewed research on the effects of other physical and emotional states on speech in light of their own analysis. Hollien argued that methods and data used in these previous studies varied too widely and thus could not be used for comparison with the present case but provided no specifics. Hollien's main criticism of the use of recording-interval comparisons was that the analyses focused on a very small sample (the phrases "*Exxon Valdez*" and "thirteen and sixteen") of the available speech data. Hollien took further issue with the IU researchers' assumption that low vocal jitter correlated with high stress (National Transportation Safety Board, 1990, p. 249); specifically, Hollien questioned both the experimental and the logical bases for this assumption (the IU researchers cited Brenner, Shipp, Doherty, & Morrissey, 1985, in regard to lower jitter measurements in emergency situations). Finally, Hollien cited the following concessions by the IU researchers: first, they conceded that there were "gaps in the previous research." Second, they also conceded a "lack of breadth and depth of existing knowledge," and third, they acknowledged the "limitations in the type and quality of the measurements" (National Transportation Safety Board, 1990, p. 251–252).

Hollien stressed that his discussion centered not on the question of intoxication in Hazelwood's case, but rather on the question of determining intoxication directly (and solely) from acoustic-phonetic measurements of the speech signal. That is, at issue here was whether or not the scientific evidence bore out the conclusions drawn by the research groups associated with the NTSB investigation. In general, Hollien believed it "hazardous" to determine intoxication from speech and voice analysis alone, due to the variation of specific parameters and possible attribution of changes to other causes. Specific criticisms raised by Hollien regarding the researchers' determination of intoxication were: (a) overestimation of the strength of support of previous research on alcohol and speech, especially in cases outside of the laboratory, that is, under field conditions; (b) the assumption that it was unnecessary to use controlled speech samples for comparison; (c) failure to consider more fully other physical or emotional states as possible causes or to obtain information pertinent to these; (d) reliance on "subjective impressions, very limited analysis and/or extensive analyses of very brief text-dependent samples"(i.e., in the ARF, NTSB staff, and IU analysis, respectively; Hollien, 1993, p. 103).

In the end, Hollien concluded that the speech and voice data did not support the findings of the NTSB and its consultants that Hazelwood was intoxicated around the time of the grounding. Although Hollien had no substantial disagreement with the actual analysis procedures employed nor did he find any suggestion of ethical impropriety, he did consider the evidence to have been misinterpreted and the conclusions drawn to have been unsubstantiated.

8.3.4 Hollien versus Tanford et al.

Consideration of Tanford et al. (1991) and Hollien (1993) reveals the widely divergent conclusions that can be drawn from pretty much the same set of data and acoustic analyses. As Hollien said, the issue here was not generally whether or not Hazelwood was intoxicated, but rather specifically whether or not the speech samples and acoustic-phonetic measurements could be used to make this determination. Hollien believed that the data did not support the conclusions drawn by the three research groups or the findings of the NTSB. In fact, these conclusions and findings contradicted the testimony of eyewitnesses, as well as Hazelwood's eventual acquittal on charges of operating a vessel while intoxicated. Still, a question that should be addressed is whether Tanford et al. and Hollien were completely at odds in regard to this evidence or this type of evidence in determining intoxication.

It was Hollien's opinion "that determination of inebriation solely from analysis of a person's speech and voice seems hazardous" (1993, p. 102), and that this indeterminacy was due to wide variability in speech cues (e.g., speaking rate, misarticulation, lowered FØ) and because of "confusion" with other physical states. It should not be concluded, however, that Hollien believed the entire enterprise of alcohol and speech research to be hopelessly futile. Nor should we conclude that he believed that no generalizations would ever be discovered. First, Hollien believed, with Klingholz et al. (1988) that at least some of the variability (or even outright inconsistency) was attributable to differences or deficiencies in research design. Klingholz et al. (1988) cited four methodological deficiencies in earlier experimental studies of alcohol: (a) lack of objective BAC measurement, (b) BACs that were so high that intoxication was obvious and acoustic analysis therefore superfluous, (c) small numbers of subjects, and (d) solely qualitative acoustic analyses. To these, Hollien added (e) lack of control for drinking habits, (f) lack of consideration of increasing versus decreasing BACs, (g) lack of study of the effects of effort, (h) lack of employment of blind controls, and (i) lack of contrast of intoxication with other physiological and psychological states. These methodological deficiencies, however, should not be fatal to the claim that alcohol produces consistent effects on speech nor to the conception of a research program investigating these effects. As Hollien noted in a number of places, the analysis techniques employed by the three research groups in the *Exxon Valdez* case were all well-established, scientifically sound ones. Note that of the above criticisms, only one (the last cited by Klingholz et al.) is directed toward speech and voice analysis itself.

Second, although the research program on alcohol and speech conducted at the University of Florida and headed by Hollien (discussed in section 7.24) has addressed a number of the methodological problems cited above and adjusted procedures accordingly, the analyses themselves are, in fact, highly similar or in some cases even identical to those conducted in previous research. Thus, of the three presentations mentioned in section 7.24, one examined procedural concerns and perception tasks (Hollien & Martin, 1995); a second fundamental frequency and articulation changes (Alderman et al., 1995); and a third speaking rate for both a reading passage and a diadochokinetic task (DeJong et al., 1995). Perception experiments of various types have been conducted by Andrews et al. (1977), Pisoni et al. (1986), Klingholz et al. (1988), Pisoni and Martin (1989), and Künzel et al. (1992). Fundamental frequency (including changes and variability measures) has been examined in a number of studies, including Pisoni et al. (1985), Klingholz et al. (1988), Behne and Rivera (1990), Künzel et al. (1992), and Watanabe et al. (1994). Changes in articulation and speaking rates have been examined in a large number of studies. Considering the speech measures broadly, the use of these analysis techniques indicates that recent researchers have not completely abrogated the speech parameters and speech-scientific analyses used in previous research, even among those critical of previous research (and specifically the investigations undertaken in the matter of the *Exxon Valdez*).

Neither the published scientific literature nor the state of current research can thus be construed to indict speech science in general or acoustic-phonetic analysis in particular as an unreasonable way to approach the study of the effects of alcohol on speech. Examination of these research procedures had remained outside the legal area in the 1990 Alaska criminal trial involving Hazelwood, and as the discussion was effectively limited to academic journals, the question of the scientific validity of these types of analyses remained essentially an academic one. In 1993, however, the discussion entered the legal realm, when it was proposed that Prof. David Pisoni, of the Indiana University research group, provide expert testimony in an upcoming civil suit involving thousands of individuals as plaintiffs and Joseph Hazelwood, Exxon Corporation, and Exxon Shipping Company as defendants. This trial would not be heard in a state court, however, but rather in the United States District Court for the District of Alaska. This meant that the *Frye* test would be irrelevant as concerned the admissibility of novel scientific evidence; instead, the Federal Rules of Evidence and liberalized United States Supreme

Court standards set forth in *Daubert v. Merrell Dow Pharmaceuticals, Inc.,* 113 S.Ct. 2786 (1993), would be applicable.

8.3.5 The Acoustic Analyses under *Daubert*

The effect of *Frye* was to exclude novel scientific evidence from the courtroom, except when it could be shown that the technique or procedure in question had gained "general acceptance." Tanford et al. (1991) proposed that this relatively restrictive procedural rule be replaced by basic tests of scientific reliability and scientific relevance. The federal standard, as interpreted by the U.S. Supreme Court in *Daubert,* contained two such prongs. The reliability prong required that the expert's testimony be "scientific knowledge," that is, grounded in the methods and procedures of science. Further, the proposed testimony had to be supported by appropriate validation, and inferences or assertions had to be derived by a scientific method. Testimony, even by an expert, would be deemed unreliable if based on "guesswork, speculation, and conjecture" (see *Joy v. Bell Helicopter Textron, Inc.,* 999 F.2d 549 [D.C. Cir. 1993]). In assessing whether the principles underlying proposed testimony are scientifically valid, courts should consider a number of factors, including (a) whether the scientific theory has been or can be tested, (b) whether the scientific theory has been subjected to peer review and publication (although publication alone should not be the sine qua non of admissibility), (c) the known or potential error rate of the scientific technique, and (d) whether the underlying theory has received general acceptance in the scientific community (as under *Frye*).

The standard of relevance for admission of novel scientific evidence requires proper application of the proposed scientific reasoning or methodology to the facts at issue; that is, a valid scientific connection must exist to the instant inquiry. Testimony by an expert not related to any issue in the case fails this relevancy test and is thus inadmissible. In this regard, see *Flanagan v. State,* 625 So.2d 827 (Fla. 1993), in which the court said, "The courtroom is not a classroom to be used to educate the jury on an entire field only tangentially related to the issues at trial." At base of the relevancy standard is the principle that the proposed evidence must assist the trier of fact, a process described by the U.S. Supreme Court as one of "fit."

Plaintiffs in the civil trial heard in 1994 were approximately 10,000 fishermen, property owners, and Alaska natives who sought US$1.5 billion (1.5×10^9) in compensation and up to 10 times that amount in punitive damages ("Skipper Says Exxon Knew," 1994). Defendants in the trial were Joseph Hazelwood, Exxon Corporation, and Exxon Shipping Company. Immediately before the trial began, in March 1994, the defendants filed a motion *in limine,* seeking to exclude the expert report (i.e., the report from the IU researchers to the NTSB) and testimony of the plaintiffs' proposed witness, Prof. David Pisoni. The defendants proposed that such evidence was inadmissible under the standards established in *Daubert*, as well as under Rules 702, 703, and 403 of the Federal Rules of Evidence.

In their motion, the defendants contended that both plaintiffs and Prof. Pisoni claimed that the determination of intoxication by voice analysis was a reliable scientific technique despite the facts that: (a) no scientist other than Pisoni had claimed this technique to be reliable; (b) the technique had never been admitted in court before; (c) Pisoni himself had stated that the technique was inconclusive; and (d) Pisoni had deliberately withheld nonsupporting and contradictory evidence. The defendants further asserted that Prof. Pisoni had conceded either in the report to the NTSB or in deposition that (a) there was insufficient prior research into the effects of alcohol on speech; (b) other factors (e.g., fatigue) could have caused the observed speech changes; (c) the potential rate of error was not known; (d) the crudeness and poor quality of the recordings made proper laboratory analysis impossible; (e) nonsupporting or contradictory data were neither discussed nor disclosed; and (f) none of the equipment in Alaska had been inspected. The defendants further suggested that the prosecution had attempted to introduce Prof. Pisoni's findings as evidence during the Alaska criminal trial of Joseph Hazelwood in 1990, but that such evidence had been excluded after the presentation of reports and affidavits from a number of acoustic and phonetics experts. These included Louis J. Gerstman, Peter Ladefoged, and Edward Seidlick.

The defendants thus objected, "because of these numerous indicia of unreliability and untrustworthiness," to the introduction of Prof. Pisoni's report and supporting testimony, specifically on the grounds (a) "that his analysis is not scientifically valid and, therefore, will not assist the trier of fact in making a determination"; (b) "that he does not have the expertise to interpret the back-up materials to the study of Hazelwood's speech"; and (c) "that the prejudicial and confusing effects of the Pisoni report outweigh its probative value" (Defendants' Motion *in Limine*, p. 6). The first point was the most detailed and specifically addressed the admissibility of novel scientific evidence under *Daubert*; the defendants contended that Pisoni's report and testimony did not satisfy the *Daubert* criteria. The defendants thus requested exclusion under Rules 702 and 703 of the Federal Rules of Evidence, cited here.

Rule 702. Testimony by Experts
   If scientific, technical, or other specialized knowledge will assist the trier of fact to understand the evidence or to determine a fact in issue, a witness qualified as an expert by knowledge, skill, experience, training, or education, may testify thereto in the form of an opinion or otherwise.

Rule 703. Bases of Opinion Testimony by Experts
    The facts or data in the particular case upon which an expert bases an opinion
    or inference may be those perceived by or made known to the expert at or before
    the hearing. If of a type reasonably relied upon by experts in the particular field
    in forming opinions or inferences upon the subject, the facts or data need not
    be admissible in evidence.

The defendants argued specifically that Prof. Pisoni's report and testimony
would not assist the court and therefore should not be admitted as evidence,
first, because the results were inconclusive, and second, because they did
not constitute "scientific . . . knowledge." In support of the first argument,
the defendants cited a number of instances in which Pisoni or his colleagues
admitted that their results (both specific and general) were inconclusive.
These included citations from K. Johnson et al. (1990, p. 236): "[T]hese
data are, in the final analysis, inconclusive"; National Transportation Safety
Board (1990, p. 228): "[T]he rate of occurrence of this pattern or the
reliability of a decision based on observations such as these is not known";
Pisoni and Martin (1989, p. 586): "[M]ore research will be needed to assess
the probabilities of given changes as well as the contribution of general and
idiosyncratic effects"; and Tanford et al. (1991, p. 590): "Analyses of Captain Hazelwood's speech cannot prove that he was alcohol-impaired at the
time of the *Exxon Valdez* accident." The defendants concluded that these
"admissions" warranted exclusion, because the findings were inconclusive
and would thus fail to assist the court in determining the intoxication issue.
Instead, they would "encourage the jury to speculate or infer that Joseph
Hazelwood may have been intoxicated at the time of the grounding," thus
prejudicing Hazelwood and the other defendants.

A second argument for excluding Prof. Pisoni's report and testimony
under *Daubert* was that the report to the NTSB was not based on "scientific
knowledge" (such as provided for in Federal Rule of Evidence 702). The
motion cited five factors suggested by the *Daubert* court when considering
novel scientific evidence and determining whether proposed testimony constitutes "scientific knowledge": (a) whether the theory or technique can be
and has been tested; (b) whether the theory or technique has been subjected
to peer review and publication; (c) the known or potential rate of error;
(d) the existence and maintenance of standards controlling the technique's
operation; and (5) "general acceptance" (all 113 S.Ct. at 2796–97). The
defendants argued that none of these factors favored consideration of the
report and proposed testimony as "scientific knowledge." First, they argued
that the findings were untestable, because of an inadequate explanation
of the methods employed and because of "subjective" and "unblinded"
measurement techniques. Further, they argued, some of the "data and back-
up material" no longer existed, including (a) the specific version of the

software used in analyzing the speech samples for the NTSB report; (b) "voice spectrographs" [sic] of Hazelwood's pronunciation of *s;* and (c) other computer data used in the analysis.

Second, the motion argued that publication was no indication that the methodology and conclusions regarding the analysis of Hazelwood's voice were reliable. In *Daubert,* the Supreme Court had proposed peer review and publication as a pertinent consideration, but had also said that "Publication (which is but one element of peer review) is not a *sine qua non* of admissibility; it does not necessarily correlate with reliability" [113 S.Ct. at 2797]. The analysis of the Hazelwood tapes had appeared in four places: National Transportation Safety Board (1990), Pisoni et al. (1991), K. Johnson et al. (1990), and Tanford et al. (1991). The defendants argued that only K. Johnson et al. (1990) had appeared in a peer-reviewed *scientific* publication. Tanford et al. (1991) had appeared in a criminology journal, and Pisoni et al. (1991) had appeared in a nonreviewed conference proceedings. The IU report in the NTSB appendix (1990) was not peer reviewed.

Third, the defendants argued that the "Pisoni report has a high, indeed immeasurable, potential rate of error." This argument was based primarily on potential confounding of intoxication effects with effects due to other physiological and emotional states, such as stress, fatigue, fear, and depression.

Fourth, the defendants' motion argued that the methodology used in the analysis was deficient. Three specific factors were cited. First, the voice samples were said to be "crude and insufficient for the purposes of conducting a laboratory analysis of Hazelwood's voice" (p. 16). The gist of this point was that the Coast Guard system could not have produced recordings of sufficient quality for the analyses actually performed (e.g., rate and pitch). Second, none of the equipment had been inspected to determine proper maintenance and calibration. This included all the relevant equipment in Alaska, as well as the video cassette recorder used to tape the televison interview with Joseph Hazelwood (used as an additional baseline condition by the IU researchers). Third, the defendants argued that Prof. Pisoni had ignored nonsupporting data. Specifically, they stated that Pisoni had failed to consider all of the occurrences of *s* on the tape recordings when assessing changes affecting that sound. They further asserted that in some instances, the IU researchers had "withheld" nonsupporting or even contradictory computer-generated analyses of voice pitch, resorting instead to "unblind" manual calculations.

Fifth, the defendants argued for inadmissibility on the grounds that it "had not been generally accepted by the scientific community." Although the Supreme Court had overturned the general acceptance standard in *Daubert,* the court nevertheless proposed that it "can yet have a bearing on the inquiry" [113 S.Ct. at 2797]. The motion cited Pisoni's concession that "his technique" had not gained "substantial acceptance" and would thus be inadmissible under a general acceptance standard. The defendants further argued that voice identification using speech spectrograms was controversial and had been rejected by various courts, and that Pisoni's analyses were even more controversial and unreliable.

The motion's second major contention was that Prof. Pisoni did "not have the expertise to testify with respect to the analysis conducted on the Hazelwood speech samples." This argument was based on the observation that Pisoni, during his pretrial deposition, was unable to interpret fully a number of documents (called "back-up materials" in the motion) generated by his laboratory; these included handwritten notes, graphs, tables, and graphic displays of acoustic data. The motion argued that Pisoni's inability to interpret these materials would unduly prejudice the defendants, because (a) the defendants and their experts would thus be unable to interpret the materials; (b) the defendants' experts would be unable to provide comment on Pisoni's methodology and conclusions in the absence of an adequate explanation of the analysis procedures; and (c) the defendants would be hampered in their ability to cross-examine Prof. Pisoni at trial.

A second prong of this argument concerned the extent of Prof. Pisoni's actual participation in the analysis (called an "experiment" in the motion). Prof. Pisoni had reported at the deposition that all of the hands-on analyses for the NTSB report had been performed by laboratory staff technicians, specifically Dr. Keith Johnson and Mr. Robert Bernacki. The motion characterized this as a "lax attitude" especially in light of the statement in Tanford et al. (1991) that "[the law] requires that human beings be accounted for. If an expert relies on lab technicians or graduate students, they must be shown to be reliable and properly trained" (Tanford et al., 1991, p. 600).

The third and final major point of the motion spoke to Rule 403 of the Federal Rules of Evidence, cited here:

> Rule 403. Exclusion of Relevant Evidence on Grounds of Prejudice, Confusion, or Waste of Time
>
> Although relevant, evidence may be excluded if its probative value is substantially outweighed by danger of unfair prejudice, confusion of the issues, or misleading the jury, or by considerations of undue delay, waste of time, or needless presentation of cumulative evidence.

In fact, the defendants argued that the probative value of the proposed testimony by Pisoni was "nonexistent" on the grounds that Pisoni had testified that it was not possible to determine intoxication from "voice spectrograph [*sic* in motion *in limine*] analysis." Additionally, the motion argued that Pisoni had stated that acoustic analysis of the type conducted for the NTSB report could not distinguish the effects of alcohol from other physical or emotional states. The defendants further reiterated that the potential error rate for the analysis technique was high, and that the conclusion that Hazelwood had been intoxicated was "based solely on speculation and not evidence," and they argued that allowing Prof. Pisoni's testimony would give a false sense of validity and thus improperly sway the jury. Finally, the defendants' motion argued that admitting Prof. Pisoni's testimony would require an undue amount of time for the jury to be educated in various aspects of that testimony, including its level of probative value.

In response to the defendants' motion *in limine,* the plaintiffs filed on 18 April 1994 a memorandum of opposition to the motion. They argued that in asserting that Pisoni's analysis could not prove intoxication "conclusively," the defendants had misstated Pisoni's opinion, misrepresented the nature of opinion testimony, and ignored applicable standards of admissibility.

The opposition to the motion *in limine* first summarized the substance of Pisoni's reports and testimony, which include explications of (a) the scientific knowledge serving as the underlying bases of the analysis, including the published literature; (b) the methodology and procedures used in the analysis; (c) the derivation of physical measurements from the speech recordings; and (d) the principles, reasoning, methodology, and published data from which Pisoni concluded that intoxication was the most likely explanation of the physical measurements. The underlying scientific knowledge was based on the observed correlation between alcohol intoxication and impairment of motor control and coordination and the principle that speech production is a complex phenomenon requiring multiple levels of motor control. The specific analysis of Captain Hazelwood's speech was based on an underlying scientific basis of previous research in speech production and in the verification of a correlation between alcohol and speech established by other researchers.

The plaintiffs further argued that the methodologies and procedures used in the specific analysis were widely used and valid in the field of speech science. Specifically, the analysis relied on the application of acoustic-phonetic methodology, aided by recent advances in acoustical engineering and in digital speech processing. This methodology had been shown to be scientifically valid in the analysis of various disturbances of speech arising from physical states. The plaintiffs stated that Pisoni had followed established scientific procedures in the specific analysis, relying on two assistants, Keith Johnson and Robert Bernacki.

The plaintiffs' third point described the derivation of measurements from the several audio recordings available. The plaintiffs noted that the request for analysis had come from the NTSB and was based on Prof. Pisoni's existing national recognition as a speech researcher with two relevant scientific publications describing controlled laboratory studies of alcohol effects on speech, showing statistically significant correlations between alcohol and speech. The plaintiffs further noted that five groups of radio transmissions

were analyzed and that Pisoni had identified in those recordings words that
were repeated in similar prosodic contexts: *Exxon Valdez, thirteen and
sixteen,* and *sea* or *see.* The plaintiffs argued that the objective physical
measurements obtained by Pisoni were highly consistent with those patterns
of speech exhibited by intoxicated subjects in laboratory studies. They further noted that analysis of Captain Hazelwood's speech in the television
interview from March 1990 and in videotapes of his deposition showed the
speech in those contexts to be consistent with the speech in the tape recording
of the radio transmission 33 hr prior to the grounding. The measurements
from these three samples thus served as "baseline" measurements that could
be used for relative comparisons with other speech samples at the time
of the grounding. The plaintiffs argued finally that measurements from
comparable tokens of the same words or phrases were objective and scientifically reliable, noting that Johnson and Bernacki had made independent
measurements and that comparison of these measurements were within
acceptable margins of error.

   The plaintiffs' fourth point explained the scientific foundations for Pisoni's conclusions and opinion. Briefly, this was the consistency in speech
patterns between those in the scientific literature and those in the tape
recordings of Captain Hazelwood's speech. Further, the plaintiffs noted that
Pisoni had conducted an analysis of the speech within the context of other
possible causes of the observed changes, such as stress and fatigue; in each
case, due consideration of the known effects of these causes led to their
elimination as possible candidates. However, the plaintiffs did concede the
point that Pisoni could not eliminate the *remote* [emphasis in original memo-
randum] possibility that a complex interaction of conditions and circumstances could have been at the base of the observed speech pattern changes.
Nevertheless, the plaintiffs noted Pisoni's contention that the simplest hypothesis to explain the observed patterns of speech entailed that (a) Captain
Hazelwood was not intoxicated when the [−33] recording was made;
(b) Captain Hazelwood was intoxicated when the [−1], [0], and [+1] recordings were made; and (c) Captain Hazelwood was "substantially, but not
completely, recovered" when the [+9] recording was made.

   The plaintiffs' memorandum next addressed the admissibility of Pisoni's
report and testimony. The plaintiffs argued three points: (a) that Pisoni's
testimony met the current requirements for the admission of expert testimony; (b) that the applicable *Daubert* standards supported the admission
of Pisoni's testimony; and (c) that the balancing test under Rule 403 of the
Federal Rules of Evidence supported the admission of Pisoni's testimony.

   The plaintiffs described briefly both the pre-*Daubert* test of admissibility
(i.e., *Frye*) and the new test embodied in the Federal Rules of Evidence and
in the Supreme Court's decision in *Daubert.* They noted the two-pronged
standard noted above for the application of Rule 702 of the Federal Rules

of Evidence: reliability (i.e., the subject of the proposed testimony must be "scientific knowledge" grounded in the methods and procedures of science and more than mere subjective belief) and relevance (i.e., the proposed evidence or testimony must assist the trier of fact to understand the evidence or determine a fact in issue). The plaintiffs noted that "the focus of the court's inquiry into admissibility 'must be solely on principles and methodology, not on the conclusions that they generate' [*Daubert v. Merrell Dow Pharmaceuticals, Inc.*, 113 S. Ct. 2786, 2793 (1993)]." The plaintiffs noted that the defendants were in this regard misdirecting attention to "conclusiveness," adding that this was properly the function of the jury.

Under *Daubert*, Pisoni's report and testimony would have to be both reliable and relevant. In reference to the proposed testimony's reliability, the plaintiffs argued that it would pertain to "scientific knowledge" as required under *Daubert*. The plaintiffs noted that *Daubert* did not require "absolute certainty" for proposed testimony to meet the "scientific knowledge" standard and to be therefore admissible: "It would be unreasonable to conclude that the subject of scientific testimony must be 'known' to a certainty; arguably there are no certainties in science" [113 S. Ct. 2786, 2795 (1993)]. Rather, the standard requires inferences and assertions to be derived by the scientific method, and the plaintiffs argued that Pisoni's report and proposed testimony were in fact derived by established scientific methods and scientifically valid reasoning. The plaintiffs further argued that the defendants were free to disagree with Pisoni's conclusions and to cross-examine and rebut, but also that the arguments would go to weight, not to admissibility.

The plaintiffs further argued that in addition to being scientifically reliable, the report and proposed testimony were also relevant, in that they would assist the jury to understand the evidence and determine the fact in issue. In this instance, the plaintiffs claimed, the physical evidence to be considered by the jury consisted of the audiotape recordings of the radio transmissions, and the fact in issue was the question of Captain Hazelwood's intoxication. The plaintiffs argued that because Pisoni's measurements were objective and reliable, and because these measurements were consistent with a hypothesis of intoxication, Pisoni's report and testimony would in fact assist the jury. The plaintiffs further noted the defendants' assertion that in the absence of absolutely conclusive evidence, Pisoni's report and proposed testimony would be of no assistance to the jury. The plaintiffs countered this assertion by asserting themselves that such reasoning had been rejected both by the courts and by the advisory committee notes to the Federal Rules of Evidence. These were construed to indicate that any single piece of evidence need not be in itself conclusive proof to be admissible; on this point, Rule 401 of the Federal Rules of Evidence is relevant:

Rule 401. Definition of "Relevant Evidence"

"Relevant evidence" means evidence having any tendency to make the existence of any fact that is of consequence to the determination of the action more probable or less probable than it would be without the evidence.

The plaintiffs cited two commentary statements from the *Notes of Advisory Committee on 1972 Proposed Rules, Rule 401*: "A brick is not a wall" and "it is not to be supposed that every witness can make a home run," as well as this from *United States v. Clifford*, 704 F.2d 86, 90 (3rd Cir. 1983): "a piece of evidence. . . need not conclusively prove a fact beyond a reasonable doubt to be admissible."

The plaintiffs second major argument was that the *Daubert* factors, so far as applicable, supported admitting Pisoni's testimony. In this they addressed the four "general observations" noted previously from the Supreme Court's decision in *Daubert* regarding expert opinion: (a) testing, (b) peer review and publication, (c) potential error rates, and (d) degree of acceptance. First, the plaintiffs asserted that Pisoni's underlying methodology, principles, and reasoning could be and had been tested. They noted that Pisoni's methodology and analysis procedures were in common use, having been validated previously as reliable. The scientific bases of Pisoni's conclusions were to be found in various disciplines, including physiology, psychology, medicine, and speech science, and worked according to the well-established principle that alcohol affects motor functioning, which in turn affects speech motor control. Evidence that this principle was well established was to be found in the use of speech as a preliminary determinant of intoxication in roadside sobriety testing and the use of speech as an evidentiary indicium of intoxication in drunk driving trials.

Second, the plaintiffs asserted that Pisoni's theory and technique had been subjected to peer review and publication, citing first the peer review occurring subsequent to the submission of K. Johnson et al. (1990) to *Phonetica* and second the implicit peer review occurring subsequent to the appearance of the article in the journal. The plaintiffs noted that *Phonetica* was a distinguished, widely circulated serial, and that subsequent to the appearance of the article, Pisoni was invited by the Human Factors Society (now the Human Factors and Ergonomics Society) to present his findings at its symposium; the report was subsequently published in the symposium proceedings. Additionally, the plaintiffs noted that the only published response from the scientific community had come from Hollien (1993), who had substantially endorsed Pisoni's methodology and analysis procedures (although he did take issue with the final conclusions).

The third prong of the plaintiffs' argument on the basis of *Daubert* factors concerned the potential rate of error of the methods and procedures, which the plaintiffs said was very low. They pointed out that the basis for Pisoni's testimony involved precise laboratory procedures used generally in speech analysis. They further asserted that the defendants had repeatedly mischaracterized Pisoni's procedures by calling it a "test," implying that these procedures were comparable to, for example, chemical tests used to assess alcohol concentrations in body fluids. The plaintiffs pointed out that whereas these tests measured molecular alcohol, Pisoni's testimony constituted an inferential opinion, based on objective and quantifiable measurements of behavioral data.

The plaintiffs further noted that copies of the relevant audio recordings had been in the possession of the defendants' experts since 1990, but that no attempt had been made to conduct an independent analysis or to replicate Pisoni's measurements. They characterized as "pure diversion" the defendants' arguments that it was not possible to replicate Pisoni's measurements and argued that the failure of the defendants' experts to attempt replication implied acceptance of the scientific reliability of Pisoni's analyses.

The defendants had cited a number of court cases in which expert testimony had been excluded as similar to the instant case, that is, *Viterbo v. Dow Chemical Co.,* 826 F.2d 420 (5th Cir. 1987); *O'Conner v. Commonwealth Edison Co.,* 13 F.3d 1090 (7th Cir. 1994); and *Maddy v. Vulcan Materials Co.,* 737 F. Supp. 1528 (D. Kan. 1990). The plaintiffs claimed that these cases were irrelevant and unhelpful, because the situations were not comparable. Specifically, the plaintiffs asserted that in each of these cases, the testimony was not based on scientific analysis, but rather on unsupported and subjective speculation. The defendants, of course, had asserted that Pisoni's proposed testimony was just that: unsupported and subjective speculation.

In their fourth point, the plaintiffs addressed the question of the degree of acceptance of the underlying methodology and principles by the relevant scientific community. Here they reiterated a point made earlier, that the relevant published scientific literature contained no challenges to Pisoni's methods, procedures, or findings (but cf. Hollien, 1993).

Finally, the plaintiffs argued that Rule 403 of the Federal Rules of Evidence supported the admission of Pisoni's testimony. The defendants had argued that Pisoni's testimony should be excluded under Rule 403, because its probative value was substantially outweighed by the danger of unfair prejudice. The plaintiffs claimed that defendants had not demonstrated prejudice, and that their request under Rule 403 was based on the erroneous argument that voice spectrographic analysis could not alone indicate a person's intoxication. The plaintiffs noted that this argument was contradicted by the advisory committee notes to the Federal Rules of Evidence and had also been rejected by the courts, for example in *United States v. Brady,* 595 F.2d at 363. The defendants had claimed that admission of Pisoni's testimony would give it an aura of scientific infallibility, but the plaintiffs argued that such evidence should be admitted if the jury would be aided in understanding the evidence and if the jury was properly instructed on the weight to be accorded opinion testimony such as Pisoni's. Thus, the plaintiffs argued, the question went to weight, not to admissibility.

The defendants had also proposed that admission of Pisoni's testimony would be a "waste of time" (as per Rule 403), since this would require educating the jury on both the underlying scientific basis of Pisoni's testimony as well as the deficiencies of that testimony. The plaintiffs argued that although judicial economy was important, nevertheless it should be overridden where proper determination of factual issues was concerned.

8.4 SUMMARY AND DISCUSSION

The grounding of the *Exxon Valdez* and the subsequent spill of tremendous amounts of crude oil into Prince William Sound was a major U.S. domestic news events of 1989, and although we do not wish to exaggerate either the role that speech analysis played in the entire story or our understanding of all of the legal niceties surrounding the admission of novel scientific evidence, it does represent the movement of basic science into a fairly well-known real-world situation. Although the speech data and subsequent analyses played virtually no role in either the criminal trial or the civil trial that arose from this incident, it nevertheless remains true that the audiotape recordings of radio transmissions between Captain Hazelwood and the Coast Guard Vessel Traffic Center were the sole objective physical evidence from the time around that of the grounding. Although the NTSB placed a good deal of stock in the speech analyses performed independently by three groups of scientists, the NTSB findings carried no legal weight in the subsequent lives of the individuals and corporate entities on either side of the ensuing legal fights. In the civil trial, it was up to the court to decide on the admissibility of the type of evidence discussed here, and in the end, the U.S. District Court judge decided that the proposed report and testimony of Prof. Pisoni did not meet the standards set forth in *Daubert* and ruled that it should be excluded.

CHAPTER 9

Conclusions

9.0 INTRODUCTION

As mentioned previously, the research dealing with alcohol and speech is scattered throughout the published literature from a variety of disciplines, and one of the main purposes of the present work has been to gather as much of this as possible in one place.

We have identified three main historical periods in the research literature on alcohol and speech, which informs our division of the literature in Chapters 5 through 7. The earliest period, ranging from Dodge and Benedict (1915) through Dunker and Schlosshauer (1964), was characterized as a "medical" era in this research, including psychiatry and psychology. In the literature, speech is considered within a constellation of signs and symptoms indicative of alcohol consumption. In the second period, ranging from Stein (1966) to Sobell et al. (1982), there appear more works in the literature that deal specifically with speech effects, but at the same time, the distribution of disciplines is more eclectic than in the earliest period. Behavioral evidence was wide ranging and included examination of articulatory errors and speech dysfluencies, response latencies, amounts of verbalization, syntactic complexity, disinhibition of verbal behavior, and changes in the acoustic signal. Publication sites were equally varied, including journals in the fields of speech pathology, linguistics, psychology, psychiatry, and alcohol studies.

Whereas the first two periods extend over approximately 70 years, the final period we have identified is just somewhat over 10 years, but more than half the literature appearing on the subject of alcohol and speech has appeared from 1985 to 1996. Despite the large amount of research reflected in the literature, this latter period, ranging from Pisoni et al. (1985) to

Cummings et al. (1996) has been much less eclectic than the previous one, and there has been a decided trend toward laboratory-based instrumental analysis when approaching the question of alcohol's effects on speech. For the most part, these analyses have been acoustic, but there have been other approaches, for example, the one physiological study by K. Johnson et al. (1993).

In view of the multiplicity of disciplines contributing to research on alcohol and speech, one might expect a wide variety of results, and this is indeed true. Reported changes in speech due to alcohol range from slower reaction times to increased variability in fundamental frequency, but in general, by whatever measure, alcohol does clearly and reliably produce a number of changes on speech and the speech signal, and these results are summarized in the following section.

9.1 SUMMARY OF RESULTS AND GENERAL CONCLUSIONS

A general result from the research on alcohol and speech is that subjects perform behavioral tasks more slowly under alcohol than without alcohol. Dodge and Benedict (1915), for instance, found a slight increase in response latencies when subjects were shown printed words and asked to say them aloud as quickly as possible. Likewise, Hollingworth (1923) found slowed performance on a color-naming task; Moskowitz and Roth (1971) reported increased response latencies on an object naming task; Sobell and Sobell (1972) found that subjects required a longer time to read a passage; and Künzel et al. (1992) reported a decrease in speaking rate.

Second, the number of speech errors increases with alcohol over a nonalcohol condition. These include a wide range of specificity, from the very broad to the very narrow. In the first instance, Jetter (1938a, 1938b) reported in broad terms "speech abnormalities" as indicative of intoxication in both clinical subjects and volunteers. At a somewhat more detailed level, Forney and Hughes (1961) measured omissions, insertions, mispronunciations, "spasms (stammers)," and prolongations (although alcohol did not appear to have a significant effect on these measures). Zaimov (1969) reported measurements for a number of types of errors, including omissions, substitutions, and repetitions, and these were further differentiated by linguistic level (segment, syllable, word) and by whether the error appeared to be based on sound or on meaning. Lester and Skousen (1974) reported a higher incidence of sound substitutions after ingestion of alcohol than before. Finally, the most detailed analyses of this type were those that measured specific acoustic parameters; these will be discussed below.

Third, listeners, both experienced and naive, are able to reliably perceive differences between speech produced with alcohol and speech produced without. In the study reported in Andrews et al. (1977), for instance, listeners who were naive to the alcohol conditions obtaining judged talkers speaking without alcohol to be more efficient, reasonable, self-confident, scholarly, artistic, theatrical, and less untrained. In a number of studies (Klingholz et al., 1988; Künzel et al., 1992; Pisoni and Martin, 1989), listeners were able to determine either which of two presented sentences was produced under alcohol (discrimination) or whether or not a single sentence presented in isolation was produced under alcohol (identification).

Fourth, alcohol exerts an effect on motor control of the speech organs, resulting in a number of changes in articulation that are observable in the acoustic signal. The use of instrumentation to examine and measure changes in the speech acoustic signal resulting from alcohol consumption has been characteristic of research on alcohol and speech since the 1980s. As mentioned in Chapter 3, the radiated acoustic speech signal from a talker's lips is the result of a complex interplay among three subsystems: respiratory, phonatory, and articulatory. Most of the changes in the acoustic signal that have been studied in depth by instrumental methods correspond to changes in either articulation or phonation. There has been very little explicit examination of the effects of alcohol on respiratory aspects of speech production.

The phenomenon of slurred speech is best considered a characteristic of alcohol's effect on articulatory processes rather than phonatory or respiratory ones. Prior to 1985, the literature contains only two instrumental acoustic studies: Lester and Skousen (1974) and Fontan et al. (1978). Although these studies lacked some of the sophistication (both in methodology and instrumentation) of later studies, many of the results described here are consistent with those later reported in the 1980s and 1990s. Lester and Skousen, for instance, found that both vowels and consonants were lengthened, and that a number of substitutions obtained, including devoicing of final obstruents, palatalization of alveolar fricatives, and incomplete or absent stop closure in affricates. Likewise, Fontan et al. also found inappropriate lengthening in vowels and frication of stop consonants.

Instrumental analysis of alcohol-affected speech became the preferred methodology in the early- to mid-1980s. Much of this interest can be attributed to the development and widespread availability of fast, accurate digital signal processing techniques. Beginning with Pisoni et al. (1985), the use of computers for any combination of acquisition, storage, retrieval, processing, and analysis of data became the norm rather than the exception. The use of computers allowed researchers to collect a larger number of speech samples from a larger number of subjects with realistic expectations that data could be analyzed in a timely fashion.

Results from these more recent studies demonstrated that the effects of alcohol on speech production mechanisms yielded instrumentally identifiable, reliable changes in the speech acoustic signal. Articulatory changes included incomplete stop closures in affricates (Pisoni et al., 1985); nasalization of oral vowels and denasalization of nasal consonants (Künzel et al, 1992); lowering of F2 and F3 (Behne & Rivera, 1990); consonant cluster reduction (Braun, 1991); incomplete articulations (Künzel et al., 1992).

Two parameters, speaking rate and fundamental frequency, were examined in quite a number of studies. A general finding was that durations increased and speaking rates decreased, and these occurred across a number of different linguistic levels. Pisoni et al. (1985) found that stop closure durations increased; Behne et al. (1991) that word and sentence durations increased; Künzel (1992) that both the number and duration of pauses increased; Künzel et al. (1992) that segmental durations increased and speaking tempo decreased; DeJong et al. (1995) that durations for both a reading task and a diadochokinetic repetition task increased; and Dunlap et al. (1995) that sentence durations in a shadowing task increased. In short, increased durations and the resulting decrease in speech tempo contribute to the listener's impression that speech produced under alcohol is slower and more drawn out.

Also investigated in a number of studies was fundamental frequency, one of the acoustic correlates of pitch. Alcohol produces changes in mean fundamental frequency as well as increases in its variability, but research results regarding a specific direction of change are equivocal at this time. On the one hand, Behne and Rivera (1990) and Künzel et al. (1992) reported a general increase in mean fundamental frequency following alcohol consumption. On the other hand, Watanabe et al. (1994) and Alderman et al. (1995) reported increases. Change of fundamental frequency in one direction or another was thus a consistent finding, but even more consistent was the increase in variation in fundamental frequency; Pisoni et al. (1985), Klingholz et al. (1988), and Künzel et al. (1992) all reported increases in fundamental frequency variability from the nonalcohol to the alcohol condition. Peak-to-peak perturbations in fundamental frequency, or "jitter," also increased, as reported by K. Johnson et al. (1990, 1993), Künzel et al. (1992), Niedzielska et al. (1994), Watanabe et al. (1994), and Cummings et al. (1996).

A wide variety of other techniques and measurements have been used, which are discussed more fully in Chapter 4 and in greater detail in Chapters 5 through 7. These include direct observation methods (e.g., Künzel et al., 1992; Watanabe et al., 1994); electropalatography and electroglottography (K. Johnson et al., 1993); clinical voice measures (e.g., Eysholdt, 1992; Niedzielska et al., 1994); and several acoustic measures (e.g., Cummings et al., 1996; Klingholz, et al., 1988). Because these techniques were used in only a few instances, results are quite tentative and await data from many more subjects for confirmation.

On the whole, however, the collective body of research on alcohol and speech has demonstrated the existence of identifiable, measurable, and reliable markers of alcohol consumption in the speech acoustic signal. These changes can be understood within the context of what is currently known about speech production and the motor-control mechanisms of sound generation in the human vocal tract (Stevens, 1964).

9.2 ALCOHOL, SPEECH, AND IMPAIRMENT

As we have just noted, the experimental evidence published in the research literature supports the proposition that alcohol exerts identifiable, measurable, and reliable changes on speech production and the resulting acoustic signal. Within certain limits, then, the types of analyses of speech that have been carried out in research laboratories can serve to identify particular acoustic markers of alcohol consumption or alcohol intoxication. A practical question that naturally arises is whether the speech signal alone contains a sufficient number of these markers to indicate relevant levels of alcohol intoxication. In other words, can some form of speech analysis serve in a capacity similar to chemical analysis (e.g., blood analysis, breath analysis) for the identification of alcohol in the body. This question was addressed in a specific context in our discussion of the *Exxon Valdez* grounding in Chapter 8; here we address some other general issues that concern this question.

9.2.1 Intoxication versus Impairment

As the element *-toxic-* indicates, the earliest uses of the words *intoxicate* and its various derivatives such as *intoxicated* and *intoxication* were concerned with poisons and their administration. Use of *intoxicate* with the transitive verbal meaning of "to poison" is first cited by the *Oxford English Dictionary* (*OED*) (Murray, Bradley, Craigie, & Onions, 1933; hereafter cited as OED) for the year 1530: "I intoxycat, I poyson with venyme" (*Palsgr.*, 592/2). For *intoxicated* ("imbued with poison"), the first citation is from 1558: "If a man be . . . hurte with anie intoxicated weapon, ye must wryng wel the bloud out of the wounde" (Warde tr. *Alexis' Secr.* (1568) 20 a); and for *intoxication* ("the act of poisoning; administration of poison; killing by poison; the state of being poisoned; an instance of this"), the first citation is from 1548: "Either by pensyvenes of hearte, or by intoxicacion of poison . . . within a few daies the Quene departed oute of this transitorie lyfe" (Hall *Chron.*, 3 *Rich. III* (1809) 407). Although upon reflection, these meanings concerning poison and poisoning are relatively transparent, nevertheless all of them are listed by the OED as obsolete meanings (except, in some cases, in medical parlance). The now more familiar meanings of these words, that is, those concerning postalcohol states, are newer, but not much newer. The first OED citation for *intoxicate* with the meaning of "to stupefy, tender unconscious or delirious, to madden or deprive of the ordinary use of the senses or reason, with a drug or alcoholic liquor; to inebriate, made drunk" is from 1598: "It . . . goeth down very pleasantly, intoxicating weake braines" (Hakluyt *Voy.* I.97). Similarly, the first citation for *intoxicated* ("stupefied or having the brain affected with a drug or alcoholic liquor; inebriated, drunk") is from 1576: "Some so full of wine, and intoxicated with Bacchus berries" (Fleming, *Panopl. Epist.* 290); and for *intoxication* ("the action of rendering stupid, insensible, or disordered in intellect, with a drug or alcoholic liquor; the making drunk or inebriated; the condition of being so stupefied or disordered") from 1646: "The prevalent intoxication is from the spirits of drink dispersed into the veynes and arteries" (Sir T. Browne *Pseud. Ep.* II.vi 101).

It is these specific alcohol-related meanings that inform our understanding of *intoxicated* in such uses as the following (Indiana Code 9-30-5-2): "A person who operates a vehicle while intoxicated commits a Class A misdemeanor." However, such legal proscriptions do not appear to depend on the mere state of intoxication (either excitement or stupefaction), but rather on the resulting inability to operate the vehicle safely. Thus, the definition of *intoxication* in *Black's Law Dictionary* (Black, 1979) specifically mentions an inability to act in a prudent, cautious manner:

> *Intoxication:* Term comprehends situation where, by reason of drinking intoxicants, an individual does not have the normal use of his physical or mental faculties, thus rendering him incapable of acting in the manner in which an ordinarily prudent and cautious man, in full possession of his faculties, using reasonable care, would act under the conditions. *Hendy v. Geary,* 105 R.I. 419, 252 A.2d 435, 441.

One word that now enjoys widespread use to describe this operational aspect of intoxication as regards safety issues is *impaired*. In general, *impair* means to diminish, make worse, or injure, but *impaired* is also used to refer to the specific effects of alcohol ingestion, as in this decision regarding an Indiana law proscribing "driving under the influence":

> 'Under the influence of intoxicating liquor' within statute proscribing driving in such condition, are words in common use and well understood by the laity as referring to the impaired condition of thought and action, and the loss of normal control of one's faculties to a marked degree, caused by drinking intoxicating liquors. (*Shorter v. State,* 1955, 122 N.E.2d 847, 234 Ind. 1)

Beyond the explicit characterization of postalcohol conditions as constituting impairment, in some uses, the word *impaired* alone implicitly refers specifically to alcohol effects: the 1976 supplement to the *OED* (Burchfield, 1976) added this meaning of *impaired*: "Of a driver or his driving: adversely affected by the influence of alcohol or narcotics." The citations, dating back to 1951, are all from Canadian sources (although this use also appears to be current in the United States). This citation from 1972 refers explicitly to driving but not at all to alcohol: "A police spokesman said the car received only slight damage. The driver was arrested and charged with impaired driving" (*Evening Telegram* [St. John's, Newfoundland, Canada] 24 June 1/1); similarly, from 1974: "A snowmobile operator was one of five persons assessed penalties ranging from $175 to $200 each in county court Tuesday on impaired driving charges" (*Kingston Whig-Standard* (Ontario, Canada) 16 Jan. 5/4).

9.2.2 Alcohol Testing

A good deal of the literature on alcohol and speech since the mid-1980s (i.e., those works discussed in Chapter 7) has been conducted against a background of safety, legal, and forensic issues. The original impetus for Pisoni et al. (1985) and other research reports emanating from the same project (conducted under contract with General Motors Research Laboratories) was the attempt to gauge the feasibility of developing an automobile safety-interlock system that would respond to changes in speech and voice caused by alcohol consumption. Similarly, many of the researchers involved in the study reported in Künzel et al. (1992) were affiliated with the German *Bundeskriminalamt*, a law enforcement agency. Furthermore, reports such as Klingholz et al. (1988) and K. Johnson et al. (1993) specifically discuss their research in the context of the development of detection methods and devices for identifying impairment due to alcohol consumption.

Although the studies we have discussed here have addressed the question of a relationship between alcohol intoxication and changes in the speech signal, practical applications of any results must also address the relationship between *impairment* and changes in the speech signal. Because in practical applications, *impairment* will refer to impairment of the ability to perform specific tasks safely, consideration of changes in speech and voice would have to be tied to varying degrees of impairment. For example, per se laws that refer to specific blood- or breath-alcohol concentrations (BACs or BrACs) are predicated on the principle that at that alcohol level, all (or most) persons suffer sufficient impairment of their ability to operate a vehicle safely. In general, when specific degrees of impairment need to be expressed (e.g., in statutes), these are given in terms of specific BACs or BrACs, and reliable methods of measuring these from small amounts of body fluids have been developed.

It is still the case, however, that different per se rules or laws will be applicable in different situations, depending on the specific task in question. In vehicular traffic, for instance, and for whatever reason, BAC or BrAC thresholds are not always uniform for different modes of transportation (e.g., automobiles vs. boats). Whereas tests based on body fluid samples are able to differentiate these thresholds to a desired degree of accuracy (in part because statutes are often written with the analysis technology in mind), it is not clear at the present time that analysis of speech and voice can do the same thing. With the development of reliable, quickly responding, and relatively noninvasive devices for measuring BrAC, the correlations most attempted in the recent literature on alcohol and speech have been with BAC or BrAC. Nevertheless, as a review of the relevant literature will show, correlations of this kind were not always perfect, and in some cases, they were quite imperfect.

The two main spheres in which alcohol (and drug) testing play a role at present are vehicular traffic and workplaces ("readiness-to-perform" testing). The extent to which speech analysis can play a routine role in these areas will depend greatly upon the extent to which speech changes can be correlated with degree of impairment, either directly or through those tests of alcohol concentration now widely (although not always universally) accepted, such as BrAC and BAC measurement. In nonroutine cases, the scientific evidence, as discussed in Chapters 5 through 7, appears strong enough to at least make a good case. Recall that in the *Exxon Valdez* case, speech recordings were the only physical evidence available from immediately prior to and immediately after the grounding. When no other physical records are available, speech recordings remain viable materials for analysis.

9.3 FUTURE RESEARCH

The trend noted in Chapter 7 toward instrumental analysis in alcohol and speech research can be expected to continue for some time. As mentioned earlier, the increasing availability of computers and digital speech processing techniques has put this type of analysis within the reach of an increasing number of researchers with varying financial resources. Ongoing developments can be expected to occur in many areas of speech science, including acoustic analysis (e.g., Cummings et al., 1996) and physiological measures (e.g., K. Johnson et al., 1993).

Although these relative end stages of research on alcohol and speech are constantly improving, and researchers would be wise to keep abreast of these developments, it would be fatal to any research program in particular and the entire enterprise in general to ignore alcohol-dosing methodology. A look at Chapters 5 through 7 should reveal two striking aspects of research on alcohol and speech. First, there is a great amount of variability and individual differences across subjects, and second, almost all of the research undertaken in the period since 1985 has been conducted by speech scientists. Prior to 1985, there were many more alcohol researchers and medical professionals involved in this research problem than after this time.

The problem of individual variability is not limited to alcohol and speech research but to alcohol research in general. First, there is wide variation in BAC and BrAC responses to administered alcohol doses, and second, there is wide variation in behavioral responses on the one hand to doses or BACs/BrACs on the other. Causes of individual differences in alcohol research are not perfectly understood, but a better understanding of the pharmacokinetics of alcohol can only result in a better understanding of the sources of individual variability and ways to control it or at least account for it. It is therefore incumbent on speech scientists, who now appear to be conducting the majority of the research on alcohol and speech, to remain current on developments in alcohol research in general and pharmacokinetic considerations specifically. The ease with which a wide variety of acoustic analyses can be performed on a computer at relatively low cost should not thereby convince the speech scientist that he or she is also able to prescribe alcohol doses accurately (and safely) or to operate a breath-alcohol analysis device. This means that all laboratory personnel must be at least well trained or ideally experts or specialists: it is one thing for an alcohol researcher to turn on a tape recorder; it is an altogether different thing for a speech scientist to administer an intoxicating, potentially addictive drug to college students.

Although the collective body of results from the research literature discussed here does point toward a constellation of identifiable, reliable speech and voice markers of alcohol intoxication, it is also nevertheless true that from a medical or pharmacological point of view, not a single study in the entire literature on alcohol and speech has been truly replicated. That is, although many of the speech and voice results appear to be potentially robust, the real relationship between alcohol and the observed changes cannot be definitely known until not only results, but also specific methodologies (particularly dosimetry and achieved BACs/BrACs), are replicated. The speech scientists who have conducted recent research on alcohol and speech are some of the best in the field, and their studies have contributed a great deal to our fundamental knowledge of possible variations in the speech signal, but this research also has the potential for contributing much to our knowledge of alcohol effects in general.

The search for an analysis system to detect alcohol consumption and impairment through cues in the speech signal, somewhat along the lines of breath-alcohol analysis devices, should not be considered beyond our reach, but a number of the researchers discussed here (e.g., Klingholz, Künzel, K. Johnson) have seriously questioned the feasibility of developing such a system. It must be remembered that most of the research reviewed here is very good science, and that as in much of science, the analyses are to a large extent interpretive; that is, interpretation of results such as those thus far obtained is not a matter of reading numbers from an LED (light-emitting diode) display on a handheld device, but rather a matter of bringing to bear a sound, reliable scientific foundation and methodology. The provision of this foundation should be the immediate goal of future research on alcohol and speech. We are just beginning to get a handle on this very complex problem as we move to the second decade of modern instrumental research on the effects of alcohol on speech motor control and acoustics.

Speech Materials for Indiana University/General Motors Research Laboratories Studies

Monosyllabic words (204): badge, belk, bilk, bing, book, booth, breathe, bulk, bush, theme, chaff, chap, cheese, chest, chief, chin, choose, chops, clang, clash, clasp, cleave, cliff, clings, clog, clots, cob, cook, coop, could, crisp, culp, cult, dab, death, deep, ding, dodge, doom, dub, dune, feast, felt, fez, fig, foot, foot's, fun, fuzz, gap, gasp, gin, give, god, good, goose, guest, gulp, hasp, hatch, heath, help, hood, hoof, hook, hulk, jam, jeeps, jest, jog, jots, judge, juice, kelp, kilt, knelt, knob, leave, lips, lisp, lodge, look, loom, loops, love, mash, mesh, milk, mob, moose, moot, mops, move, nest, news, niece, nook, noose, nudge, palp, please, plebe, pledge, plod, plop, plot, plug, plume, pooch, posh, pulp, push, puss, put, puts, rasp, reach, rib, roof, rook, rough, says, scalp, seethe, sheath, sheathe, shoes, shook, shoots, shops, should, shove, silk, smash, smelt, smith, smooch, smooth, smudge, smug, smut, soot, soothe, soup, stash, stilt, sting, stock, stood, stoops, stop, stuff, such, sulk, talk, teeth, teethe, than, that, that's, thatch, thief, them, then, these, thieve, thing, things, this, thud, thug, thus, took, tooth, tots, touch, tube, van, vast, vat, veldt, vest, vet, vets, vim, wasp, watch, weave, wedge, welt, whelp, wisp, with, would, wreath, wreathe, zag, zen, zest, zig, zing, zip, zips, zoom

Spondees (38): airplane, backbone, bathtub, birthday, buckwheat, cookbook, daybreak, drawbridge, duckpond, earthquake, eggplant, football, footstool, hardware, headlight, hedgehog, horseshoe, hotdog, inkwell, lifeboat, mushroom, northwest, nutmeg, oatmeal, platform, scarecrow, schoolboy, seahorse, shipwreck, sundown, starlight, toothbrush, washboard, whitewash, wildcat, windmill, woodchuck, woodwork

Tongue Twisters: 1. Brother Sam sits on the seesaw. 2. Don's dog didn't eat food. 3. Zelda's zipper was easy to close. 4. Lyn held the little doll. 5. Nan and her two cousins had fun. 6. Tom tied a tighter knot. 7. Sue roasted duck for supper. 8. Dad patted the black cat that sat beside the hat. 9. Five violets cover the seven groves. 10. She showed the shiny, splashing fish. 11. Fifty-five and a half pounds of fish. 12. Chuck and Charlie watched the championship match. 13. John changed Jim and Jack's badge. 14. She feeds three geese peas, beets, and wheat. 15. Ten men came when Hane rang.

Isolated Sentences (from Borden, 1971): 1. The mother is sweeping the kitchen. 2. The girl is making a peanut butter and jelly sandwich. 3. There are grapes and oranges on the table. 4. There are some matches on the stove. 5. The little girl is talking on the telephone. 6. It's hard to lift a lot of dishes. 7. There's a knife and a spoon. 8. The boy's in his pajamas. 9. He's brushing his teeth with a toothbrush. 10. His sister is washing her face. 11. The father is shaving with a razor. 12. The mother and child are sleeping. 13. She's putting stamps on three letters. 14. She got some presents for her birthday. 15. She's saying thank you for the sweater. 16. Here's a shirt and a pair of pants. 17. The kids are throwing snowballs. 18. He's zipping his jacket. 19. She's putting on her gloves. 20. The boy has two shovels. 21. There's a sled. 22. The garbage cans are by the garage. 23. There are bicycles in the garage. 24. That's a school. 25. There's a flag. 26. There's a pencil on the desk. 27. There are some books on the chair. 28. There's smoke coming from the chimney. 29. The boy is building with blocks. 30. This boy is making valentines with scissors and paste. 31. It's the month of February. 32. There are five cats. 33. They have whiskers. 34. They scratch the baskets. 35. They play with the string. 36. A new leaf is on the tree. 37. The bird has a nest. 38. Spring is here. 39. He caught a big fish. 40. It's hard to grasp a frog. 41. There's a bridge. 42. She's splashing in the ocean. 43. To smell a flower you breathe in. 44. The spider spins a lovely web. 45. The squirrel is on a box. 46. That's a wasp. 47. There are snakes at the zoo. 48. There's a giraffe in a cage. 49. There are some zebras. 50. The mouse is eating the cheese. 51. The colt is thirsty. 52. He's drinking some milk. 53. They have a bed of straw. 54. That smiling boy is first in line. 55. That's a rooster. 56. The baby is looking at his shoe. 57. This engine has to be fixed. 58. There's a taxi. 59. The boy is watching TV. 60. The girl is swinging and laughing. 61. That's a clown. 62. He has a yellow mouth with yellow lips. 63. He has red cheeks. 64. There's Casper the Friendly Ghost. 65. He's flying away from the Earth. 66. There are stars in the sky.

Grandfather Passage (see Darley et al., 1975; 9 sentences, 132 words): You wish to know all about my grandfather. Well, he is nearly ninety-three years old. He dresses himself in an ancient black frock coat usually minus several buttons, yet, he still thinks as swiftly as ever. A long flowing beard clings to his chin giving those who observe him a pronounced feeling of utmost respect. When he speaks his voice is just a bit cracked and quivers a trifle. Twice each day he plays skillfully and with zest upon our small organ. Except in the winter when the ooze or snow or ice prevents he slowly takes a short walk in the open air each day. We have often urged him to walk more and smoke less but he always answers "banana oil." Grandfather likes to be modern in his language.

Victory Garden Passage (12 sentences, 202 words): In order to demonstrate as many good gardening techniques as possible, I've planted quite an assortment of beans from time to time in the Victory Garden. Our best crop is the bush or snap bean. One year we planted several varieties of pole beans in addition to the bush varieties, and the bush beans won the contest hands down. Bush beans grow and are gathered quickly so that they rarely have disease or pest difficulties. Pole beans, however, grow over a long season and are apt to get unsightly foliage due to diseases that attack the leaves. Broccoli, cabbage, and cauliflower are all members of the cabbage family. They mature at greatly different rates, cauliflower growing the slowest. I plant the first of my broccoli, cabbage, and cauliflower seeds in March. I only need about a dozen green plants. I set the pots in the bright warmth of the greenhouse or hotbed and when the seedlings get one inch tall I transfer them to individual places in six-packs. They grow very quickly in indoor heat, so later I move the six-packs to the cold frame. They will continue to grow there and will be ready for the open ground in April.

Rainbow Passage (from Fairbanks, 1960; 19 sentences, 332 words): When the sunlight strikes raindrops in the air, they act like a prism and form a rainbow. The rainbow is a division of white light into many beautiful colors. These take the shape of a long round arch, with its path high above, and its two ends apparently beyond the horizon. There is, according to legend, a boiling pot of gold at one end. People look, but no one ever finds it. When a man looks for something beyond his reach, his friends say he is looking for the pot of gold at the end of the rainbow. Throughout the centuries men have explained the rainbow in various ways. Some have accepted it as a miracle without physical explanation. To the Hebrews it was a token that there would be no more universal floods. The Greeks used to imagine that it was a sign from the gods to foretell war or heavy rain. The Norsemen considered the rainbow as a bridge over which the gods passed from earth to their home in the sky. Other men have tried to explain the phenomenon physically. Aristotle thought that the rainbow was caused by a reflection of the sun's rays by the rain. Since then physicists have found that it is not reflection, but refraction by the raindrops which causes the rainbow. Many complicated ideas about the rainbow have been formed. The difference in the rainbow depends considerably upon the size of the water drops, and the width of the colored band increases as the size of the drops increases. The actual primary rainbow observed is said to be the effect of superposition of a number of bows. If the red of the second bow falls upon the green of the first, the result is to give a bow with an abnormally wide yellow band, since red and green lights when mixed form yellow. This is a very common type of bow, one showing mainly red and yellow, with little or no green or blue.

Reading Text for Wiesbaden Studies

Der Nordwind und die Sonne ("The Northwind and the Sun"): Einst stritten sich Nordwind und Sonne, wer von ihnen beiden wohl der Stärkere wäre, als ein Wanderer, der in einen warmen Mantel gehüllt war, des Weges daher kam. Sie wurden einig, daß derjenige für den Stärkeren gelten sollte, der den Wanderer zwingen würde, seinen Mantel auszuziehen. Der Nordwind blies mit aller Macht, aber je mehr er blies, desto fester hüllte sich der Wanderer in seinen Mantel ein. Endlich gab der Nordwind den Kampf auf. Nun erwärmte die Sonne die Luft mit ihren freundlich Strahlen, und schon nach wenigen Augenblicken zog der Wanderer seinen Mantel aus. Da mußte der Nordwind zugeben, daß die Sonne von ihnen beiden der Stärkere war.

Speech Materials for Swartz (1992)

[d]: 1. What did Beth do last weekend? 2. It's not beneath Dooley's chair. 3. I saw a moth do long flights. 4. Has Faith Doolen been here yet? 5. It was the ninth due last week.

[t]: 6. He said earth tools are needed. 7. The fourth tulip is yellow. 8. I've lived up north too long now. 9. You said Heath Tulidge is here? 10. This month two little boys go.

References

Abercrombie, D. (1967). *Elements of general phonetics*. Edinburgh: Edinburgh University Press.

Adams, A. J., & Brown, B. (1975). Alcohol prolongs time course of glare recovery. *Nature* (London), *257*, 481–483.

Alajouanine, T., Ombredane, A., & Durant, M. (1939). *Le syndrome de désintégration phonétique dans l'aphasie*. Paris: Masson.

Alderman, G. A., Hollien, H., Martin, C., & DeJong, G. (1995). Shifts in fundamental frequency & articulation resulting from intoxication [Abstract]. *Journal of the Acoustical Society of America, 97*, 3363–3364 (Abstract).

American Medical Assocation Committee on Medicolegal Problems. (1970). *Alcohol and the impaired driver: A manual on the medicolegal aspects of chemical tests for intoxication with supplement on breath/alcohol tests*. Chicago: American Medical Association.

Ammons, R., & Ammons, C. (1962). *The quick test*. Missoula: University of Montana Press.

Anderson, T. E., Schweitz, R. M., & Snyder, M. B. (1983). *Field evaluation of a behavioral test battery for DWI* (NHTSA Report No. DOT HS-806 475). Washington, DC: National Highway Transportation Safety Administration, Office of Driver and Pedestrian Research.

Andrews, M. L., Cox, W. M., & Smith, R. G. (1977). Effects of alcohol on the speech of non-alcoholics. *Central States Speech Journal, 28*, 140–143.

Andrews, M. L., & Smith, R. G. (1976). Perceptions of auditory components of stuttered speech. *Journal of Communication Disorders, 9*, 121–128.

Aronson, A. E. (1990). *Clinical voice disorders: An interdisciplinary approach* (3rd ed.). New York: Thieme Medical Publishers.

Ashton, H. (1987). *Brain systems, disorders, and psychotropic drugs*. Oxford, England: Oxford University Press.

Babor, T. F., Mendelson, J. H., Gallant, B. A., & Kuehnle, J. C. (1978). Interpersonal behavior in a group discussion during marijuana intoxication. *International Journal of the Addictions, 13*, 89–102.

Babor, T. F., Mendelson, J. H., Uhly, B., & Kuehnle, J. C. (1978). Social effects of marijuana use in a recreational setting. *International Journal of the Addictions, 13*, 947–959.

Babor, T. F., Meyer, R. E., Mirin, S. M., McNamee, H. B., & Davies, M. (1976). Behavior and social effects of heroin self-administration and withdrawal. *Archives of General Psychiatry, 33,* 363–367.

Babor, T. F., Rossi, A. M., Sagotsky, G., & Meyer, R. E. (1974a). Group behavior: Patterns of smoking. In: J. H. Mendelson, A. M. Rossi, & R. E. Meyer (Eds.), *The use of marijuana: A psychological and physiological inquiry* (pp. 47–59). New York: Plenum Press.

Babor, T. F., Rossi, A. M., Sagotsky, G., & Meyer, R. E. (1974b). Group behavior: Verbal interaction. In: J. H. Mendelson, A. M. Rossi, & R. E. Meyer (Eds.), *The use of marijuana: A psychological and physiological inquiry* (pp. 61–72). New York: Plenum Press.

Baken, R. J. (1987). *Clinical measurement of speech and voice.* Boston: College-Hill Press.

Balint, I. (1961). Die Rolle des Alkohols bei Betriebsunfällen. *Zentralblatt für Arbeitsmedizin, Arbeitsschutz, Prophylaxie und Ergonomie, 11,* 60–63.

Bárány, E. H., & Halldén, U. (1947). The influence of some central nervous system depressants on the reciprocal inhibition between the two retinae as manifested in retinal rivalry. *Acta Physiologica Scandinavica, 14,* 298–316.

Batt, R. D. (1989). Absorption, distribution, and elimination of alcohol. In: K. E. Crow & R. D. Batt (Eds.), *Human metabolism of alcohol, Vol I: Pharmacokinetics, medicolegal aspects, and general interest* (pp. 3–8). Boca Raton, FL: CRC Press.

Beam, S. L., Gant, R. W., & Mecham, M. J. (1978). Communication deviations in alcoholics: A pilot study. *Journal of Studies on Alcohol, 39,* 548–551.

Behne, D. M., & Rivera, S. M. (1990). Effects of alcohol on speech: Acoustic analysis of spondees. *Research on Speech Perception, 16,* 263–291.

Behne, D. M., Rivera, S. M., & Pisoni, D. B. (1991). Effects of alcohol on speech: Durations of isolated words, sentences and passages. *Research on Speech Perception, 17,* 285–301.

Belt, B. L. (1969). *Driver eye movement as a function of low alcohol concentrations.* Columbus: The Ohio State University, Driving Research Laboratory.

Berkow, R. (Ed.) (1992). *The Merck manual of diagnosis and therapy* (16th ed). Rahway, NJ: Merck & Co.

Berry, M. S., & Pentreath, V. W. (1980). The neurophysiology of alcohol. In M. Sandler (Ed.), *Psychopharmacology of Alcohol* (pp. 43–72). New York: Raven Press.

Bishop, K. (1990, April 6). Leaps of science create quandaries on evidence. *New York Times,* p. B6.

Black, H. C. (1979). *Black's law dictionary* (5th ed.). St. Paul, MN: West Publishing Company.

Blomberg, L.-H., & Wassén, A. (1962). The effect of small doses of alcohol on the 'optokinetic fusion limit.' *Acta Physiologica Scandinavica, 54,* 193–199.

Borden, G. J. (1971). *Some effects of oral anesthesia upon speech: A perceptual and electromyographic analysis.* Doctoral dissertation, City University, New York.

Borden, G. J., & Harris, K. S. (1984). *Speech science primer: Physiology, acoustics, and perception of speech* (2nd ed.). Baltimore and London: Williams & Wilkins.

Borden, G. J., Harris, K. S., & Raphael, L. J. (1994). *Speech science primer: Physiology, acoustics, and perception of speech* (3d ed.). Baltimore and London: Williams & Wilkins.

Borkenstein, R. F., & Smith, H. W. (1961). The Breathalyzer and its application. *Medicine, Science and the Law, 1,* 13–22.

Braun, A. (1991). Speaking while intoxicated: Phonetic and forensic aspects. *Proceedings of the XIIth International Congress of Phonetic Sciences, Aix-en-Provence* (Vol. 4, pp. 146–149). Aix-en-Provence: Université de Provence.

Brenner, M. & Cash, J. R. (1991). Speech analysis as an index of alcohol intoxication—The Exxon Valdez accident. *Aviation, Space, and Environmental Medicine, 62,* 893–898.

Brenner, M., Shipp, T., Doherty, E. T., & Morrissey, P. (1985). Voice measures of psychological stress–Laboratory and field data. In I. R. Titze & R. C. Scherer (Eds.), *Vocal fold physiology: Biomechanics, acoustics and phonatory control* (pp. 239–248). Denver, CO: The Denver Center for the Performing Arts.

Broca, P. (1861). Remarques sur le siège de la faculté du langage articulé; suivies d'une observasion d'aphémie (perte de la parole). *Bulletin de la Société Anatomique de Paris, 36,* 330–357.

Broca, P. (1863). Localisation des fonctions cérébrales: Siège du langage articulé. *Bulletin de la Société d'Anthropologie de Paris, 4,* 200–202.

Browman, C. P. & Goldstein, L. (1986). Towards an articulatory phonology. *Phonology Yearbook, 3,* 219–252.

Browman, C. P. & Goldstein, L. (1989). Articulatory gestures as phonological units. *Phonology, 6,* 201–251.

Browman, C. P. & Goldstein, L. (1992). Articulatory phonology: An overview. *Phonetica, 49,* 155–180.

Burchfield, R. W. (Ed.). (1976). *A supplement to the Oxford English dictionary.* Oxford, England: The Clarendon Press.

Burns, M., & Moskowitz, H. (1977). *Psychophysical tests for DWI* (NHTSA Report No. DOT HS-802 424). Washington, DC: National Highway Transportation Safety Administration.

Cahalan, D., Cisin, I. H., Crossley, H. M. (1969). American drinking practices: A national survey of drinking behavior and patterns (Monograph No. 6). New Brunswick, NJ: Rutgers Center of Alcohol Studies.

Carrow-Woolfolk, E. (1974). *Carrow elicited language inventory.* Austin, TX: Learning Concepts.

Catford, J. C. (1977). *Fundamental problems in phonetics.* Edinburgh: Edinburgh University Press.

Chardon, G., Boiteau, H., & Bogaert, E. (1959). Etude de l'action de très faibles doses d'alcool sur l'activité nerveuse supérieure. *Annales de Médecine Légale, Criminologie, Police Scientifique et Toxicologie, 39,* 462–472.

Chevrie-Muller, C., Dordain, M., & Gremy, F. (1970). Etude phoniatrique clinique et instrumentale des dysarthries. II. Résultat chez les malades présentant des syndromes bulbaires et pseudo-bulbaires. *Revue Neurologique, 122,* 123–138.

Chevrie-Muller, C., & Grappin-Gilette, M. L. (1971). Etude oscillographique des consonnes occlusives orales chez les sujets infirmes moteurs cérébraux (essai d'interprétation physio- pathologique de troubles de l'articulation chez les infirmes moteurs cérébraux). *Revue de Laryngologie, Otologie, Rhinologie, 92,* 492–534.

Chiba, T., & Kajiyama, J. (1941). *The vowel: Its nature and sructure.* Tokyo: Tokyo–Kaiseikan Publishing.

Chu, N.-S. (1983). Effects of ethanol on rat cerebellar Purkinje cells. *International Journal of Neuroscience, 21,* 265–277.

Collins, P. J. (1980). A comparison of the oral syntactic performance of alcoholic and non-alcoholic adults. *Language and Speech, 23,* 281–288.

Colquhoun, W. P. (1962). Effets d'une faible dose d'alcool et certains autres facteurs sur la performance dans une tâche de vigilance. *Bulletin du Centre d'Études et Recherches Psychotechniques, 11,* 27ff.

Colton, R. H., & Conture, E. G. (1990). Problems and pitfalls of electroglottography. *Journal of Voice, 4,* 10–24.

Colton, R. H., & Casper, J. K. (1990). *Understanding voice problems: A physiological perspective for diagnosis and treatment.* Baltimore: Williams & Wilkins.

Crow, K. E., & Batt, R. D. (Eds.). (1989). *Human metabolism of acohol* (3 vols.). Boca Raton, FL: CRC Press.

Cummings, K. E. (1992). *Analysis, synthesis, and recognition of stressed speech.* Doctoral dissertation, Georgia Institute of Technology, Atlanta.

Cummings, K. E., Chin, S. B., & Pisoni, D. B. (1996). *Analysis of the glottal excitation of intoxicated versus sober speech: A first report.* Paper presented at the 131st meeting of the Acoustical Society of America, Indianapolis, IN.

Cummings, K. E., & Clements, M. (1990, April). Analysis of glottal waveforms across stress styles. *Proceedings of the International Conference on Acoustics, Speech, and Signal Processing, 1,* 301–304.

Cummings, K. E., & Clements, M. (1992, March). Improvements to and applications of analysis of stressed speech using glottal waveforms. *Proceedings of the International Conference on Acoustics, Speech, and Signal Processing, 2,* 25–28.

Cummings, K. E., & Clements, M. (1993, April). Application of the analysis of glottal excitation of stressed speech to speaking style modification. *Proceedings of the International Conference on Acoustics, Speech, and Signal Processing, 2,* 207–210.

Cummings, K. E., & Clements, M. (1995). Glottal models for digital speech processing: A historical survey and new results. *Digital Signal Processing: A Review Journal, 5,* 21–42.

Darley, F. L., Aronson, A. E., & Brown, J. R. (1975). *Motor speech disorders.* Philadelphia: Saunders.

Davis, S. B. (1976). *Computer evaluation of laryngeal pathology based on inverse filtering of speech* (SCRL Monograph No. 13). Santa Barbara, CA: Speech Communications Research Lab.

DeJong, G., Hollien, H., Martin, C., & Alderman, G. A. (1995). Speaking rate and alcohol intoxication [Abstract]. *Journal of the Acoustical Society of America, 97,* 3364.

Denes, P. B., & Pinson, E. N. (1993). *The speech chain: The physics and biology of spoken language* (2nd ed.). New York: Freeman.

Dickson, D. R., & Maue-Dickson, W. (1982). *Anatomical and physiological bases of speech.* Boston: Little, Brown.

Dildy-Mayfield, J. E., & Leslie, S. W. (1991). Mechanism of inhibition of N-methyl-D-aspartate-stimulated increases in free intracellular Ca^{2+} concentration by ethanol. *Journal of Neurochemistry, 56,* 1536–1543.

Docter, R. F., Naitoh, R., & Smith, J. C. (1966). Electroencephalographic changes and vigilance behavior during experimentally induced intoxication with alcoholic subjects. *Psychosomatic Medicine, 28,* 605–615.

Dodge, R. & Benedict F. G. (1915). *Psychological effects of alcohol: An experimental investigation of moderate doses of ethyl alcohol on a related group of neuromuscular processes in man* (Publication No. 232). Washington, DC: Carnegie Institution of Washington.

Donegan, P. J. & Stampe, D. (1979). The study of natural phonology. In D. A. Dinnsen (Ed.), *Current approaches to phonological theory* (pp. 126–173). Bloomington: Indiana University Press.

Dordain, M., Degos, J. D., & Dordain G. (1971). Troubles de la voix dans l'hémiplégie gauche. *Revue de Laryngologie, Otologie, Rhinologie, 92,* 178–188.

Dordain, M. & Dordain, G. (1972). L'épreuve du (A) tenu au cours des tremblements de la voix (tremblement idiopathique et dyskinésie volitionelle, leurs rapports avec la dysphonie spasmodique). *Revue de Laryngologie, Otologie, Rhinologie, 93,* 167–182.

Drew, G. C., Colquhoun, W. P., & Long, H. A. (1958). Effect of small doses of alcohol on a skill resembling driving. *British Medical Journal, 2,* 993–999.

Dubowski, K. M. (1985). Absorption, distribution, and elimination of alcohol: Highway safety aspects. *Journal of Studies on Alcohol, Supplement, 10,* 98–108.

Dubowski, K. M. (1986). Recent developments in alcohol analysis. *Alcohol, Drugs and Driving: Abstracts and Reviews, 2,* 13–46.

Dubowski, K. M. (1991). *The technology of breath–alcohol analysis* (DHHS Publication No. (ADM)92–1728). Rockville, MD: U.S. Department of Health and Human Services.

Dunker, E. & Schlosshauer, B. (1964). Irregularities of the laryngeal vibratory pattern in healthy and hoarse persons. In D. W. Brewer (Ed.), *Research potentials in voice physiology* (*International Conference at Syracuse, 1961*) (pp. 151–184). [Syracuse:] State University of New York.

Dunlap, J. D., Pisoni, D., Bernacki, R. H., & Rose, R. J. (1995). *Alterations in speech production following alcohol challenge: A marker of acute susceptibility?* Poster presented at the annual meeting of the Research Society on Alcoholism, Steamboat Springs, CO.

Eighth Special Report to the U.S. Congress on Alcohol and Health from the Secretary of Health and Human Services. (1993, September). Rockville, MD: U.S. Department of Health and Human Services, Public Health Service, National Institutes of Health, National Institute on Alcohol Abuse and Alcoholism.

Eysholdt, U. (1992). Stroboscopic findings and clinical voice changes under acute alcohol intoxication/Aspects stroboscopiques et cliniques des perturbations vocales sous intoxication éthylique aiguë. *Bulletin d'Audiophonologie, 8,* 53–62.

Fabré, P. (1957). Un procédé électrique percutané d'inscription de l'accolement glottique au cours de la phonation: Glottographie de haute fréquence. Premiers résultats. *Bulletin de l'Académie Nationale de Médecine (Paris), 141,* 66–69.

Fairbanks, G. (1960). *Voice and articulation drillbook* (2nd ed.). New York: Harper & Row.

Fant, G. (1960). *Acoustic theory of speech production.* The Hague: Mouton.

Fisher, H. B., & Logemann, J. A. (1971). *Fisher-Logemann test of articulation competence.* Boston: Houghton-Mifflin.

Fletcher, S. G. (1978). *The Fletcher time-by-count test of diadochokinetic syllable rate.* Tigard, OR: C. C. Publications.

Fontan, M., Bouanna, G., Piquet, J. M., & Wgeux, F. (1978). Les troubles articulatoires chez l'éthylique. *Lille Médical, 23,* 529–542.

Forney, R. B. (1971). General pharmacology of alcohol [Abstract]. *American Pharmaceutical Association Academy of Pharmaceutical Sciences, 1,* 28–29.

Forney, R. B. & Hughes, F. W. (1961). Delayed auditory feedback and ethanol: Effect on verbal and arithmetical performance. *Journal of Psychology, 52,* 185–192.

Forney, R. B., Hughes, F. W., Harger, R. N., & Richards, A. B. (1964). Alcohol distribution in the vascular system: Concentration of orally administered alcohol in blood from various points in the vascular system, and in rebreathed air, during absorption. *Quarterly Journal of Studies on Alcohol, 25,* 205–217.

Forshee, J. C., & Nusbaum, H. C. (1984). An update on computer facilities in the Speech Research Laboratory. *Research on Speech Perception, 10,* 453–462.

Franklin, C. L., & Gruol, D. L. (1987). Acute ethanol alters the firing pattern and glutamate response of cerebellar Purkinje neurons in culture. *Brain Research, 416,* 205–218.

Franks, H. M., Hensley, V. R., Hensley, W. J., Starmer, G., & Teo, R. K. C. (1975). The relationship between alcohol dosage and performance decrement in humans. *Journal of Studies on Alcohol, 37,* 284–297.

Fregly, A. R., Bergstedt, M., & Graybiel, A. (1967). Relationships between blood alcohol, positional alcohol nystagmus and postural equilibrium. *Quarterly Journal of Studies on Alcohol, 28,* 11–21.

Fry, D. B. (1979). *The physics of speech.* Cambridge, England: Cambridge University Press.

Gay, T., Lindblom, B., & Lubker, J. (1981). Production of bite-block vowels: Acoustic equivalence by selective compensation. *Journal of the Acoustical Society of America, 69,* 802–810.

Gianelli, P. C. (1980). The admissibility of novel scientific evidence: *Frye v. United States,* a half-century later. *Columbia Law Review, 80,* 1197–1250.

Givens, B. S., & Breese, G. R. (1990). Electrophysiological evidence that ethanol alters function of medial septal area without affecting lateral septa function. *Journal of Pharmacology and Experimental Therapeutics, 253,* 95–103.

Gleason, H. (1961). *An introduction to descriptive linguistics* (2nd ed.). New York: Holt.

Goldman-Eisler, F. (1968). *Psycholinguistics: Experiments in Spontaneous Speech.* London and New York: Academic Press.

Goodwin, D., Othmer, E., Halikas, J., & Freeman, F. (1970). Loss of short-term memory as a predictor of the alcoholic 'blackout.' *Nature* (London), 227, 201–202.

Gough, H. G. (1969). *Manual for the California psychological inventory.* Palo Alto, CA: Consulting Psychologists Press.

Grassegger, H. (1994). Libri: H. J. Künzel, A. Braun, U. Eysholdt: Einfluss von Alkohol auf Sprache und Stimme. *Phonetica, 51,* 239–240.

Green, D. M., & Swets, J. A. (1966). *Signal detection theory and psychophysics.* New York: Wiley.

Gremy, F., Chevrie-Muller, C., & Garde, E. (1967). Etude phoniatrique clinique et instrumentale des dysarthries. I. Technique, résultat chez les malades présentant un syndrome cérébelleux. *Revue Neurologique, 116,* 401–426.

Griffiths, R. R., Stitzer, M., Corker, K., Bigelow, G. E., & Liebson, I. (1977). Drug produced changes in human social behavior: Facilitation by d-amphetamine. *Pharmacology, Biochemistry and Behavior, 7,* 365–372.

Grüner, O. (1955). Alkohol und Aufmerksamkeit. Ihre Bedeutung im motorischen Verkehr. *Deutsche Zeitschrift für die Gesamte Gerichtliche Medizin, 44,* 187–195.

Grüner, O. (1959). Konstitutionelle Unterschiede der Alkoholwirkung. *Deutsche Zeitschrift für die Gesamte Gerichtliche Medizin, 49,* 84–90.

Grüner, O., Ludwig, O., & Domer, H. (1964). Zur Abhängigkeit alkoholbedingter Aufmerksamkeitsstörungen vom Blutalkoholwert bei niedrigen Konzentrationen. *Blutalkohol, 3,* 445–452.

Guedry, F. E. J., Gilson, R. D., Schroeder, D. J., & Collins, W. E. (1975). Some effects of alcohol on various aspects of oculomotor control. *Aviation, Space, and Environmental Medicine, 46,* 1008–1013.

Haertzen, C. A. (1966). Development of scales based on patterns of drug effects, using the Addiction Research Center Inventory (ARCI). *Psychological Reports, 18,* 163–194.

Haggard, H. W. & Jellinek, E. M. (1942). *Alcohol explored.* Garden City, NY: Doubleday.

Harger, R. N. & Hulpieu, H. R. (1956). Chapter Two: The pharmacology of alcohol. In G. N. Thompson (Ed.), *Alcoholism* (pp. 103–232). Springfield, IL: Charles C. Thomas.

Hartocollis, P. & Johnson, D. M. (1956). Differential effects of alcohol on verbal fluency. *Quarterly Journal of Studies on Alcohol, 17,* 183–189.

Hecker, M. H. L., & Kreul, E. J. (1971). Descriptions of the speech of patients with cancer of the vocal folds. Part I. Measures of fundamental frequency. *Journal of the Acoustical Society of America, 49,* 1275–1282.

Heffner, R.-M. S. (1950). *General phonetics.* Madison: University of Wisconsin Press.

Heise, H. A. (1934). Specificity of test for alcohol in body fluids. *American Journal of Clinical Pathology, 4,* 182–188.

Higgins, S. T. & Stitzer, M. L. (1986). Acute marijuana effects on social conversation. *Psychopharmacology, 89,* 234–238.

Higgins, S. T. & Stitzer, M. L. (1988). Effects of alcohol on speaking in isolated humans. *Psychopharamacology, 95,* 189–194.

Hirano, M. (1974). Morphological structure of the vocal cord as a vibrator and its variations. *Folia Phoniatrica, 26,* 89–94.

Hirano, M. (1981). *Clinical examination of voice.* Vienna and New York: Springer-Verlag.

Hiraoka, N., Kitzoe, Y., Ueta, H., Tanaka, S., & Tanabe, M. (1984). Harmonic-intensity analysis of normal and hoarse voice. *Journal of the Acoustical Society of America, 76,* 1648–1651.

Hollien, H. (1985). *Pilot study of intoxication effects on voice* [Report]. Gainesville, FL: IASCP [Institute for Advanced Study of the Communication Processes].

Hollien, H. (1990). *The acoustics of crime: The new science of forensic phonetics.* New York: Plenum Press.

Hollien, H. (1993). An oilspill, alcohol and the captain: A possible misapplication of forensic science. *Forensic Science International, 60,* 97–105.

Hollien, H., Michel, J., & Doherty, E. T. (1973). A method for analyzing vocal jitter in sustained phonation. *Journal of Phonetics, 1,* 85–91.

Hollien, H., & Martin, C. (1995). Interrelationships between ethanol intoxication and speech [Abstract]. *Journal of the Acoustical Society of America, 97,* 3363.

Hollien, H., & Martin, C. A. (1996). Conducting research on the effects of intoxication on speech. *Forensic Linguistics: The International Journal of Speech, Language and the Law, 3,* 107–127.

Hollingworth, H. L. (1923). The influence of alcohol. *Journal of Abnormal Psychology and Social Psychology, 18,* 204–237.

Horii, Y. (1979). Fundamental frequency perturbation observed in sustained phonation. *Journal of Speech and Hearing Research, 22,* 5–19.

Hughes, F. W., & Forney, R. B. (1964). Comparative effect of three antihistiminics and ethanol on mental and motor performance. *Clincal Pharmacology and Therapeutics, 5,* 414–421.

Hunt, W. A. (1985). *Alcohol and biological membranes.* New York: Guilford Press.

Huntley, M. S. (1970). *Effects of alcohol and fixation-task demands upon human reaction time to achromatic targets in the horizontal meridian of the visual field.* Doctoral dissertation, University of Vermont, Burlington.

International Phonetic Association. (1989). Report on the 1989 Kiel convention. *Journal of the International Phonetic Association, 19,* 67–80.

Jellinek, E. M. & MacFarland, R. A. (1940). Analysis of psychological experiments on the effects of alcohol. *Quarterly Journal of Studies on Alcohol, 1,* 272–371.

Jetter, W. W. (1938a). Studies in alcohol I: The diagnosis of acute alcoholic intoxication by a correlation of clinical and chemical findings. *American Journal of the Medical Sciences, 196,* 477–487.

Jetter, W. W. (1938b). Studies in alcohol II: Experimental feeding of alcohol to non-alcoholic individuals. *American Journal of the Medical Sciences, 196,* 487–493.

Johnson, K., Pisoni, D. B., & Bernacki, R. H. (1989). Report to the NTSB: Analysis of speech produced by the captain of the Exxon Valdez. *Research on Speech Perception, 15,* 1–9.

Johnson, K., Pisoni, D. B., & Bernacki, R. H. (1990). Do voice recordings reveal whether a person is intoxicated? A case study. *Phonetica, 47,* 215–237.

Johnson, K., Southwood, M. H., Schmidt, A. M., Mouli, C. M., Holmes, A. T., Armstrong, A. A., Critz-Crosby, P., Sutphin, S. M., Crosby, R., McCutcheon, M. J., & Wilson, A. S. (1993). *A physiological study of the effects of alcohol on speech and voice.* Paper presented at the 22nd annual Symposium on the Care of the Professional Voice at the Voice Foundation.

Johnson, W., Boehmler, R. M., Dahlstrom, W. G., Darley, F. L., Goodstein, L. D., Kools, J. A., Neelley, J. N., Prather, W. F., Sherman, D., Thurman, C. G., Trotter, W. D., Williams, D., & Young, M. A. (1959). *The Onset of Stuttering: Research Findings and Implications.* Minneapolis: University of Minnesota Press.

Johnson, W., Darley, F., & Spriesterbach, D. C. (1963). *Diagnostic methods in speech pathology*. New York: Harper & Row.

Jones, A. W. (1989). Measurement of alcohol in blood and breath for legal purposes. In K. E. Crow & R. D. Batt (Eds.), *Human metabolism of alcohol: Vol. I. Pharmacokinetics, medicolegal aspects, and general interest* (pp. 71–99). Boca Raton, FL: CRC Press.

Jones, B. M. (1973). Memory impairment on the ascending and descending limbs of the blood alcohol curve. *Journal of Abnormal Psychology, 82*, 24–32.

Jones, K. L., & Smith, D. W. (1973). Recognition of the fetal alcohol syndrome in early infancy. *Lancet, 2*, 999–1001.

Jones, K. L., Smith, D. W., Ulleland, C. N., & Streissguth, A. P. (1973). Pattern of malformation in offspring of chronic alcoholic mothers. *Lancet, 1*, 1267–1271.

Kahane, J., & Folkins, J. (1984). *Atlas of speech and hearing anatomy*. Columbus, OH: Charles E. Merrill.

Kalant, H. (1971). Absorption, diffusion, distribution, and elimination of ethanol: Effects on biological membranes. In B. Kissin & H. Begleiter (Eds.), *The biology of alcoholism, Vol. 1: Biochemistry* (pp. 1–62). New York: Plenum Press.

Karl, J. H. (1989). *Digital signal processing*. San Diego, CA: Academic Press.

Kasuya, H., Ogawa, S., Mashima, K., & Ebihara, S. (1986). Normalized noise energy as an acoustic measure to evaluate pathologic voice. *Journal of the Acoustical Society of America, 80*, 1329–1334.

Kawi, A. A. (1961). Psychological and physiological changes at the intravenously induced slurred speech threshold for ethyl alcohol. *Journal of Clinical and Experimental Psychopathology & Quarterly Review of Psychiatry and Neurology, 22*, 7–17.

Kent, R. D., & Moll, K. L. (1975). Articulatory timing in selected consonant sequences. *Brain and Language, 2*, 304–323.

Kent, R. D. & Read, C. (1992). *The acoustic analysis of speech*. San Diego, CA: Singular Publishing.

Khanna, J. M., LeBlanc, A. E., & Mayer, J. M. (1989). Alcohol pharmacokinetics and forensic issues: A commentary. In K. E. Crow & R. D. Batt (Eds.), *Human metabolism of alcohol: Vol. I. Pharmacokinetics, medicolegal aspects, and general interest* (pp. 59–70). Boca Raton, FL: CRC Press.

Kissin, B., & Begleiter, H. (Eds.) (1971). *The biology of alcoholism: Vol. 1. Biochemistry*. New York and London: Plenum Press.

Kissin, B., & Begleiter, H. (Eds.) (1972). *The biology of alcoholism: Vol. 2. Physiology and behavior*. New York and London: Plenum Press.

Kissin, B., & Begleiter, H. (Eds.) (1974). *The biology of alcoholism: Vol. 3. Clinical pathology*. New York and London: Plenum Press.

Kitajima, K. (1981). Quantitative evaluation of the noise level in the pathologic voice. *Folia Phoniatrica, 33*, 115–124.

Klatt, D. H. (1975). Voice onset time, frication, and aspiration in word-initial consonant clusters. *Journal of Speech and Hearing Research, 18*, 686–706.

Klingholz, F., Penning, R., & Liebhardt, E. (1988). Recognition of low-level alcohol intoxication from speech signal. *Journal of the Acoustical Society of America, 84*, 929–935.

Kobayashi, M. (1974). Effects of small doses of alcohol on the eye movements of drivers. In *Proceedings of the Sixth International Conference on Alcohol, Drugs and Traffic Safety* (pp. 313–318). Toronto, Ont: Addiction Research Foundation.

Koenig, W., Dunn, H. K., & Lacy, L. Y. (1946). The sound spectrograph. *Journal of the Acoustical Society of America, 18,* 19–49.

Koike, Y. (1973). Application of some acoustic measures for the evaluation of laryngeal dysfunction. *Studia Phonologica, 7,* 17–23.

Kozhevnikov, V. A., & Chistovich, L. A. (1965). *Speech: Articulation and perception* [English translation of *Rech: Artikulyatsiya i Vospriyatiye*] (Joint Publications Research Service Report No. 30,543). Washington, DC: U.S. Department of Commerce, Joint Publications Research Service.

Kuehn, D. P., Lemme, M. L., &, Baumgartner, J. M. (Eds.). (1989). *Neural bases of speech, hearing, and language.* Boston: College-Hill Press.

Künzel, H. J. (1985). Praxis der forensischen Sprechererkennung. *Kriminalistik, 3,* 120–126.

Künzel, H. J. (1987). *Sprechererkennung: Grundzüge forensischer Sprachverarbeitung.* Heidelberg, Germany: Kriminalistik-Verlag.

Künzel, H. J. (1988). Zum Problem der Sprecheridentifizierung durch Opfer und Zeugen. *Goltdammers Archiv für Strafrecht, 5,* 215–224.

Künzel, H. J. (1990, February). Influence of alcohol on speech and language. Paper presented at the 42nd Annual Meeting of the American Academy of Forensic Sciences, Cincinnati, OH.

Künzel, H. J. (1992). Produktion und Perzeption der Sprache alkoholisierter Sprecher. In H. J. Dingeldein & R. Lauf (Eds.), *Phonetik und Dialektologie: Joachim Göschel zum 60. Geburtstag* (pp. 27–53). Marburg, Germany: Philipps-Universität-Bibliothek Marburg.

Künzel, H. J., Braun, A. & Eysholdt, U. (1992). *Einfluss von Alkohol auf Sprache und Stimme.* Heidelberg, Germany: Kriminalistik-Verlag.

Ladefoged, P. (1993). *A course in phonetics* (3rd ed.). New York: Harcourt Brace Jovanovich.

Ladefoged, P., & Broadbent, D. E. (1957). Information conveyed by vowels. *Journal of the Acoustical Society of America, 29,* 98–103.

Laver, J. (1979). The description of voice quality in general phonetic theory (Work in Progress, Vol. 12, pp. 30–52). Edinburgh: Edinburgh University, Department of Lingusitics. (Reprinted in J. Laver, pp. 184–208, 1991) [Citations in text are to the reprint]

Laver, J. (1980). *The phonetic description of voice quality.* Cambridge, England: Cambridge University Press.

Laver, J. (1991). *The gift of speech: Papers in the analysis of speech and voice.* Edinburgh: Edinburgh University Press.

Laver, J. (1994). *Principles of phonetics.* Cambridge, England: Cambridge University Press.

Laver, J., & Trudgill, P. (1979). Phonetic and linguistic markers in speech. In K. R. Scherer & H. Giles (Eds.), *Social markers in speech* (pp. 1–32). Cambridge, England: Cambridge University Press, and Paris: Editions de la Maison des Science de l'Homme. (Reprinted in J. Laver, pp. 235–264, 1991) [Citations in text are to the reprint]

Lawton, M. P., & Cahn, B. (1963). The effects of diazepam (Valium) and alcohol on psychomotor performance. *Journal of Nervous and Mental Disease, 136,* 550–554.

Leake, C. D., & Silverman, M. (1971). The chemistry of alcoholic beverages. In B. Kissin & H. Begleiter (Eds.), *The biology of alcoholism: Vol. 1. Biochemistry* (pp. 575–612). New York and London: Plenum Press.

Lee, L. L. (1974). *Developmental sentence analysis: A grammatical assessment procedure for speech and language clinicians.* Evanston, IL: Northwestern University Press.

Lemme, M. L., Kuehn, D. P., & Baumgartner, J. M. (1989). Studying the nervous system: Communication science perspective. In D. P. Kuehn, M. L. Lemme, & J. M. Baumgartner (Eds.), *Neural bases of speech, hearing, and language* (pp. 1–24). Boston: College-Hill Press.

Lemoine, P., Harouseau, H., Borteryu, J. T., & Menuet, J.-C. (1968). Les enfants des parents alcooliques. Anomalies observées à-propos de 127 cas. *Ouest Médical, 21,* 476–482.

Lennard, H., Jarvik, M.D., & Abramson, H. A. (1956). Lysergic acid diethylamide (LSD-25): XII. A preliminary statement of its effects upon interpersonal communication. *Journal of Psychology 41,* 185–198.

Lennard, H. L., Epstein, L. S., Katzung, B. G. (1967). Psychoactive drug action and group interaction processes. *Journal of Nervous and Mental Disease, 145,* 68–78.

Lenneberg, E. H. (1967). *Biological foundations of language.* New York: Wiley.

Lester, L. & Skousen, R. (1974). The phonology of drunkenness. In A. Bruck, R. Fox, & M. W. LaGaly (Eds.), *Papers from the parasession on natural phonology* (pp. 233–239). Chicago, IL: Chicago Linguistic Society.

Lieberman, P. (1977). *Speech physiology and acoustic phonetics: An introduction.* New York: Macmillan.

Lin, A. M., Freund, R. K., & Palmer, M. R. (1991). Ethanol potentiation of GABA-induced electrophysiological responses in cerebellum: Requirement for catecholamine modulation. *Neuroscience Letters, 122,* 154–158.

Linnoila, M. (1974). Effect of drugs and alcohol on psychomotor skills related to driving. *Annals of Clinical Research, 6,* 7–18.

Love, R. J., & Webb, W. G. (1986). *Neurology for the speech–language pathologist.* Boston: Butterworth.

Lovinger, D. M., White, G., & Weight, F. F. (1989). Ethanol inhibits NMDA-activated ion current in hippocampal neurons. *Science, 243,* 1721–1724.

Lundquist, F., & Wolthers, H. (1958). The kinetics of alcohol elimination in man. *Acta Pharmacologica et Toxicologica, 14,* 265–289.

Lyons, J. (1977). *Semantics* (2 vols.). Cambridge, England: Cambridge University Press.

MacAndrew, C. (1965). The differentiation of male alcoholic outpatients from nonalcoholic psychiatric outpatients by means of the MMPI. *Quarterly Journal of Studies on Alcohol, 26,* 238–246.

Machover, K. (1949). *Personality projection in the drawing of the human figure.* Springfield, IL: Charles C. Thomas.

Martin, R., LeBreton, R., & Roche, M. (1957). Variations individuelles du comportement sous l'influence des doses moyennes d'alcool éthylique. *Annales du Medicine Legale, 37,* 56– 70.

Martin, W. R., Sloan, J. W., Sapira, J. D., & Jasinski, D. R. (1971). Physiologic, subjective, and behavioral effects of amphetamine, methamphetamine, ephedrine, phenmetrazine, and methylphenidate in man. *Clinical Pharmacology and Therapeutics, 12,* 245–258.

Mayfield, D., McLeod, G., Hall, P. (1974). The CAGE questionnaire: Validation of a new alcoholism screening instrument. *American Journal of Psychiatry, 131,* 1121–1123.

McDavid, R. I., & Muri, J. T. (1967). *Americans speaking.* Champaign, IL: National Council of Teachers of English.

McGuire, M. T., Stein, S., & Mendelson, J. H. (1966). Comparative psycho-social studies of alcoholic and nonalcoholic subjects undergoing experimentally induced ethanol intoxication. *Psychosomatic Medicine, 28,* 13–26.

Mellanby, E. (1919). *Alcohol: Its absorption into and disappearance from the blood under different conditions* (Medical Research Committee Special Report Series No. 31). London: Oxford University Press.

Meyer, H. H. & Gottlieb, R. (1914). *Die experimentelle Pharmakologie als Grundlage der Artzneibehandlung: ein Lehrbuch für Studierende und Ärzte* (3rd rev. ed.). Berlin: Urban & Schwarzenberg.

Michaelis, L., & Menten, M. L. (1913). Die Kinetik der Invertinwirkung. *Biochemische Zeitschrift, 49,* 333–369.

Mishler, E., & Waxler, N. (1968). *Interaction in families.* New York: Wiley.

Mizoi, Y., Fukunaga, T., & Adachi, J. (1989). The flushing syndrome in Orientals. In K. E. Crow & R. D. Batt (Eds.), *Human metabolism of alcohol: Vol. II. Regulation, enzymology, and metabolites of ethanol* (pp. 219–229). Boca Raton, FL: CRC Press.

Monnier, D. (1956). Un nouvel appareil de dépistage de l'alcoolisme: Le Breathalyzer. *Revue Internationale de Criminologie et de Police Technique, 10,* 1–6.

Montagu, A. (1958). *Man: His first million years.* New York: New American Library.

Mortimer, R. G. (1963). Effect of low blood-alcohol concentrations in simulated day and night driving. *Perceptual and Motor Skills, 17,* 399–408.

Mortimer, R. G., & Sturgis, S. P. (1972). *Effects of alcohol on driving skills* (National Institute on Alcohol Abuse and Alcoholism). Ann Arbor, MI: Highway Safety Research Institute.

Moskowitz, H., Daily, J., & Henderson, R. (1979). The Mellanby effect in moderate and heavy drinkers. In I. R. Johnson (Ed.), *Alcohol, Drugs and Traffic Safety* (pp. 139ff). Canberra: Australian Government Publishing Service.

Moskowitz, H., & Murray, J. (1976). Alcohol and backward masking of visual information. *Quarterly Journal of Studies on Alcohol, 37,* 40–45.

Moskowitz, H. & Roth, S. 1971. Effect of alcohol on response latency in object naming. *Quarterly Journal of Studies on Alcohol, 32,* 969–975.

Müller, J. (1848). *The physiology of the senses, voice and muscular motion with the mental faculties* (W. Baly, Trans.). London: Walton and Maberly.

Murray, H. A. (1943). *Thematic apperception test: Examiner's manual.* Cambridge, MA: Harvard University Press.

Murray, J. A. H., Bradley, H., Craigie, W. A., & Onions, C. T. (Eds.). (1933). *Oxford English dictionary.* Oxford, England: Clarendon Press.

Nash, H. (1962). *Alcohol and caffeine: A study of their psychological effects.* Springfield, IL: Charles C. Thomas.

Natale, M., Kanzler, M., Jaffe, J., & Jaffe, J. (1980). Acute effects of alcohol defensive and primary-process language. Results with three human volunteers. *International Journal of the Addictions, 15,* 1055–1067.

National Transportation Safety Board. (1990). *Marine accident report—Grounding of the U.S. Tankship EXXON VALDEZ on Bligh Reef, Prince William Sound, near Valdez, Alaska, March 24, 1989* (Report No. NTSB/MAR-90/04). Washington, DC: U.S. Government Printing Office.

Netsell, R. (1982). Speech motor control and selected neurologic disorders. In: S. Grillner, B. Lindblom, J. Lubker, & A. Persson (Eds.), *Speech motor control* (pp. 247–261). New York: Pergamon Press. (Reprinted in *A neurobiologic view of speech production and the dysarthrias,* pp. 33–52, by R. Netsell, 1986, San Diego, CA: College-Hill Press) [Citations in text are to the reprint]

Netsell, R., Kent, R., & Abbs, J. (1980). *The organization and reorganization of speech movements.* Paper presented at the Society for Neuroscience, Cincinnati, OH.

Newman, H., Fletcher, E., & Abramson, M. (1942). Alcohol and driving. *Quarterly Journal of Studies on Alcohol, 3,* 15–30.

Niedzielska, G., Pruszewicz, A., & Swidzinski, P. (1994). Acoustic evaluation of voice in individuals with alcohol addiction. *Folia Phoniatrica et Logopaedica, 46,* 115–122.

Oldfield, R. C. & Wingfield, A. (1965). Response latencies in naming objects. *Quarterly Journal of Experimental Psychology, 17,* 273–281.

Oppenheim, A. V., & Schafer, R. W. (1975). *Digital signal processing.* Englewood Cliffs, NJ: Prentice-Hall.

Palmer, M. R., VanHorne, C. G., Harlan, J. T., & Moore, E. A. (1988). Antagonism of ethanol effects on cerebellar Purkinje neurons by the benzodiazepine inverse agonists RO 15-4513 and FG 7124: Electrophysiological studies. *Journal of Pharmacology and Experimental Therapeutics, 247,* 1018–1024.

Penfield, W., & Roberts, L. (1959). *Speech and brain—mechanisms.* Princeton, NJ: Princeton University Press.

Peters, F. H. (Ed.). (1957). *Aristotle's selections.* New York: Fine Editions Press.

Pihkanen, T., & Kauko, O. (1962). The effects of alcohol on the perception of musical stimuli. *Annales Medicinae Experimentalis et Biologia Fenniae, 40,* 275–285.

Pisoni, D. B., Hathaway, S. N., & Yuchtman, M. (1985). *Effects of alcohol on the acoustic-phonetic properties of speech: Final report to GM Research Laboratories.* (SRL Technical Note No. 85-03). Bloomington: Indiana University.

Pisoni, D. B., Johnson, K., & Bernacki, R. H. (1991). Effects of alcohol on speech. In *Proceedings of the Human Factors Society* (pp. 694–698). Santa Monica, CA: Human Factors Society.

Pisoni, D. B. & Martin, C. S. (1989). Effects of alcohol on the acoustic-phonetic properties of speech: Perceptual and acoustic analyses. *Alcoholism: Clinical and Experimental Research, 13,* 577–587.

Pisoni, D. B., Yuchtman, M., & Hathaway, S. N. (1986). Effects of alcohol on the acoustic-phonetic properties of speech. In Society of Automotive Engineers (Ed.),

Alcohol, Accidents, and Injuries (pp. 131–150). Warrendale, PA: Society of Automotive Engineers.

Pliner, P., & Cappell H. (1974). Modification of affective consequences of alcohol. *Journal of Abnormal Psychology, 83,* 418–425.

Pohorecky, L. A. (1977). Biphasic action of ethanol. *Neuroscience and Biobehavioral Reviews, 1,* 231–240.

Pokorny, A. D., Miller, B. A., & Kaplan, H. B. (1972). The brief MAST: A shortened version of the Michigan Alcoholism Screening Test. *American Journal of Psychiatry, 129,* 342–348.

Pruszewicz, A., Obrebowski, A., Swidzinski, P., Demenko, G., Wika, T., & Wojciechowska, A. (1991). Usefulness of acoustic studies on the differential diagnostics of organic and functional dysphonia. *Acta Oto-Laryngologica, 111,* 414–419.

Pullum, G. K., & Ladusaw, W. A. (1986). *Phonetic symbol guide.* Chicago: University of Chicago Press.

A question recurs: Was Hazelwood drunk? (1990, February 25). *New York Times* (Associated Press).

Rabiner, L. W., & Gold, B. (1975). *Theory and application of digital signal processing.* Englewood Cliffs, NJ: Prentice-Hall.

Rauschke, J. (1954). Leistungsprüfung bei an- und abfallendem Blutalkoholgehalt unter besonderen Bedingungen. *Deutsche Zeitschrift für die Gesamte Gerichtliche Medizin, 43,* 27–37.

Reiss, D., & Salzman, C. (1973). Resilience of family processes. *Archives of General Psychiatry, 28,* 425–433.

Rizzo, P. (1957). Ricerche sulle modificazioni della frequenza critica degli stimoli luminosi indotte dall'ingestioni di alcool etilico. *Rivista di Medicina Aeronautica, 20,* 249–261.

Rogers, J., Siggins, G. R., Schulman, J. A., & Bloom, F. E. (1979). Physiological correlates of ethanol intoxication, tolerance, and dependence in rat cerebellar Purkinje cells. *Brain Research, 196,* 183–198.

Romano, J., Michael, M., Jr., & Merritt, H. H. (1940). Alcoholic cerebellar degeneration. *Archives of Neurology and Psychiatry, 44,* 1230–1236.

Rosen, L., & Lee, C. (1976). Acute and chronic effects of alcohol use on organization process in memory. *Journal of Abnormal Psychology, 85,* 309–317.

Rossing, T. (1982). *The science of sound.* Reading, MA: Addison-Wesley.

Ryback, R. S. (1971). The continuum and specificity of the effects of alcohol on memory. *Quarterly Journal of Studies of Alcohol, 32,* 995–1016.

Santamaria, J. N. (1989). The effects of ethanol and its metabolism on the brain. In K. E. Crow & R. D. Batt (Eds.), *Human metabolism of alcohol: Vol. III. Metabolic and physiological effects of alcohol* (pp. 35–47). Boca Raton, FL: CRC Press.

Schmidt, I., & Bingel, A. G. A. (1953). *Effect of oxygen deficiency and various other factors on color saturation thresholds* (U.S.A.F. School of Aviation Medical Project Report 21-31-0021). Washington, DC: United States Air Force.

Schroeder, M. R. (1968). Period histogram and product spectrum: New methods for fundamental frequency measurement. *Journal of the Acoustical Society of America, 43,* 829–834.

Seedorf, H. H. (1956). Effects of alcohol on the motor fusion reserves and stereopsis as well as on the tendency to nystagmus. *Acta Ophthalmologica, 34,* 273–280.

Selzer, M. L., Vinokur, A., & Van Rooijen, L. A. (1975). A self-administered Short Michigan Alcoholism Screening Test (SMAST). *Journal of Studies on Alcohol, 36,* 117–126.

Seventh Special Report to the U.S. Congress on Alcohol and Health From the Secretary of Health and Human Services, January 1990. (1990). Rockville, MD: U.S. Department of Health and Human Services; Public Health Service; Alcohol, Drug Abuse, and Mental Health Administration; National Institute on Alcohol Abuse and Alcoholism.

Skipper says Exxon knew of alcoholism. (1994, May 13). *New York Times* (Associated Press), p. A8.

Smith, C. (1992). *Media and apocalypse: News coverage of the Yellowstone forest fires, Exxon Valdez oil spill, and Loma Prieta earthquake* (Contributions to the Study of Mass Media and Communications, No. 36). Westport, CT: Greenwood Press.

Smith, R. C., Parker, E. S, & Noble, E. P. (1975). Alcohol's effect on some formal aspects of verbal social communication. *Archives of General Psychiatry, 32,* 1394–1398.

Sobell, L. C. & Sobell, M. B. (1972). Effects of alcohol on the speech of alcoholics. *Journal of Speech and Hearing Research, 15,* 861–868.

Sobell, L. C., Sobell, M. B., & Coleman, R. F. (1982). Alcohol-induced dysfluency in nonalcoholics. *Folia Phoniatrica, 34,* 316–323.

Starmer, G. A. (1989). Effects of low to moderate doses of ethanol on human driving-related performance. In K. E. Crow & R. D. Batt (Eds.), *Human metabolism of alcohol: Vol. I. Pharmacokinetics, medicolegal aspects, and general interest* (pp. 101–130). Boca Raton, FL: CRC Press.

Stein, D. R. (1966). Linguistic analysis of the speech of a selected group of former alcoholics: A research note. *Quarterly Journal of Studies on Alcohol, 27,* 106–109.

Stevens, K. N. (1964). Acoustical aspects of speech production. In W. O. Fenn & H. Rahn (Eds.), *Handbook of Physiology: Sec. 3. Respiration* (Vol. I., pp. 347–355). Washington, DC: American Physiological Society.

Stevens, K. N., & House, A. S. (1955). Development of a quantitative description of vowel articulation. *Journal of the Acoustical Society of America, 27,* 484–493.

Stevens, K. N., & House, A. S. (1961). An acoustical theory of vowel production and some of its implications. *Journal of Speech and Hearing Research, 4,* 303–320.

Stitzer, M. L., Griffiths, R. R., Bigelow, G. E., & Liebson, I. A. (1981a). Social stimulus factors in drug effects in human subjects. In T. Thompson & C. E. Johanson (Eds.), *Behavioral pharmacology of human drug dependence* (NIDA Research Monograph 37, DHHS Publication No. (ADM) 81-1137, pp. 130–154). Washington, DC: U.S. Department of Health and Human Services.

Stitzer, M. L. Griffiths, R. R., Bigelow, G. E., & Liebson, I. (1981b). Human social conversation: Effects of ethanol, secobarbital and chlorpromazine. *Pharmacology Biochemistry and Behavior, 14,* 353–360.

Stitzer, M. L., McCaul, M. E., Bigelow, G. E., & Liebson, I. A. (1984). Hydromorphone effects on human conversational speech. *Psychopharmacology, 84,* 402–404.

Stone, B. M. (1984). Paper and pencil tests—sensitivity to psychotropic drugs. *British Journal of Clinical Pharmacology, 18* (Suppl.), 15S–20S.

Sturtevant, R. P., & Sturtevant, F. M. (1989). Circadian variation in rates of ethanol metabolism. In K. E. Crow & R. D. Batt (Eds.), *Human metabolism of alcohol: Vol. I. Pharmacokinetics, medicolegal aspects, and general interest* (pp. 23–39). Boca Raton, FL: CRC Press.

Sunshine, I., & Hodnett, N. (1971). Methods for the determination of ethanol and acetaldehyde. In B. Kissin & H. Begleiter (Eds.), *The biology of alcoholism: Vol. 1. Biochemistry* (pp. 545–573). New York and London: Plenum Press.

Suzdak, P. D., & Paul, S. M. (1987). Ethanol stimulates GABA receptor-mediated Cl- ion flux in vitro: Possible relationship to the anxiolytic and intoxicating actions of alcohol. *Psychopharmacology Bulletin, 23*, 445–451.

Swartz, B. L. (1988). *Intrasubject variability in voice onset time as a function of alcohol induced changes in physiological state.* Doctoral dissertation, Michigan State University, East Lansing.

Swartz, B. L. (1992). Resistance of voice onset time variability to intoxication. *Perceptual and Motor Skills, 75*, 415–424.

Swets, J. A. (1986a). Indices of discrimination or diagnostic accuracy: Their ROCs and implied models. *Psychological Bulletin, 99*, 100–117.

Swets, J. A. (1986b). Form of empirical ROCs in discrimination and diagnostic tasks: Implications for theory and measurement of performance. *Psychological Bulletin, 99*, 181–198.

Takahashi, H. & Koike, Y. (1975). Some perceptual dimensions and acoustical correlates of pathologic voices. *Acta Otolaryngologica, Supplement, 338*, 1–24.

Talland, G. A., Mendelson, J. H., & Ryack, P. (1964). Experimentally induced chronic intoxication withdrawal in alcoholics. V. Tests of attention. *Quarterly Journal of Studies on Alcohol, 2* (Suppl.), 74–86.

Tanford, J. A., Pisoni, D. B., & Johnson, K. (1991). Novel scientific evidence of intoxication: Acoustic analysis of voice recordings from the Exxon Valdez. *Journal of Criminal Law and Criminology, 82*, 579–609.

Taylor, J. A. (1951). The relationship of anxiety to the conditioned eyelid response. *Journal of Experimental Psychology, 4*, 81–92.

Taylor, J. A. (1953). A personality scale of manifest anxiety. *Journal of Abnormal and Social Psychology, 48*, 285–290.

Tharp, V., Burns, M., & Moskowitz, H. (1981). *Development and field test of psychophysical tests for DWI arrest* (National Highway Traffic Safety Administration Report No. DOT HS-805 864). Washington, DC: The Administration.

Thorndike, E. L., & Lorge, I. (1944). *The teacher's word book of 30,000 words.* New York: Columbia University Press.

Titze, I. (1990). Interpretation of the electroglottographic signals. *Journal of Voice, 4*, 1–9.

Trager, G. (1958). Paralanguage: A first approximation. *Studies in Linguistics, 13*, 1–12.

Trojan, F. (1955). Zur Grundlegung einer "Entwicklungsphonetik." *Folia Phoniatrica, 7*, 99–115.

Trojan, F. & Kryspin-Exner, K. (1968). The decay of articulation under the influence of alcohol and paraldehyde. *Folia Phoniatrica, 20*, 217–238.

Valdez jurors face basic questions. (1990, March 20). *New York Times* (Associated Press), p. A15.

van den Berg, J. (1958). Myoelastic-aerodynamic theory of voice production. *Journal of Speech and Hearing Research, 1,* 227–244.

Verriest, G., & Laplasse, D. (1965). New data concerning the influence of ethyl alcohol on human visual thresholds. *Experimental Eye Research, 4,* 95–101.

von Wartburg, J.-P. (1989). Pharmacokinetics of alcohol. In K. E. Crow & R. D. Batt (Eds.), *Human metabolism of alcohol: Vol. I. Pharmacokinetics, medicolegal aspects, and general interest* (pp. 9–22). Boca Raton, FL: CRC Press.

von Wright, J., & Mikkonen, V. (1970). The influence of alcohol on the detection of light signals in different parts of the visual field. *Scandanavian Journal of Psychology, 11,* 167–175.

Wallgren, H. & Barry, H., III. (1970). *Actions of alcohol* (2 vols.). Amsterdam: Elsevier.

Warrington, S. J., Ankier, S. I., & Turner, P. (1984). An evaluation of possible interactions between ethanol and trazodone or amitriptyline. *British Journal of Clinical Pharmacology, 18,* 549–557.

Watanabe, H., Shin, T., Matsuo, H., Okuno, F., Tsuji, T., Matsuoka, M., Fukaura, J., & Matsunaga, H. (1994). Studies on vocal fold injection and changes in pitch associated with alcohol intake. *Journal of Voice, 8,* 340–346.

Watson, P. E. (1989). Total body water and blood alcohol levels: Updating the fundamentals. In K. E. Crow & R. D. Batt (Eds.), *Human metabolism of alcohol: Vol. I. Pharmacokinetics, medicolegal aspects, and general interest* (pp. 41–56). Boca Raton, FL: CRC Press.

Wernicke, C. (1874). *Der aphasische Symptomencomplex.* Breslau, Poland: Cohn & Weigert.

Widmark, E. M. P. (1932). *Die theoretischen Grundlagen und die praktische Verwendbarkeit der gerichtlich-medizinischen Alkoholbestimmung.* Berlin, Wien: Urban & Schwarzenberg. (Translated as: *Principles and Applications of Medicolegal Alcohol Determination.* Davis, CA: Biomedical Publications, 1981).

Wilkinson, I. M. S., & Kime, R. (1974). Alcohol and human eye movements. *Transactions of the American Neurological Association, 99,* 38–41.

Williams, G. D., & DeBakey, S. F. (1992). Changes in levels of alcohol consumption: United States, 1983 to 1988. *British Journal of Addiction, 87,* 643–648.

Wilson, M. (1963). A standardized method for obtaining a spoken language sample. *Journal of Speech and Hearing Research, 12,* 95–102.

Wist, E. R., Hughes, F. W., & Forney, R. B. (1967). Effect of low blood alcohol level on stereoscopic acuity and fixation disparity. *Perceptual and Motor Skills, 24,* 83–87.

Wolff, P. (1979). *Theoretical issues in the development of motor skills* (Symposium on Developmental Disabilities in the Pre-School Child) Chicago: Johnson & Johnson Baby Products.

Wong, D. Y., Markel, J. D., & Gray, A. H., Jr. (1979). Least squares glottal inverse filtering from the acoustic speech waveform. *IEEE Transactions on Acoustics, Speech, and Signal Processing, ASSP-27* (4), pp. 350–355.

Woodworth, R. S., & Wells, F. L. (1911). *Association tests* (Psychological Monographs No. 57, Vol. XIII, No. 5). Princeton, NJ: Psychological Review Company.

Yumoto, E. (1987). Qualitative assessment of the degree of hoarseness. *Journal of Voice, 1,* 310–314.

Yumoto, E., Gould, W. J., & Baer, T. (1982). The harmonics-to-noise ratio as an index of the degree of hoarseness. *Journal of the Acoustical Society of America, 71,* 1544–1550.

Yumoto, E., Sasaki, Y., & Okamura, H. (1984). Harmonics-to-noise ratio and psychophysical measurement of the degree of hoarseness. *Journal of Speech and Hearing Research, 27,* 2–6.

Zaimov, K. (1969). Die Sprachstörungen als Kriterium der Bewußtseinstrübungen. *Psychiatrie, Neurologie, und Medizinische Psychologie, 21,* 218–225.

Zemlin, W. R. (1988). *Speech and hearing science anatomy and physiology* (3rd ed.). Englewood Cliffs, NJ: Prentice Hall.

Glossary

Abduction Moving away from the median plane of the body, such as the vocal folds; cf. **Adduction.**

Adduction Moving toward the median plane of the body, such as the vocal folds; cf. **Abduction.**

ADH Alcohol dehydrogenase, primary enzyme involved as a catalyst in the oxidation of alcohol to acetaldehyde.

Afferent Conducting nerve impulses toward a cell body or toward the central nervous system; cf. **Efferent.**

Acoustic Pertaining to hearing or sound.

Acoustic-Phonetics The branch of phonetics concerned with speech as a physical signal.

Affricate Consonant speech sound produced with a stop-like closure followed by a fricative-like release.

Airstream mechanism The source and direction of airflow used in producing speech sounds. Sources include the lungs (producing a pulmonic airstream mechanism), the larynx (glottalic airstream mechanism), or the soft palate (velaric airstream mechanism). An ingressive airstream mechanism moves air toward the lungs; an egressive airstream mechanism moves air away from the lungs toward the outside air.

Alcohol (as used in this book) A clear, colorless, volatile liquid (chemical formula CH_3CH_2OH) having industrial applications but especially as used in beverages prepared for human consumption; also called ethanol, ethyl alcohol, grain alcohol.

ALDH Aldehyde dehydrogenase, primary enzyme involved in the oxidation of acetaldehyde to acetic acid.

Alveolar (1) Pertaining to the alveolar ridge (also called alveolar arch), the border of the upper jaw with sockets to hold teeth, especially speech sounds produced by articulation of the tongue tip and the alveolar ridge. (2) Pertaining to alveoli (sing. alveolus), the air cells of the lungs, especially air emanating from the deeper parts of the lungs during respiration.

Alveopalatal Relating to the back of the alveolar ridge, especially a consonant formed by articulation of the tongue blade and the back of the alveolar ridge.

Amplitude The displacement magnitude of a sound wave.

Aphasia A loss (complete or partial) of language ability associated with injury to the brain.

Approximant A speech sound formed by relatively close positioning of articulators without the formation of a passage sufficiently narrow to cause turbulence, including glides and liquids (q.v.).

Arterial blood Blood going from the heart to the tissues.

Articulation The positioning of speech organs, so as to produce an obstruction or characteristic shape in the vocal tract for the production of a speech sound. Participating speech organs are called articulators.

Ataxia Inability to coordinate voluntary muscle movements due to disorders of the nervous system, particularly lesions of the cerebellum.

Axon A thin, cylindrical process of a neuron that conducts impulses away from the cell body.

Backness Parameter in the description of speech sounds referring to the position of the tongue dorsum on a horizontal scale.

Baseline measure A measure or observation taken before administration of an experimental treatment (e.g., alcohol) for comparison with posttreatment measures or observations to determine treatment effects.

Bilabial A consonant formed by articulation of the upper and lower lips.

Blood-alcohol concentration (BAC) The concentration of alcohol in whole blood, usually expressed as units weight of alcohol per volume of blood. Common expressions include grams alcohol per 100 ml blood (percent or %), milligrams alcohol per milliliter blood (or grams alcohol per liter blood) (per mille or ‰), and milligrams alcohol per 100-ml blood (mg%). Used as a measure of expo-

sure of the brain to alcohol and therefore indirectly as a measure of degree of alcohol intoxication; cf. **Breath-alcohol concentration**.

Breath-alcohol concentration (BrAC) The concentration of alcohol in breath, more specifically, in expired alveolar air, usually expressed as units weight of alcohol per volume of breath. Expression often converted to equivalent expression of blood alcohol concentration, in order, for example, to facilitate cross-study comparison or to satisfy statutory requirements; cf. **Blood-alcohol concentration**.

Buccal Pertaining to the cheeks, or sometimes more generally, the mouth.

Central nervous system (CNS) That part of the nervous system consisting of the brain and the spinal cord.

Cepstrum analysis Analysis based on a Fourier transform of the power spectrum of a signal.

Cerebellum A portion of the brain located dorsal to the pons and dorsal to and overhanging the medulla oblongata. Important for the synergic control of skeletal muscles and coordination of voluntary muscular movements.

Cerebral hemisphere One of the roughly symmetrical halves of the cerebrum.

Cerebrum The large anterior and superior part of the brain, consisting of two roughly symmetrical hemispheres, the basal ganglia, and the rhinencephalon.

Click A speech sound produced with a velaric ingressive airstream mechanism.

Consonant A speech sound produced with a relatively constricted vocal tract causing radical obstruction of airflow; cf. **vowel**.

Content analysis Linguistic analysis based on semantic and pragmatic considerations, rather than purely structural considerations.

Contralateral Pertaining to the opposite side of a midline.

Control A standard used to establish the validity of observations and conclusions of an experimental procedure, especially a condition in which a subject is not exposed to a treatment or condition to which an experimental subject is exposed.

Cortex The outer layer of gray matter of the cerebrum and cerebellum.

Cortical Relating to the cortex, especially the cerebral cortex.

Decussation Crossing of nerve fibers to the opposite side of the nervous system.

Delayed auditory feedback (DAF) Artificially produced (e.g., through a tape recorder and headphones) delay in hearing one's own speech.

Dendrite A branching process of a neuron that conducts nerve impulses toward the cell body.

Diadochokinesis The ability to perform rapid repetitions of simple patterns of oppositional muscle contractions. Nonspeech measures include finger tapping; a common oral or speech measure is rapid repetition of the syllables [pʌ], [tʌ], or [kʌ], or the sequence [pʌtʌkʌ]. Diminished or absent ability is called *adiadochokinesia* or *dysdiadochokinesia*.

Digital signal processing (DSP) The representation, storage, and analysis of a signal (such as a speech acoustic signal) in digitized form (i.e., as discrete values).

Diphthong A vowel sound in which there is a change in quality within a single syllable; cf. **Monophthong**.

Distillation A process in which substances are vaporized and then condensed by cooling, especially the distillation of volatile alcohol from nonvolatile water in the production of alcoholic beverages.

Duodenum The upper part of the small intestine from the pylorus to the jejunum.

Dysarthria A speech or articulatory disorder resulting from insult to the neural mechanisms that regulate speech movements.

Edema Condition in which body tissues contain an excess amount of tissue fluid.

Efferent Conducting nerve impulses away from a cell body or away from the central nervous system toward the periphery; cf. **Afferent**.

Ejective A speech sound produced with a glottalic egressive airstream mechanism.

Electroglottography (EGG) An indirect method of investigating vocal fold adduction by measuring the degree of conductance for an electrical current flowing between electrodes placed on opposite sides of the neck.

Electropalatography (EPG) Method of analyzing lingual-palatal contact using a pseudo-palate fitted with electrodes.

Fermentation An enzymatically controlled anaerobic decomposition of carbohydrates, especially the decomposition of sugars to carbon dioxide and ethanol.

Filter A device (or program) that allows the passage of energy at some frequencies and blocks the transmission of energy at other frequencies. Filters may transmit only lower frequencies (low-pass filter), higher frequencies (high-pass filter), only frequencies within a relatively narrow range (band-pass filter), or frequencies outside a relatively narrow range (band-reject filter).

Fluency Continuous, smooth, facile production of speech.

Formants Resonances of the vocal tract.

Fourier analysis The analysis of a complex wave into its constituent sine waves.

Frequency The number of completed vibration cycles in a given period of time. Generally measured in Hertz (Hz) (i.e., cycles per second [cps]).

Fricative A consonant formed by positioning two articulators in such a way that a narrow passage between them is formed so that air passing through will produce friction and a noisy, turbulent airflow.

Fundamental frequency The lowest frequency component of a complex periodic signal, especially the first harmonic of a human voice, corresponding to the lowest periodic component of vocal-fold vibration; cf. **Pitch.**

GABA (gamma-aminobutyric acid) A type of inhibitory neurotransmitter.

Glide A consonant speech sound displaying vowel-like characteristics (i.e., formant structure) but also dynamic changes in vocal tract configuration.

Glottis The opening between the vocal folds.

Gyrus (pl. gyri) One of the convolutions of the cerebral hemispheres; cf. **Sulcus.**

Height Parameter in the description of speech sounds referring to the position of the tongue dorsum on a vertical scale.

Ileum Lower three-fifths of the small intestine from the jejunum to the ascending colon.

Implosive A speech sound produced with a glottalic ingressive airstream mechanism.

Interdental A speech sound produced by articulating the tongue tip with both the upper and lower teeth.

Intraperitoneal Within the peritoneal cavity (i.e., the region surrounded by a serous membrane containing all of the abdominal organs except the kidneys).

Ipsilateral Pertaining to the same side of a midline.

Jejunum The second part of the small intestine from the duodenum to the ileum.

Jitter Involuntary short-term perturbation in fundamental frequency or fundamental period; usually measured as cycle-to-cycle variation, using various algorithms.

Labiodental A speech sound produced by articulating the lower lip against the upper teeth.

Larynx Modified cartilage located at the upper end of the trachea, consisting of structural cartilage, muscles, membranes, and the vocal folds.

Liquid An articulatory category referring to *l*-sounds and *r*-sounds.

Lingual Pertaining to the tongue.

Mandible The lower jaw.

Manner (of articulation) A parameter in the description of consonant speech sounds referring to the type of obstruction in the vocal tract. See **Stop, Fricative, Affricate, Nasal, Liquid, Glide.**

Maxilla The upper jaw.

Mellanby effect State of lower concentration of alcohol in venous blood compared to arterial blood during active absorption and before equilibration.

Metabolism Physical and chemical changes taking place within an organism.

Monophthong A vowel sound without a change in quality within a single syllable; cf. **Diphthong.**

Morphology The branch of linguistics dealing with word formation.

Myoelastic-aerodynamic theory A theory of voice production (phonation) proposing that vocal-fold vibration is activated by the pulmonic airstream rather than by individual nerve impulses, and that the frequency of vibration can be changed by using the muscles to change the elasticity and tension of the vocal folds.

Nasal Pertaining to the nose, especially (1) to the paired cavities communicating with the nostrils anteriorially and the nasopharynx posteriorly, or (2) to speech sounds produced with a lowered velum (open velopharyngeal port), allowing resonance either in the nasal cavities alone or in both the nasal cavities and the oral cavity.

Neuron A specialized cell in the nervous system, consisting of a cell body, an axon, and dendrites.

Neurotransmitter A chemical messenger released by an excited or stimulated nerve cell that travels across a synapse and binds to a receptor on a postsynaptic nerve cell, triggering chemical and electrical changes in that cell.

Nystagmus Involuntary jerking of the eye.

Obstruent A linguistic category of speech sounds that includes the stops, fricatives, and affricates; cf. **Sonorant.**

Oral Pertaining to the mouth, especially (1) to the mouth as a resonating cavity, and (2) to sounds produced with a closed velopharyngeal port; cf. **Nasal.**

Oscillograph Instrument that displays waveforms (i.e., changes in amplitude [or pressure variations] over time).

Palatal Pertaining to the palate.

Palate The roof of the mouth. Generally viewed as consisting of the more anterior hard palate, which is a bony plate and separates the oral cavity from the nasal cavity, and the more posterior soft palate (also called the velum), a muscular valve between the oral and nasal cavitites.

Parenternal Situated or occurring outside of the intestines.

Peripheral nervous system (PNS) Those parts of the nervous system lying outside of the brain and spinal cord.

Per se alcohol limit A statutory prohibition against operating a motor vehicle with a specified blood- or breath-alcohol concentration. Under this type of statute, the presence of alcohol in the body in the specified amount (by whichever measure) constitutes in itself a violation of the statute.

Pharmacodynamics The effects of drugs on the body when introduced into it.

Pharmacokinetics The effects of the body on drugs introduced into it (i.e., the absorption, distribution, metabolism, and elimination of drugs by the body).

Pharynx That section of the alimentary canal between the mouth and the esophagus: the throat, consisting of the nasopharynx, the oropharynx, and the laryngopharynx.

Phonation The imposition of periodicity or quasi-periodicity on airflow at the larynx by means of the vibration of the vocal folds.

Phonetics The study of the production and perception of speech sounds.

Phoniatrics The study of the voice, its disorders, and treatment of its disorders.

Phonology The study of the sound system of a language or of the sound systems of languages.

Pitch The perception of frequency, especially the perception of the vocal fundamental frequency on a scale ranging from low to high.

Placebo A preparation used in a controlled experiment that does not contain the test substance (e.g., alcohol), used to test the effects of the test substance.

Place (of articulation) A parameter for the description of consonant speech sounds referring to the location of the constriction used to obstruct the airstream.

Plasma The liquid part of the blood, consisting of serum and protein substances in solution.

Purkinje cells Large neurons located in the cerebellum.

Pylorus Orifice at the bottom of the stomach opening into the duodenum.

Reaction time The time interval between presentation of a stimulus and initiation of a response.

Resonant A sonorant (q.v.) sound.

Respiration Breathing.

Response latency The time interval between presentation of a stimulus and initiation of an overt response.

Retroflex A speech sound produced with the tongue tip raised and retracted.

Saccadic eye movements Rapid conjugate shifts of gaze to follow a target.

Sequela (pl. sequelae) A condition following or resulting from a disease or administration of a drug.

Serum The watery portion of blood remaining after coagulation.

Shadowing An experimental method for elicitation of speech in which subjects hear utterances (usually through headphones) and then repeat the utterance as soon as possible.

Shimmer Involuntary short-term perturbation in amplitude; usually measured as cycle-to-cycle variation, using various algorithms.

Sibilant A category of fricative sounds having higher acoustic energy at higher frequencies than other fricatives; the sibilant fricatives are the voiced and voiceless alveolar and alveopalatals.

Slurred speech Clinical or legal sign of intoxication characterized by imprecise speech articulation; incorrect production of consonants and vowels; and rate, pitch, and intensity deviations.

Slurred speech threshold The point during administration of a drug at which a subject exhibits slurring of speech.

Sonorant A linguistic category comprising vowels, glides, liquids, and nasals.

Sonority The loudness of a sound relative to other sounds that have the same pitch, stress, and duration.

Source—filter theory Theory of acoustic speech production that posits a source of acoustic energy (phonation) that is modified by a filter or filters (supralaryngeal cavity).

Source function The origin of spectral energy for a signal, especially the origin of acoustic energy for the production of a speech sound.

Spectrographic analysis Analysis of an acoustic signal (including speech) in terms of frequency and intensity as a function of time. A spectrograph is the instrument used to perform the analysis, and a spectrogram is the visual display produced. The spectrogram displays frequency on the ordinate, time on the abscissa, and intensity on the gray scale.

Spectrum A display of a signal showing energy or intensity as a function of frequency.

Spondee A metrical foot or a word containing two long or stressed syllables (e.g., *doghouse, football*).

Stop A consonant produced by bringing two articulators together, such that airflow behind the articulation is completely occluded momentarily, and then releasing the occlusion suddenly; also called a *plosive*.

Sulcus (pl. sulci) A groove-like depression on the surface of the brain. Also called a *fissure*; cf. **Gyrus**.

Synapse The juncture between two neurons, consisting of the presynaptic nerve, the postsynaptic nerve, and the

synaptic gap or cleft (i.e., a narrow gap between the neurons).

Syntax The branch of linguistics dealing with the arrangement of words into phrases, clauses, and sentences.

Tongue A fleshy process located on the floor of the mouth, highly moveable and used for taste, mastication, and deglutition, but especially for the formation of a large number of speech sounds in humans. Consists anatomically of, from posterior to anterior, a dorsum, constituting the major mass of the tongue; a blade; and an apex or tip.

Tracking Adjustment of an instrument or machine to maintain a desired value (compensatory tracking) or to follow a moving reference marker (pursuit tracking).

Transfer Function The contribution of a filter of a source function to a resulting signal, especially, the contribution of the vocal tract and its resonances to the resulting speech sound.

Uvula The fleshy appendage constituting the posterior-most part of the soft palate.

Velum see **Palate**.

Venous blood Unaerated blood moving toward the heart; cf. **Arterial blood**.

Vital capacity The total volume of air that can be expelled from the lungs after maximum inspiration.

Vocal attack The mode of vocal-fold vibration initiation, including (1) hard, glottal, or stopped attack; (2) even or static attack; and (3) breathy attack.

Vocal folds Paired bands of muscular and membranous tissue situated dorsoventrally in the larynx and free along their medial edges. Proper positioning and sufficient airflow causes them to vibrate periodically or quasi-periodically, producing a phonatory airstream used for speech.

Voice onset time (VOT) The time interval between a supralaryngeal event, such as the release of a stop consonant, and the onset of periodic voicing of a following vowel.

Voice quality Perception of the complexity of phonation modified by articulation and cavity resonation.

Voicing A linguistic parameter referring to the presence or absence of vocal-fold vibrations accompanying the production of a speech sound. Sounds produced with vocal vibrations are termed *voiced,* whereas those produced without vibration are *voiceless.*

Vowel A speech sound produced with a relatively unconstricted vocal tract (i.e., without radical obstruction of the airflow); cf. **consonant.**

Waveform A two-dimensional display of an acoustic signal that plots amplitude as a function of time.

Widmark's factor beta The rate of descent of blood-alcohol concentration after equilibration (i.e., the slope of the descending portion of the blood alcohol curve).

Widmark's factor rho "Factor by which the body weight must be reduced in order to obtain the theoretical body mass which would have the same alcohol concentration as the blood" (Watson, 1989).

Subject Index

Printed in the United States
By Bookmasters